P9-AQX-647

Handbook of Pediatric Hematology and Oncology

Handbook
of Pediatric
Hematology
and Oncology

Children's Hospital & Research Center Oakland

Caroline A. Hastings, MD

Pediatric Hematology and Oncology
Children's Hospital & Research Center Oakland
Oakland, CA, USA

Joseph C. Torkildson, MD, MBA

Pediatric Hematology and Oncology
Children's Hospital & Research Center Oakland
Oakland, CA, USA

Anurag K. Agrawal, MD

Pediatric Hematology and Oncology
Children's Hospital & Research Center Oakland
Oakland, CA, USA

Second edition

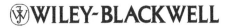

A John Wiley & Sons, Ltd., Publication

This edition first published 2012 © 2012 by John Wiley & Sons, Limited.

Wiley-Blackwell is an imprint of John Wiley & Sons, formed by the merger of Wileys global Scientific, Technical, and Medical business with Blackwell Publishing.

Registered office: John Wiley & Sons, Ltd, The Atrium, Southern Gate, Chichester, West Sussex, PO19 8SQ, UK

Editorial offices: 9600 Garsington Road, Oxford, OX4 2DQ, UK

The Atrium, Southern Gate, Chichester, West Sussex, PO19 8SQ, UK

111 River Street, Hoboken, NJ 07030-5774, USA

For details of our global editorial offices, customer services, and for information about how to apply for permission to reuse the copyright material in this book please see our Website at www.wiley.com/wiley-blackwell

The right of the author to be identified as the author of this work has been asserted in accordance with the UK Copyright, Designs and Patents Act 1988.

All rights reserved. No part of this publication may be reproduced, stored in a retrieval system, or transmitted, in any form or by any means, electronic, mechanical, photocopying, recording or otherwise, except as permitted by the UK Copyright, Designs and Patents Act 1988, without the prior permission of the publisher.

Designations used by companies to distinguish their products are often claimed as trademarks. All brand names and product names used in this book are trade names, service marks, trademarks or registered trademarks of their respective owners. The publisher is not associated with any product or vendor mentioned in this book. This publication is designed to provide accurate and authoritative information in regard to the subject matter covered. It is sold on the understanding that the publisher is not engaged in rendering professional services. If professional advice or other expert assistance is required, the services of a competent professional should be sought.

The contents of this work are intended to further general scientific research, understanding, and discussion only and are not intended and should not be relied upon as recommending or promoting a specific method, diagnosis, or treatment by physicians for any particular patient. The publisher and the author make no representations or warranties with respect to the accuracy or completeness of the contents of this work and specifically disclaim all warranties, including without limitation any implied warranties of fitness for a particular purpose. In view of ongoing research, equipment modifications, changes in governmental regulations, and the constant flow of information relating to the use of medicines, equipment, and devices, the reader is urged to review and evaluate the information provided in the package insert or instructions for each medicine, equipment, or device for, among other things, any changes in the instructions or indication of usage and for added warnings and precautions. Readers should consult with a specialist where appropriate. The fact that an organization or Website is referred to in this work as a citation and/or a potential source of further information does not mean that the author or the publisher endorses the information the organization or Website may provide or recommendations it may make. Further, readers should be aware that Internet Websites listed in this work may have changed or disappeared between when this work was written and when it is read. No warranty may be created or extended by any promotional statements for this work. Neither the publisher nor the author shall be liable for any damages arising herefrom.

Library of Congress Cataloging-in-Publication Data

Hastings, Caroline, 1960–
    Handbook of pediatric hematology and oncology : Children's Hospital & Research Center Oakland / Caroline A. Hastings, Joseph Torkildson, Anurag Kishor Agrawal. – 2nd ed.
        p. ; cm.
    Rev. ed. of: The Children's Hospital Oakland hematology/oncology handbook / Caroline Hastings. 1st ed. c2002.
    Includes bibliographical references and index.
    ISBN 978-0-470-67088-0 (pbk. : alk. paper)
    I. Torkildson, Joseph. II. Agrawal, Anurag Kishor. III. Hastings, Caroline, 1960– Children's Hospital Oakland hematology/oncology handbook. IV. Children's Hospital Medical Center (Oakland, Calif.) V. Title.
    [DNLM: 1. Child. 2. Hematologic Diseases–Handbooks.
3. Neoplasms–Handbooks. WS 39]
    618.97′6994–dc23
                                                            2011048154

A catalog record for this book is available from the British Library.

Set in 10/12.5 pt Minon by Thomson Digital, Noida, India

Printed in the UK

Contents

Preface

The pace of change in the field of pediatric hematology and oncology is staggering. Molecular biology, genomics, and biochemistry have accelerated the accumulation of knowledge and understanding of disease states. Yet the application of this new knowledge to the individual child before you, the work of the physician, is often overwhelming, even for the most experienced practitioner. The course and prognosis for the child is often determined by the rapidity of disease onset, diagnosis, and initial treatment. What is needed is a practical, tested approach to these problems that ensures timely evaluation, competent early care, and avoidance of pitfalls that might prejudice future treatment options. This practical approach is clearly brought by spending time with the patients and their families, and observing the myriad variations that are never mentioned in the large studies or case reports.

This handbook represents the work of my colleagues at Children's Hospital & Research Center Oakland toward this endeavor. The guidelines offered here have been used to train medical students, pediatric residents, and pediatric hematology/oncology fellows for over 20 years. This handbook will give you clinical approaches for common problems in pediatric hematology and oncology, the knowledge to organize and to evaluate the care of your patients, and a framework to incorporate ever-expanding psychosocial needs, clinical studies, medical treatments, and science. All of these are essential components that make up the care of the child with cancer or a blood disease.

Caroline Hastings, M.D.
March 2012

Acknowledgments

We could not be here without the long-standing love and support of our families. On a day to day basis, the patients and their families continue to show us how to live gracefully in even the hardest of times and inspire us to continue to endeavor for improved outcomes. Our experiences have taught us the magnitude of remembering our roles: "to cure sometimes, to relieve often, to comfort always." *(Anonymous, 15th century)*

1

Approach to the Anemic Child

Anemia is the condition in which the concentration of hemoglobin or the red cell mass is reduced below normal. Anemia results in a physiological decrease in the oxygen-carrying capacity of the blood and reduced oxygen supply to the tissues. Causes of anemia are increased loss or destruction of red blood cells (RBCs) or a significant decreased rate of production. When evaluating a child with anemia, it is important to determine if the problem is isolated to one cell line (e.g., RBCs) or multiple cell lines (i.e., RBCs, white blood cells [WBCs], or platelets). When two or three cell lines are affected, it may indicate bone marrow involvement (leukemia, metastatic disease, and aplastic anemia), sequestration (i.e., hypersplenism), immune deficiency, or an immune-mediated process (e.g., hemolytic anemia and immune thrombocytopenic purpura).

Evaluation of anemia

The evaluation of anemia includes a complete medical history, family history, physical examination, and laboratory assessment. See Figure 1.1.

The diagnosis of anemia is made after reference to established normal controls for age (Table 1.1). The blood smear and red cell indices are very helpful in the diagnosis and classification of anemia. It allows for classification by the cell size (MCV, mean corpuscular volume), gives the distribution of cell size (RDW, red cell distribution width), and may give important diagnostic clues if specific morphological abnormalities are present (e.g., sickle cells, target cells, and spherocytes). The MCV, RDW, and reticulocyte count are helpful in the differential diagnosis of anemia. A high RDW, or anisocytosis, is seen in stress erythropoiesis and is often suggestive of iron deficiency or hemolysis. A normal or low reticulocyte count is an inappropriate response to anemia and suggests impaired red cell production. An elevated reticulocyte count suggests blood loss, hemolysis, or sequestration.

The investigation of anemia requires the following steps:

1. The medical history of the anemic child (Table 1.2), as certain historical points may provide clues as to the etiology of the anemia.

2. Detailed physical examination (Table 1.3), with particular attention to acute and chronic effects of anemia.

3. Evaluation of the complete blood count (CBC), RBC indices, and peripheral blood smear, with classification by MCV,

Handbook of Pediatric Hematology and Oncology: Children's Hospital & Research Center Oakland,
Second Edition. Caroline A. Hastings, Joseph C. Torkildson, and Anurag K. Agrawal.
© 2012 John Wiley & Sons, Ltd. Published 2012 by John Wiley & Sons, Ltd.

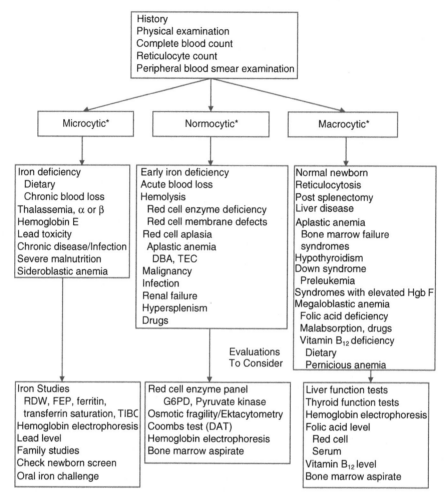

Figure 1.1 Diagnostic approach to the child with anemia. (Abbreviations: DBA, Diamond–Blackfan anemia; TEC, transient erythroblastopenia of childhood; RDW, red cell distribution width; FEP, free erythrocyte protoporphyrin; TIBC, total iron binding capacity; G6PD, glucose-6-phosphate dehydrogenase deficiency; DAT, direct antiglobulin test).
*Refer to Table 1.1 for age-based normal values.

reticulocyte count, and RBC morphology. Consideration should also be given to the WBC and platelet counts as well as their respective morphology.

4. Determination of an etiology of the anemia by additional studies as needed (see Figures 1.1, 1.2, and 1.3).

Interventions

Oral iron challenge

An oral iron challenge may be indicated in the patient with significant iron depletion, as documented by moderate-to-severe anemia and deficiencies in circulating

Table 1.1 Red blood cell values at various ages.*

Age	Hemoglobin (g/dL)		MCV (fL)	
	Mean	−2 SD	Mean	−2 SD
Birth (cord blood)	16.5	13.5	108	98
1–3 d (capillary)	18.5	14.5	108	95
1 wk	17.5	13.5	107	88
2 wk	16.5	12.5	105	86
1 mo	14.0	10.0	104	85
2 mo	11.5	9.0	96	77
3–6 m	11.5	9.5	91	74
0.5–2 y	12.0	11.0	78	70
2–6 y	12.5	11.5	81	75
6–12 y	13.5	11.5	86	77
12–18 y female	14.0	12.0	90	78
12–18 y male	14.5	13.0	88	78
18–49 y female	14.0	12.0	90	80
18–49 y male	15.5	13.5	90	80

*Compiled from the following sources: Dutcher TF. Lab Med 2:32–35, 1971; Koerper MA, et al. J Pediatr 89:580–583, 1976; Marner T. Acta Paediatr Scand 58:363–368, 1969; Matoth Y, et al. Acta Paediatr Scand 60:317–323, 1971; Moe PJ. Acta Paediatr Scand 54:69–80, 1965; Okuno T. J Clin Pathol 2:599–602, 1972; Oski F, Naiman J. Hematological Problems in the Newborn, 2nd ed., Philadelphia: WB Saunders, 1972, p. 11; Penttilä I, et al. Suomen Lääkärilehti 26:2173, 1973; and Viteri FE, et al. Br J Haematol 23:189–204, 1972. Cited in: Rudolph AM (ed). Rudolph's Pediatrics, 16th ed., Norwalk, CT: Appleton & Lange, 1977.
Abbreviation: MCV, mean corpuscular volume.

and storage iron forms (such as total iron-binding capacity [TIBC], serum iron, transferrin saturation, and ferritin). Iron absorption is impaired in certain chronic disorders (autoimmune diseases such as lupus, peptic ulcer disease, ulcerative colitis, and Crohn's disease), by certain medications (antacids and histamine-2 blockers), and by environmental factors such as lead toxicity.

Indications for an oral iron challenge include any condition in which a poor response to oral iron is being questioned, such as in: noncompliance, severe anemia secondary to dietary insufficiency (excessive milk intake), and ongoing blood loss.

Administration of an oral iron challenge is quite simple: first, draw a serum iron level; second, administer a dose of iron (3 mg/kg elemental iron) orally; third, draw another serum iron level 30 to 60 minutes later. The serum level is expected to increase by at least 100 mcg/dL if absorption is adequate. The oral iron challenge is a quick and easy method to assess appropriateness of oral iron to treat iron deficiency—a safer, cheaper yet equally efficacious method of treatment as parenteral iron.

Parenteral iron therapy

Due to the potential risks of older parenteral iron preparations (specifically high molecular weight iron dextran), a reluctance remains to use the newer and much safer formulations. The majority of safety data exists with low molecular weight (LMW) iron dextran although many practitioners have moved to newer (and perceived safer)

Table 1.2 The medical history of the anemic child.

History of	Consider
Prematurity	Anemia of prematurity (EPO responsive)
Perinatal risk factors	
Maternal illness (autoimmune)	Hemolytic anemia
Drug ingestion	Impaired production
Infections (TORCH [e.g., rubella, CMV], hepatitis)	
Perinatal problems	Acute blood loss
	Fetal–maternal hemorrhage
	Iron deficiency due to above or maternal iron deficiency
Ethnicity	
African-American	Hgb S, C; α- and β-thalassemia; G6PD deficiency
Mediterranean	α- and β-thalassemia; G6PD deficiency
Southeast Asian	α- and β-thalassemia; Hgb E
Family history	
Gallstones, cholecystectomy	Inherited hemolytic anemia, spherocytosis, elliptocytosis
Splenectomy, jaundice at birth or with illness	Inherited enzymopathy, G6PD, pyruvate kinase deficiencies
Isoimmunization (Rh or ABO)	Hemolytic disease of newborn (predisposed to iron deficiency)
Sex	
Male	X-linked enzymopathies (G6PD deficiency)
Early jaundice (<24 h of age)	Isoimmune, infectious
Persistent jaundice	Suggests hemolytic anemia
Diet (Usually > 6 mo)	
Pica (ice, dirt)	Lead toxicity, iron deficiency
Excessive milk intake	Iron deficiency
Macrobiotic diets	Vitamin B_{12} deficiency
Goat's milk	Folic acid deficiency
Drugs	
Sulfa drugs, anticonvulsants	Hemolytic anemia (G6PD deficiency)
Chloramphenicol	Hypoplastic anemia
Low socioeconomic status	
Pica	Lead toxicity, iron deficiency
Malnutrition	
Malabsorption	Anemia of chronic disease
Environmental	Iron, vitamin B_{12}, or folate deficiency, vitamin E or K deficiency
Liver disease	Shortened red cell survival
	Heinz bodies
Renal disease	Shortened red cell survival
Decreased red cell production (↓EPO)	
Infectious diseases	
Mild viral infection (acute gastroenteritis, otitis media, pharyngitis)	Transient mild decreased Hgb
Sepsis (bacterial, viral, mycoplasma)	Hemolytic anemia
Parvovirus	Anemia with reticulocytopenia (TEC)

Abbreviations: EPO, erythropoietin; TORCH, toxoplasmosis, other, rubella, cytomegalovirus, herpes simplex virus; G6PD, glucose-6-phosphate dehydrogenase deficiency; TEC, transient erythroblastopenia of childhood.

Table 1.3 Physical examination of the anemic child.

System	Clinical sign or symptom	Potential underlying disorder
Skin	Pallor	Severe anemia
	Jaundice	Hemolytic anemia, acute and chronic hepatitis, aplastic anemia
	Petechiae, purpura	Autoimmune hemolytic anemia with thrombocytopenia, hemolytic uremic syndrome, bone marrow aplasia or infiltration
	Cavernous hemangioma	Microangiopathic hemolytic anemia
HEENT	Frontal bossing, prominent malar and maxillary bones	Extramedullary hematopoiesis (thalassemia major, congenital hemolytic anemia)
	Icteric sclerae	Congenital hemolytic anemia and hyper-hemolytic crises associated with infection (red cell enzyme deficiencies, red cell membrane defects, thalassemias, hemoglobinopathies)
	Angular stomatitis	Iron deficiency
	Glossitis	Vitamin B_{12} or iron deficiency
Chest	Rales, gallop rhythm, tachycardia	Congestive heart failure, acute or severe anemia
Spleen	Splenomegaly	Congenital hemolytic anemia, infection, hematological malignancies, portal hypertension, resultant hypersplenism
Extremities	Radial limb dysplasia	Fanconi anemia
	Spoon nails	Iron deficiency
	Triphalangeal thumbs	Red cell aplasia

formulations including ferric gluconate and iron sucrose. Three additional compounds have been approved recently, 2 in Europe (ferric carboxymaltose and iron isomaltoside) and 1 in the United States (ferumoxytol). These newer agents have the potential benefit of total dose replacement in a very short and single infusion as compared to ferric gluconate and iron sucrose which require multiple doses. LMW iron dextran is approved as a total dose infusion for adults in Europe but not the United States. Due to the smaller dose generally required in pediatric patients, total iron replacement is feasible in 1 to 2 doses of LMW iron dextran. Calculation of the necessary dose is as follows:

$$\text{Dosage (mL)} = 0.0442 \times \text{LBW (kg)}$$
$$\times (\text{Hgb}_n - \text{Hgb}_o)$$
$$+ [0.26 \times \text{LBW (kg)}],$$

where

LBW = lean body weight

males: 50 kg + 2.3 kg for every inch over 5 ft in height

females: 45.5 kg + 2.3 kg for every inch over 5 ft in height

Hgb_n = desired hemoglobin (g/dL) = 12 if < 15 kg or 14.8 if > 15 kg

Hgb_o = measured hemoglobin (g/dL)

The maximum adult dose is 2 mL and each milliliter of iron dextran contains 50 mg

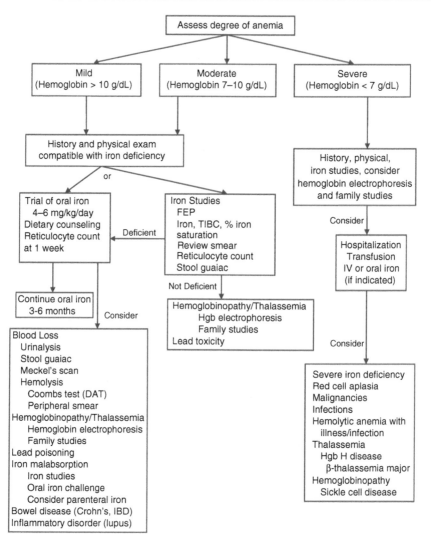

Figure 1.2 Evaluation of the child with microcytic anemia. (Abbreviations: FEP, free erythrocyte protoporphyrin; TIBC, total iron binding capacity; DAT, direct antiglobulin test; IBD, inflammatory bowel disease).

of elemental iron. Add 10 mg elemental iron/kg to replenish iron stores (chronic anemia states). Replacement may be given in a single dose, depending on the dose required. See the formulary for further information.

Severe allergic reactions can occur with iron dextran and the low molecular weight product should be preferentially utilized. A test dose (10 to 25 mg) should be given prior to the first dose with observation of the patient for 30 to 60 minutes prior to administering the remainder of the dose. A common side effect is mild to moderate arthralgias the day after drug administration, especially in patients with autoimmune disease. Acetaminophen frequently

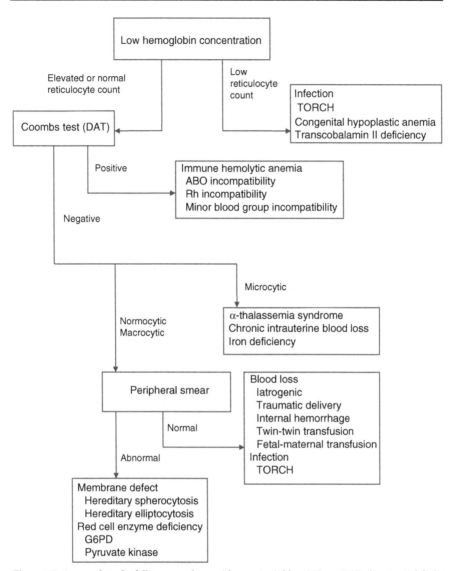

Figure 1.3 Approach to the full-term newborn with anemia. (Abbreviations: DAT, direct antiglobulin test; G6PD, glucose-6-phosphatase deficiency; TORCH, toxoplasmosis, other, rubella, cytomegalovirus, herpes simplex virus).

alleviates the arthralgias. Iron dextran is contraindicated in patients with rheumatoid arthritis.

Iron sucrose or ferric gluconate can be considered in inpatients in which multiple doses are more convenient and feasible than the outpatient setting. With continued usage and safety data, ferumoxytol will likely replace the currently used products due to the much larger maximum dose that can be given, lack of need for a test dose, and excellent side effect profile.

Erythropoietin

Recombinant human erythropoietin (EPO) stimulates proliferation and differentiation of erythroid precursors, with an increase in heme synthesis. This increased proliferation creates an increased demand in iron availability and can result in a functional iron deficiency if not given with iron therapy.

Indications for EPO include end-stage renal disease, anemia of prematurity, anemia of chronic disease, anemia associated with treatment for AIDS, and autologous blood donation. EPO use for the treatment of chemotherapy-induced anemia remains controversial and is not routinely recommended in pediatric patients (see Chapter 25).

The most common side effect of EPO administration is hypertension, which may be somewhat alleviated with changes in the dose and duration of administration.

Typical starting dose of EPO is 150 U/kg three times a week (IV) or subcutaneous (SC). CBCs and reticulocyte counts are checked weekly. Higher doses, and more frequent dosing, may be necessary. Response is usually seen within 1 to 2 weeks. Adequate iron intake (3 mg/kg/d orally or intermittent parenteral therapy) should be provided to optimize effectiveness and prevent iron deficiency.

Transfusion therapy

Children with very severe anemia (Hgb < 5 g/dL) may require treatment with red cell transfusion, depending on the underlying disease and baseline hemoglobin status, duration of anemia, rapidity of onset, and hemodynamic stability. The pediatric literature is scarce as to the best method of transfusing such patients. However, it appears to be common practice to give slow transfusions to children with cardiovascular compromise (i.e., gallop rhythm, pulmonary edema, excessive tachycardia, and poor perfusion) while being monitored in an ICU setting. Transfusions are given in multiple small volumes, sometimes separated by several hours, with careful monitoring of the vitals and fluid balance. For those children who have gradual onset of severe anemia, without cardiovascular compromise, continuous transfusion of 2 mL/kg/h has been shown to be safe and result in an increase in the hematocrit of 1% for each 1 mL/kg of transfused packed RBCs (based on RBC storage method). The hemoglobin should be increased to a normal value to avoid further cardiac compromise (i.e., Hgb 8 to 12 g/dL). Again, the final endpoint may be dependent on several factors including nature of anemia, ongoing blood loss or lack of production, baseline hemoglobin, and volume to be transfused. Care should be taken to avoid unnecessary exposure to multiple blood donors by maximal use of the unit of blood, proper division of units in the blood bank, and avoidance of opening extra units for small quantities to meet a total volume. See Chapter 5 for product preparation, ordering, and premedication. A posttransfusion hemoglobin can be checked if necessary at any point after the transfusion has been completed. Waiting for "reequilibration" is anecdotal and unnecessary.

Case study for review

You are seeing a one year old for their well child check in clinic. As part of routine screening, a fingerstick hemoglobin is recommended.

1. What questions in the history might help screen for anemia?
2. What about the physical examination?

Multiple questions in the history can be helpful. Dietary screening for excessive milk intake is important in addition to asking about intake of iron-rich foods such as green leafy vegetables and red meat. One should also ask about pica behavior such as eating dirt or ice and include questions regarding the age of the house to help screen for lead paint exposure and ingestion. Any sources of blood loss should also be explored including blood in the urine or stool as well as frequent gum or nose bleeding (more likely in an older child). Finally, family history should be explored regarding anemia during pregnancy, previous history of iron deficiency in siblings, and history of hemoglobinopathies.

Physical examination to search for anemia should be focused. Pallor, especially subconjunctival, perioral, and periungual should be checked. Tachycardia, if present, would be more consistent with acute anemia rather than well-compensated chronic anemia. Splenomegaly, sclera icterus, and jaundice may point to an acute or chronic hemolytic picture.

You do the fingerstick hemoglobin in clinic and it is 10.2 g/dL. The history is not suggestive of iron deficiency and the exam is unremarkable.

3. What are the reasonable next steps?

Depending on the prevalence of iron deficiency in your population, it would be reasonable at this point to give a 1 month trial of oral iron therapy. The family should be counseled that oral iron tastes bad and should be given with vitamin C (i.e., orange juice) and not milk to improve absorption. If there is a low likelihood of iron deficiency, a family history of thalassemia or sickle cell disease, or a suggestive newborn screen, an empiric trial of oral iron supplementation should not be performed. Similarly, if there are signs that are consistent with a hemolytic process or a significant underlying disorder, further workup should be done. In these cases, it would be correct to next perform a CBC. If there are concerns for sickle cell disease or thalassemia, it would be reasonable to also perform hemoglobin electrophoresis. If there are concerns for hemolysis, labs including reticulocyte count, total bilirubin, lactate dehydrogenase, and a direct Coombs should be performed. Finally, if there is concern for a systemic illness such as leukemia, a manual differential should be requested. Further workup for iron deficiency (ferritin and TIBC) as well as lead toxicity could be included or deferred until the anemia is better characterized utilizing the MCV and RDW on the CBC.

Suggested Reading

Auerbach M, Ballard H. Clinical use of intravenous iron: administration, efficacy, and safety. Hematology Am Soc Hematol Educ Program 338–347, 2010.

Bizzarro MJ, Colson E, Ehrenkranz RA. Differential diagnosis and management of anemia in the newborn. Pediatr Clin North Am 51:1087–1107, 2004.

Hermiston ML, Mentzer WC. A practical approach to the evaluation of the anemic child. Pediatr Clin North Am 49:877–891, 2002.

Janus J, Moerschel SK. Evaluation of anemia in children. Am Fam Physician 81:1462–1471, 2010.

Richardon M. Microcytic anemia. Pediatr Rev 28:5–14, 2007.

2 Hemolytic Anemia

Red blood cells (RBCs) normally live for about 100 to 120 days in the circulation. Hemolytic anemia results from a reduced red cell survival due to increased destruction. To compensate for a reduced RBC life span, the bone marrow increases its output of red cells, a response mediated by erythropoietin. Destruction of red cells can be intravascular (within the circulation) or extravascular (by phagocytic cells of the bone marrow, liver, or spleen). Red cell injury or destruction is associated with a transformation to a rigid or abnormal form. Altered cell deformability then leads to decreased survival. Hemolytic anemia may be inherited (thalassemias, hemoglobinopathies, red cell enzyme deficiencies, or membrane defects) or acquired (immune-mediated, associated with infection, or medication related). It can be chronic or acute. Some types of low-grade chronic hemolytic anemias can have acute exacerbations, such as a child with glucose-6-phosphate dehydrogenase (G6PD) deficiency with an exposure to fava beans or naphthalene.

Red cell membrane disorders

Hereditary spherocytosis (HS) is the most common congenital red blood cell membrane disorder. The usual patient with HS has intermittent jaundice, and hemolytic or red cell aplastic episodes associated with viral infection, splenomegaly, and cholelithiasis. However, the clinical presentation is quite variable, with most severe cases presenting in the newborn period or early childhood and milder cases presenting in adulthood.

Several membrane protein defects are responsible for HS. Most result in the instability of spectrin, one of the major red cell skeletal membrane proteins. Structural changes that result as a consequence of protein deficiency lead to membrane instability, loss of surface area, abnormal membrane permeability, and decreased red cell deformability. Metabolic depletion accentuates the defect in HS cells, which accounts for an increase in osmotic fragility after a 24-hour incubation of whole blood at 37 °C. The splenic sinusoids prevent passage of nondeformable spherocytic red cells. This explains the occurrence of splenomegaly in HS and the therapeutic effect of splenectomy.

Patients with HS have a mild-to-moderate chronic hemolytic anemia. Red cell indices reveal a normal to low mean corpuscular volume (MCV) depending on the number of microspherocytes. Cellular dehydration increases the mean corpuscular hemoglobin concentration (characteristically >36%). The red cell distribution width (RDW) is

Handbook of Pediatric Hematology and Oncology: Children's Hospital & Research Center Oakland, Second Edition. Caroline A. Hastings, Joseph C. Torkildson, and Anurag K. Agrawal.
© 2012 John Wiley & Sons, Ltd. Published 2012 by John Wiley & Sons, Ltd.

elevated because of the variable presence of microspherocytes and reticulocytes in proportion to the degree of hemolysis. The peripheral blood smear can be diagnostic with the presence of spherocytes, although this can be a normal finding in the patient with severe anemia and a resultant reticulocytosis. Osmotic fragility tests and ektacytometry studies are characteristic for HS, with increased fragility in hypotonic environments.

As with other hemolytic anemias, affected individuals are susceptible to hypoplastic crises during viral infections. Human parvovirus B19, a frequent pathogen and the organism responsible for erythema infectiosum (fifth disease), selectively invades erythroid progenitor cells and may result in a transient arrest in red cell proliferation. Recovery begins within 7 to 10 days after infection and is usually completed by 4 to 6 weeks. If the initial presentation of a patient with HS is during an aplastic crisis, a diagnosis of HS might not be considered because the reticulocyte count will be low and the peripheral blood smear may be nondiagnostic. The family history of HS should be explored; if it is positive, the patient should be evaluated for HS after recovery from the aplastic episode.

Splenectomy is often considered for patients who have had severe hemolysis requiring transfusions or repeated hospitalization. In patients with mild hemolysis, the decision to perform splenectomy should be delayed; in many cases, it is not required. For pediatric patients who have excessive splenic size, an additional consideration for splenectomy is to diminish the risk of traumatic splenic rupture. The risks of splenectomy must be considered before any clinical decision is made regarding the procedure.

Red cell survival returns to normal values after splenectomy unless an accessory spleen develops. Although an increased number of spherocytes can be seen in the peripheral blood after splenectomy and the osmotic fragility is more abnormal, the hemoglobin value is normal. Platelet counts frequently increase to more than 1000×10^9/L immediately after splenectomy but return to normal levels over several weeks. No therapeutic interventions are required for postsplenectomy thrombocytosis in patients with HS.

To minimize the risk of sepsis due to *Haemophilus influenza* and *Streptococcus pneumoniae*, the splenectomy procedure (when necessary) is often postponed until after the child's fifth or sixth birthday. Patients should be immunized against these organisms in addition to *Neisseria meningiditis* prior to splenectomy and receive penicillin prophylaxis following the procedure. The increase in penicillin-resistant strains of *S. pneumoniae* has raised questions regarding the use of prophylactic penicillin. No studies have determined the frequency of this problem in children receiving prophylactic penicillin after splenectomy.

Red cell enzyme deficiencies

Glucose is the primary metabolic substrate for the red cell. Because the mature red cell does not contain mitochondria, it can metabolize glucose only by anaerobic mechanisms. The two major metabolic pathways within the red cell are the Embden–Meyerhof pathway (EMP) and the hexose monophosphate shunt.

Red cell morphological changes are minimal in patients with red cell enzyme deficiency involving the EMP. Red cell indices are usually normocytic and normochromic. The reticulocyte count is elevated in proportion to the extent of hemolysis. Because many enzyme activities are normally increased in young red cells, a mild deficiency in one of the enzymes may be obscured by the reticulocytosis.

Pyruvate kinase (PK) deficiency is the most common enzyme deficiency in the EMP. The inheritance pattern of this disorder is autosomal recessive. Homozygotes usually have hemolytic anemia with splenomegaly, whereas heterozygotes are usually asymptomatic. The disorder is found worldwide, although it is most common in Caucasians of northern European descent. The range of clinical expression is variable, from severe neonatal jaundice to a fully compensated hemolytic anemia. Anemia is usually normochromic and normocytic, but macrocytes may be present shortly after a hemolytic crisis, reflecting erythroid hyperplasia and early release of immature red cells. The osmotic fragility of red cells is normal to slightly reduced. Diagnosis is confirmed by a quantitative assay for pyruvate kinase, by the measurement of enzyme kinetics and glycolytic intermediates, and by family studies.

Splenectomy is a therapeutic option for PK-deficient patients. As with HS, the decision should be made on the basis of the patient's clinical course. Unlike HS patients, PK-deficient patients, although they improve after splenectomy, do not have complete correction of their hemolytic anemia. As with all hemolytic anemias, these patients should have dietary supplementation with folic acid (1 mg/day) to prevent megaloblastic complications associated with relative folate deficiency. Immunization against *H. influenza*, *S. pneumonia*, and *N. meningiditis* should be given, as well as lifelong penicillin prophylaxis in the splenectomized patient.

Glucose-6-phosphate dehydrogenase (G6PD) deficiency is the most common X-linked red cell enzyme deficiency, with partial expression in the female population and full expression in the affected male population. The distribution of G6PD deficiency is worldwide, with the highest incidence in Africans and African-Americans.

Mediterraneans, American Indians, Southeast Asians, and Sephardic Jews are also affected. In African-Americans, 12% of the male population has the deficiency, 18% of the female population is heterozygous, and 2% of the female population is homozygous. In Southeast Asians, G6PD deficiency is found in approximately 6% of the male population. Most likely, the prevalence of this enzyme abnormality confers resistance to malaria, thus its geographic distribution.

Many variants of G6PD deficiency are known and have been characterized at the biochemical and molecular levels. A variant found in Mediterraneans is associated with chronic hemolytic anemia. Other variants are associated with an unstable enzyme that has normal levels in young red cells. These result in hemolysis only in association with an oxidant challenge (as found in African-Americans). In some cases of G6PD deficiency, hemolysis may be triggered by the oxidant intermediates generated during viral or bacterial infections or after ingestion of oxidant compounds. Shortly after exposure to the oxidant, hemoglobin is oxidized to methemoglobin and eventually denatured, forming intracellular inclusions called Heinz bodies that attach to the red cell membrane. This portion of the membrane may be removed by reticuloendothelial cells resulting in a "bite" cell that has a shortened survival owing to its loss of membrane components. To compensate for hemolysis, red cell production is increased and thus the reticulocyte count is increased.

Individuals with the Mediterranean or Asian forms of G6PD deficiency, in addition to being sensitive to infections and certain drugs, often have a chronic, moderately severe anemia, with nonspherocytic red cells and jaundice. Hemolysis usually starts in early childhood. Reticulocytosis is present and can increase the MCV.

When a hemolytic crisis occurs in G6PD deficiency (or favism), pallor, scleral icterus, hemoglobinemia, hemoglobinuria, and splenomegaly may be noted. Plasma haptoglobin and hemopexin concentrations are low with a concomitant rise in plasma-free hemoglobin. The peripheral smear shows the fragmented bite cells and polychromatophilic cells. Red cell indices may be normal. Special stains can detect Heinz bodies in the cells during the first few days of hemolysis.

A diagnosis of G6PD deficiency should be based on family history, ethnicity, laboratory features, physical findings, and clinical suspicion suggested by a recent exposure to oxidants with resultant acute hemolysis. The diagnosis is confirmed by a quantitative enzyme assay or by molecular analysis of the gene. Since reticulocytes may have a normal level of G6PD enzyme activity, screening tests during acute hemolysis may be falsely elevated; therefore, it is important to test once the hemolytic crisis has ended and the patient again has mature red blood cells. Treatment is directed toward supportive care during the acute event and counseling regarding prevention of future hemolytic crises. In patients with chronic hemolysis, dietary supplementation with folic acid (1 mg/day) is recommended. Use of vitamin E, 500 mg/day, may improve red cell survival in patients with chronic hemolysis.

Autoimmune hemolytic anemia

In addition to intrinsic causes of hemolytic anemia, patients may also develop an autoantibody and/or alloantibody toward their red blood cells. The underlying cause for this antibody formation is often idiopathic or due to a secondary condition including drugs, infectious syndromes, autoimmune diseases, or an oncological process. A positive direct antiglobulin test (DAT, direct Coombs) is pathognomonic for immune-mediated hemolysis with the appropriate clinical and laboratory findings (i.e.,

jaundice, scleral icterus, elevated bilirubin, and anemia with reticulocytosis). Fortunately, the majority of pediatric cases of autoimmune hemolytic anemia (AIHA) are acute and self-limited.

In the DAT, the patient's erythrocytes are washed and then incubated with specific antiglobulin antisera (usually anti-IgG and anti-C3d). Agglutination indicates a positive test. In patients with severe immune-mediated hemolytic anemia, the DAT is often strongly positive, although the strength of the reaction does not always correlate to the severity of the disease. Similarly, up to 80% of patients will have antibodies in the serum as well, measured by the indirect Coombs (indirect antiglobulin test, IAT). In the IAT, donor erythrocytes are incubated with test serum, washed, and then incubated with specific antiglobulin antisera. Agglutination again indicates a positive test. Of note, patients without symptoms of hemolysis may have a positive DAT and/or IAT; therefore, screening is only recommended in the setting of clinical and laboratory signs of hemolysis. In approximately 5% to 10% of cases, patients may have an AIHA with a negative DAT.

The initiation of autoimmunity is poorly understood. Viral syndromes are often proposed as a culprit, although causation has been hard to prove. A majority of cases of AIHA in pediatrics are due to "warm" antibodies, so named because they react at 37 °C. These are often secondary to a viral syndrome, although patients with an underlying autoimmune disease or oncological process can also present with a warm AIHA. The formation of IgG antibodies leads to extravascular hemolysis in which pieces of the red cell membrane are sequentially removed during passages through the spleen. Patients may also develop direct Coombs positive hemolytic anemia and immune-mediated thrombocytopenia (Evans syndrome).

Hemolytic disease of the newborn

Intrinsic causes of hemolytic anemia can present as jaundice in the newborn period. These syndromes must be differentiated from hemolytic disease of the newborn in which alloimmunization in the mother occurs due to foreign RBC antigens from the fetus. RBC antigens can either be major (ABO) or minor (Rh, Kell, Duffy, etc.). For ABO hemolytic disease, typically the mother is type O and the fetus is type A; anti-A antibodies subsequently produced by the mother then traverse the placenta leading to hemolytic anemia in the fetus. RhoGAM® (Rho[D] Immune Globulin) has virtually eliminated hemolytic disease in the Rh-negative (D-negative) mother with a Rh-positive (D-positive) fetus although is still possible in the mother not receiving prenatal care. Many cases of hemolytic disease of the newborn are now due to other minor RBC antigens with varying levels of clinical severity. AIHA in the mother can also lead to hemolytic disease of the newborn. In this case, maternal antibodies traverse the placenta and are transferred to the fetus. If the mother is DAT positive but does not have clinical signs of hemolytic anemia, there is usually no risk to the fetus.

Microangiopathic hemolytic anemia

Microangiopathic hemolytic anemias are due to extracorpuscular abnormalities and are not associated with antibody formation. Causes include disseminated intravascular coagulation, thrombotic thrombocytopenic purpura/hemolytic uremic syndrome, preeclampsia, malignant hypertension, valvular abnormalities, and march hemoglobinuria. In these cases, red blood cells travel through damaged blood vessels or heart valves or are damaged by the formation of an intravascular fibrin mesh due to hypercoagulability, leading to fragmentation (e.g., schistocytes) and intravascular hemolysis.

Evaluation

The evaluation of hemolytic anemia includes a thorough history assessing for evidence of chronic hemolytic anemia and possible precipitants of an acute event (see Figure 2.1).

The family history is equally important and questions to ask include:

History of newborn jaundice
Gallstones
Splenomegaly or splenectomy
Episodes of dark urine and/or yellow skin/ sclerae
Anemia unresponsive to iron supplementation
Medications
Environmental exposures
Ethnicity
Dietary history

The physical exam should be complete, but focused on:
Skin color (pallor, jaundice, and icteric sclerae)
Facial bone changes (extramedullary hematopoiesis)
Abdominal fullness and splenomegaly

The laboratory evaluation includes:
Complete blood count, RBC indices, and reticulocyte count ($\uparrow$)
Peripheral blood smear (assess for fragmented forms or evidence of inherited anemia with specific morphological abnormalities)
Bilirubin ($\uparrow$)
Coombs test, direct and indirect (to exclude antibody-mediated red cell destruction)
Urinalysis (for heme, bili)
Free plasma hemoglobin ($\uparrow$)

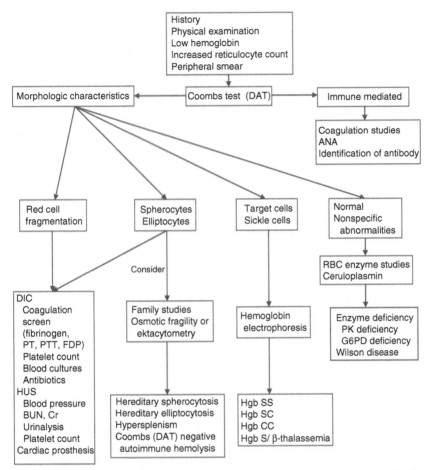

Figure 2.1 Diagnostic approach to the child with hemolytic anemia. (Abbreviations: DAT, direct antiglobulin test; ANA, anti-nuclear antibody; DIC, disseminated intravascular coagulation; PT, prothrombin time; PTT, partial thromboplastin time; FDP, fibrin degradation products; HUS, hemolytic uremic syndrome; BUN, blood urea nitrogen; Cr, creatinine; PK, pyruvate kinase; G6PD, glucose–6-phosphate dehydrogenase).

Specific tests for diagnosis may include:
Osmotic fragility
Ektacytometry
Red cell enzyme defects (G6PD and PK)
Red cell membrane defects (HS)

The osmotic fragility test is used to measure the osmotic resistance of red cells. Red cells are incubated under hypotonic conditions, and their ability to swell before lysis is determined. The osmotic fragility of red cells is increased when the surface area to volume ratio of the red cells is decreased, as in hereditary spherocytosis, in which membrane instability results in membrane loss and decreased surface area. Conversely, osmotic fragility is decreased in liver disease as the ratio of the red cell surface area to volume is increased. Ektacytometry measures the deformability of red cells subjected simultaneously to shear stress and osmotic stress.

Treatment

Therapy depends on the underlying cause of the anemia and the degree of acute hemolysis. In chronic hemolysis, such as that associated with hereditary spherocytosis, splenectomy is often recommended to decrease the degree of splenic destruction and level of anemia and to decrease the incidence of bilirubin gallstones. This therapy must be now weighed against the potential long-term complications of splenectomy including risk for infection, thrombosis, and pulmonary hypertension. In other forms of inherited anemias in which the hemolysis is more significant and even life-threatening, such as thalassemia or some forms of enzymopathies, chronic transfusion therapy is recommended. Other general measures include folic acid replacement due to high cell turnover, avoidance of oxidant chemicals and drugs, and iron chelation therapy as indicated for transfusion-related iron overload.

Immune hemolytic anemias can require more immediate and aggressive therapy. The underlying disease, if present and identifiable, warrants treatment. Additionally, the use of corticosteroids in high doses is frequently necessary. Splenectomy and immunosuppressive drugs have also been successful. Microangiopathic hemolytic anemias can also be severe and life-threatening. Treatment should again first be directed toward the primary disorder to remove the cause of trauma, if possible. Transfusions are frequently necessary and splenectomy may be needed in some patients with severe hypersplenism.

Case study for review

You are seeing a 6-year-old child in the emergency department. The family notes that the child has been jaundiced and fatigued over the last few days with a red color to the urine. Fingerstick hemoglobin at the pediatrician's office reveals a hemoglobin of 5 g/dL prior to transfer to the ED. On the basis of this history and hemoglobin, it appears that the child is suffering from a hemolytic anemia.

1. What initial lab studies will help confirm the diagnosis and also help with the initial treatment plan?

Initial lab studies should include a complete blood count with reticulocyte count. The reticulocyte count is an important first step to confirm that the patient is undergoing hemolysis, which should present with a low hemoglobin and a resultant increase in the reticulocyte count. A low reticulocyte count in this setting should lead to consideration of alternative diagnoses such as viral suppression (although one would not expect hemolysis). A complete metabolic panel as well as lactate dehydrogenase (LDH) should be done to ensure that the patient is actually suffering from jaundice (elevated total bilirubin) and hemolysis (elevated LDH and AST). A direct and indirect Coombs (DAT/IAT) is an important first step to determine if the patient is undergoing an immune or nonimmune hemolytic anemia.

The patient is noted to have a hemoglobin of 4.6 g/dL with 12.6% reticulocytes. One should first determine if the patient is having an appropriate bone marrow response to anemia by calculating the reticulocyte index (RI):

$$RI = \text{Reticulocyte count } (\%)$$
$$\times \left(\frac{\text{current hemoglobin}}{\text{expected hemoglobin}} \right)$$

In this case, the RI is $12.6\% \times (4.6/13) = 4.5$.

An $RI \geq 3.0$ is consistent with an appropriate bone marrow response to anemia, and therefore helps to rule out bone marrow dysfunction in this case. Modern blood cell analyzers have the ability to calculate the absolute reticulocyte count and the fraction of "immature" reticulocytes directly. Patients who are demonstrating an appropriate response to hemolysis will have an elevated absolute reticulocyte count and immature reticulocyte fraction; these will be low or normal in patients with an inadequate response.

Other labs include a total bilirubin of 6.7 mg/dL, LDH of 936 U/L (reference range 313 to 618 U/L), and AST of 161 U/L. DAT is noted to be positive for IgG and C3d.

2. What is the likely diagnosis?

With the positive DAT to IgG and complement and clinical and laboratory signs of hemolysis, warm antibody-mediated AIHA is the likely diagnosis. It should be noted that a positive DAT without clinical and laboratory signs of hemolysis is not sufficient for the diagnosis of AIHA.

3. What should be the initial treatment plan?

The patient is started on steroid therapy, IV methylprednisolone 1 mg/kg BID. After a couple of days, the hemoglobin has continued to decrease to 3 g/dL even though the methylprednisolone has been increased to 4 mg/kg BID and the patient is showing signs of symptomatic anemia and congestive heart failure.

4. How should your treatment change at this point?

Since the patient has a falling hemoglobin with clinical signs of cardiac instability and volume overload, the patient should be transfused. The term "least incompatible unit" has been used in the past but is a misnomer if phenotypically matched blood is given. The patient may not have a normal increase in hemoglobin with transfusion due to continued hemolysis and the potential for increased, bystander hemolysis with transfusion. Because of the cardiac instability, it is advisable to give the transfusion slowly and monitor for worsening cardiac function. Finally, a change in therapy would be advisable at this point with either intravenous immunoglobulin or a different immunosuppressant such as cyclosporine, cyclophosphamide, or rituximab (monoclonal antibody to CD20).

Suggested Reading

Garratty G. Immune hemolytic anemia—a primer. Semin Hematol 42:119–121, 2005.

3 Sickle Cell Disease

Sickle cell disease refers to a group of genetic disorders that share a common feature: hemoglobin S (Hgb S) alone or in combination with another abnormal hemoglobin. The sickle cell diseases are inherited in an autosomal codominant manner. The molecular defect in Hgb S is due to the substitution of valine for glutamic acid at the sixth position of the β-globin chain. The change of location of this substitution results in polymerization of the hemoglobin and causes the red cells to transform from deformable biconcave discs into rigid, sickle-shape cells. Hypoxia, acidosis, and hypertonicity facilitate polymer formation.

The most common combinations of abnormal hemoglobins are (1) Hgb SS, (2) Hgb SC, and (3) Hgb S with a beta-thalassemia, either $S\beta^+$ or $S\beta^0$. The most severely affected individuals have either Hgb SS or $S\beta^0$ (no normal beta-globin production). Individuals with Hgb $S\beta^+$ have decreased beta-globin production and less severe disease, whereas children who have Hgb SC have intermediate severity of disease. There is phenotypic overlap between Hgb SS and Hgb SC; some children with Hgb SC are more symptomatic than children with Hgb SS. There are many variables to expression of this hemoglobinopathy including haplotypes, Hgb F concentration, and other yet to be delineated factors. As yet, it is not possible to predict the severity of disease in advance of severe complications. Generally, children who have vaso-occlusion and other complications have a more severe course. Increased leukocyte count, decreased hemoglobin with concomitant increased reticulocytosis, as well as frequency and severity of vaso-occlusive episodes (VOEs) are associated with increased morbidity and mortality.

Alpha-thalassemia (frequency 1% to 3% in African-Americans) may be coinherited with sickle cell trait or disease. Individuals who have both α-thalassemia and sickle cell anemia are less anemic than those who have sickle cell anemia alone due to a more similar concentration of α- and β-globulins. However, α-thalassemia trait does not appear to prevent frequency or severity of vaso-occlusive complications, resulting in eventual end-organ damage.

Sickle cell disease is not uncommon and has developed due to protection from malaria in those with sickle cell trait. In African-Americans, the frequency of genetic alteration is quite high: 8% have the Hgb S gene, 4% the Hgb C gene, and 1% the β-thalassemia gene. Approximately 1 in 600 African-American infants has sickle cell anemia. Sickle cell disease also occurs in children from the Middle East, India, Central and South America, and the Caribbean.

Handbook of Pediatric Hematology and Oncology: Children's Hospital & Research Center Oakland,
Second Edition. Caroline A. Hastings, Joseph C. Torkildson, and Anurag K. Agrawal.
© 2012 John Wiley & Sons, Ltd. Published 2012 by John Wiley & Sons, Ltd.

All children who have sickle cell hemo-globinopathies have a variable degree of hemolytic anemia and vaso-occlusive tissue ischemia resulting in numerous clinical complications. Organs most sensitive to the ischemic-hypoxic injury of red cell sickling are the lungs, spleen, kidneys, bone marrow, eyes, brain, and the heads of the humeri and femurs. Sickling has both acute and long-term implications for organ function. **Cerebral vascular disease** can be subtle, causing only abnormal neuropsychological testing or it can be catastrophic, resulting in hemiparesis, coma, or death; acute **pulmonary sickling** causes lung injury leading to restrictive lung disease and eventually pulmonary hypertension; **osteonecrosis** of the femoral head can be debilitating, resulting in the need for hip replacement; untreated **retinopathy** can lead to blindness; and, sickle cell **nephropathy** can cause asymptomatic proteinuria, an early sign of the risk of eventual renal failure.

Now that newborn hemoglobinopathy testing is mandatory in most states, children are diagnosed early and receive appropriate care before they are at risk for complications. All infants who have an electrophoretic pattern of Hgb FS at birth will have some form of sickle cell disease.

Fever and infection in sickle cell disease

Susceptibility to infection is increased not only because of loss of splenic function due to infarction but also because of other acquired immunologic abnormalities. This can result in life-threatening episodes of sepsis. Recognition of this susceptibility and aggressive medical management have resulted in an increased life span for most patients.

Most children with sickle cell disease are identified at birth, started on prophylactic penicillin by age 2 months, and aggressively monitored and treated for signs of infection. However, with the increasing concern for bacterial **antibiotic resistance,** health care providers need to be vigilant when confronted with an infant or a child who has fever ($\geq$38.3 °C) and/or appears ill. Overall, *Streptococcus pneumoniae* is responsible for >80% of the morbidity of infection. In some areas of the United States, up to 50% of pneumococcal isolates are penicillin resistant. Infections can precipitate vaso-occlusive episodes and other complications of sickle cell anemia and, in this population, can quickly become fulminant. Although the American Academy of Pediatrics guidelines recommend the discontinuation of penicillin prophylaxis after 6 years of age, our institutional practice is to continue it as long as possible (until compliance becomes an issue) due to the high risk of *S. pneumoniae* infection.

Additional bacteria that cause morbidity and mortality include *Haemophilus influenzae, Neisseria meningitidis, Mycoplasma pneumoniae, Staphylococcus aureus, Salmonella* species, *Escherichia coli,* and *Streptococcus pyogenes.* The *S. pneumoniae* and *H. influenzae* vaccines have importantly resulted in a lowered case rate of sepsis from these organisms. Viral infections, particularly parvovirus B19, can cause severe aplastic crises as well as acute chest syndrome (ACS).

Infants, young children, and any patient who has a central venous catheter with a fever ($\geq$38.3 °C) should have a complete evaluation and laboratories including CBC with differential, reticulocyte count, blood culture, urinalysis, and urine culture (see Figure 3.1). A chest radiograph should also be obtained. Meningitis can occur in children with sickle cell disease but routine lumbar puncture without physical signs of

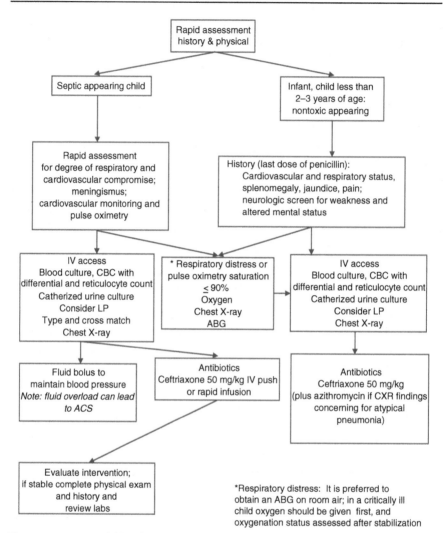

Figure 3.1 Fever in a child with sickle cell disease. (Abbreviations: IV, intravenous; CBC, complete blood count; LP, lumbar puncture; ABG, arterial blood gas; CXR, chest x-ray; ACS, acute chest syndrome).

meningitis is not warranted. Urosepsis is common in sickle cell patients of all ages. All infants (up to 2 to 3 years of age) should be admitted and cultures followed for 48 to 72 hours. These patients should not be discharged during this time even if they appear well and are afebrile. Some practitioners would recommend complete evaluation in all patients with a fever.

Children with a documented fever should have the same workup as infants, although admission is not required if they are well appearing, with reassuring labs and chest radiograph, and follow-up can be reasonably guaranteed. Acute chest syndrome should be high on the differential in all children with fever. While physical examination is essential, 60% of pulmonary infiltrates in children with sickle cell disease and fever will be missed on exam alone, therefore chest radiography is essential. If there is another possible source of infection, appropriate cultures should be obtained. If a child appears to be ill, has a temperature of 38.3 °C or higher, or has an elevated WBC with a left shift, treatment should be immediate with parenteral antibiotics and close monitoring, preferably in a hospital setting. Of note, studies have shown that the higher the temperature, the more likely the risk for bacterial sepsis. If there is difficulty with intravenous (IV) access, ceftriaxone can be given intramuscular (IM) while access is being obtained.

Children who do not appear septic, in whom there is a low index of suspicion, and who are older than 2 to 3 years of age (per institutional preference), can be treated as outpatients with IV/IM ceftriaxone while awaiting culture results, only if close monitoring can be assured (parents can be contacted by telephone and daily evaluation is easily done while still febrile). If all cultures are negative after 2 to 3 days and the child is afebrile without clinical symptoms, the antibiotics and follow-up can be discontinued.

All patients who appear ill should be hospitalized and treated for presumed infection. Many children will develop increasing symptoms after being evaluated and hospitalized. Acute chest syndrome commonly occurs after hydration and is frequently precipitated by a vaso-occlusive pain episode.

Vaso-occlusive episodes

The bones and joints are the major sites of pain in sickle cell disease. In trabecular bones, such as the vertebrae, infarction can occur and eventually lead to collapse of the vertebral plates and compression. The classic radiographic appearance is of "fish mouth" disc spaces and the "step" sign (a depression in the central part of the vertebral body). Back pain is a common symptom in sickle cell disease, likely as a result of recurrent infarction and vertebral compression. Infarction in the long bones can cause swelling and edema in the overlying soft tissues. It may be difficult to differentiate VOE from acute osteomyelitis. Although uncommon, infection should be considered. Osteomyelitis may be ruled out by close clinical observation, blood cultures, and occasionally, aspiration of the affected area. Plain radiographs are not helpful in the early stages of infection and bone scans may not differentiate a simple infarct from osteomyelitis.

Dactylitis, or hand-foot syndrome, refers to painful swelling of the hands and feet. This is seen exclusively in infants and children (<5 years of age). It presents with pain, low-grade fever, and diffuse nonpitting edema of the dorsum of the hands and feet, which extends to the fingers. One or more extremities may be affected at one time. Radiographic changes (periostitis and subperiosteal new bone formation with periosteal elevation) may appear 1 week or more after the clinical presentation. Therapy is analgesics, hydration, and parental reassurance. Although the swelling or radiographic changes may persist for weeks, the syndrome is almost always self-limited. Transfusions and antibiotics are not necessary, unless there is concern for infection or the medical condition worsens.

Occasionally, there is a precipitating event such as hypoxia (obstructive sleep apnea), fever, viral illness, or dehydration that leads to the vaso-occlusive episode. Few children have frequent pain episodes; it should not be taken for granted that each of these episodes is similar, and a source for each painful event should be sought. If the pain changes or is very persistent, the child should be reevaluated. If a young child has a symptom that is interpreted as pain, such as refusal to walk or a limp, also consider that the cause may be due to an acute CNS event.

The most common type of pain is musculoskeletal pain. The pain may be of any configuration: isolated, multifocal, symmetric, migratory, or associated with erythema or swelling. There can be low-grade fevers, possibly associated with other clinical symptoms. It can sometimes be difficult to distinguish pain from an infection, synovitis, or other pathological process.

Children are frequently seen with **abdominal pain**. A surgical abdominal problem needs to be considered. Children who have sickle cell anemia have a high incidence of cholecystitis. Also consider pancreatitis, urinary tract infection, pelvic inflammatory disease, and pneumonia presenting as abdominal pain. Ileus and acute chest syndrome are frequent complications of abdominal vaso-occlusive episodes.

Vaso-occlusive episodes can last for many days. *Do not assume that the episode is controlled when the acute administration of analgesia is effective.* Children with these symptoms may have a medical problem that needs aggressive treatment beyond therapy for their pain. A vaso-occlusive episode is a diagnosis of exclusion. The pain needs to be treated while there is a workup for potential other causes of pain beyond the vaso-occlusive episode itself.

A reliable tool should be used to assess a child's level of pain. The assessment should be modified depending on the age and developmental level of the child, and the pain tool should be able to rate both subjective and objective aspects of the child's pain. Physicians should be familiar with their use and refer to them when assessing children and adolescents with pain.

High-risk factors for complications other than VOE in children with pain:
- Fever $\geq 101°F$ (38.3°C) and signs of infection
- Acute pulmonary symptoms (chest pain, hypoxia, abnormal ausculatory exam)
- Persistent vomiting
- Pain that is unusual for the patient
- Severe abdominal pain
- Extremity weakness or loss of function
- Any neurological symptoms
- Severe headache
- Acute joint swelling

Pain management

Following are the recommendations for the management of vaso-occlusive events. However, many children and adolescents need individualized care plans for their routine treatment.

Outpatient
Mild pain
- Increase fluids to 1 to 1.25× maintenance. Water, fruit juice, and fruit drinks as well as decaffeinated soda are recommended.
- Acetaminophen without codeine (15 mg/kg q4 to 6 hours) orally should be tried prior to using acetaminophen with codeine (1.0 mg codeine/kg q4 to 6 hours). For many children, acetaminophen alone is not sufficient for vaso-occlusive pain.
- Ibuprofen (10 mg/kg q6 to 8 hours) orally should be used routinely, every 8 hours even if pain is temporarily controlled.
- Rest and heat to the area of pain.
- Relaxation and biofeedback exercises, such as positive visualization and meditation.

Severe pain
- IV hydration: bolus to correct fluid losses, then IV with D5W 1/2 NS at 1 to 1.25× maintenance (IV + PO). Use caution not to overhydrate, especially if there are any

pulmonary symptoms (overhydration can lead to pulmonary edema and precipitate acute chest syndrome). **Note that if the patient does not appear volume depleted, an IV fluid bolus is not routinely required.**

- Analgesics (IV): Morphine: 0.1 to 0.15 mg/kg/dose q3 to 4 hours. In children <2 years who have not been exposed to narcotic analgesics, 0.05 to 0.1 mg/kg should be used. The pharmacokinetics of morphine differs between individual children and doses must be titrated for individual patients. Both underdosing and overdosing need to be avoided. **Careful management is required! Previous medication history is often a good starting place.**

- Ketorolac: (child) IV: 1 mg/kg/load, then 0.5 mg/kg q6 hours (max 30 mg); (adult) IV: 30 to 60 mg/load, then 15 to 30 mg/kg q6 hours. **GI bleeding** has been reported, and an H2 blocker such as ranitidine is required if ketorolac is given IV. Morphine and ketorolac can be given simultaneously or in succession for the initial treatment of pain in children. Added to narcotic therapy, ketorolac increases analgesia and has a narcotic sparing effect. **Ketorolac is very useful in pain control, but should not be used for more than 5 days.** There are numerous other analgesic medications that have been used to treat sickle cell pain.

Upon presentation to the clinic or emergency room, the child or adolescent should be rapidly assessed and treated for pain. Initially, both morphine and ketorolac should be given at the maximum recommended doses. If the pain returns, repeat the parenteral narcotic dose; it is unlikely that oral analgesics will be successful if this regimen is not effective. If pain relief can be achieved and maintained for 3 hours, administer an oral narcotic and observe for 1 hour. If this regimen is successful, give a prescription of narcotic and nonsteroidal anti-inflammatory medications for several days (10 to 15 doses). There should be follow-up within 72 hours. If this regimen is not successful, if other symptoms develop with hydration, or a fever develops, the patient should be admitted and observed.

Inpatient

As noted above, the administration of narcotics to acutely ill patients requires careful monitoring. A plan for pain management is defined on admission and followed for the duration of hospitalization. In addition to whirlpool therapy, warm packs, and biofeedback therapy (as available), routine care includes:

Management

- Correct acute losses due to dehydration. Do not overhydrate children who have pulmonary symptoms.
- Total fluid intake (IV + PO) should be 1 to 1.25× daily maintenance fluids; do not overhydrate.
- Monitor daily weight, record strict intake and output (I&O), and observe for signs of fluid overload.
- Encourage ambulation, sitting up in bed, and taking deep breaths.
- Incentive spirometry, 10 times an hour, every hour while awake.

Analgesics

- Pain medication should be administered on a fixed-time schedule, with an interval that does not extend beyond the duration of the analgesic effect. Do not give narcotics on a PRN basis except for when the patient is ready for discharge.
- Titration schedules (requires a written plan, close observation, and a flow sheet to monitor effectiveness; sedation and hypoventilation can lead to hypoxia and increased sickling and pain).
- Patient-controlled analgesia (PCA). This is the method of choice for controlling pain in children who are ≥7 years of age or older.

PCA protocols may be hospital specific. Generally, there is an initial bolus (0.1 mg/kg morphine), and an on-demand dose (0.01 to 0.04 mg/kg morphine) with a 10 to 20 minute lock out, and a 1 hour maximum of 0.1 to 0.15 mg/kg of morphine. At night, there may be a need for a continuous low-dose infusion (0.01 to 0.02 mg/kg/h morphine) without changing the 1 hour lock out.

Side effects of narcotics include respiratory depression, nausea, vomiting, pruritus, hypotension, constipation, inappropriate secretion of anti-diuretic hormone, and change in seizure threshold. Low-dose naloxone drip has been used for severe pruritus and urinary retention due to morphine. The most common side effects of nausea, vomiting, and pruritus resolve over time. IV or PO diphenhydramine may be used safely in this setting and can have a synergistic positive effect with morphine. Meperidine should not be substituted for morphine. The metabolites of meperidine can accumulate and cause seizures, especially if used over a longer period at high doses. A plan for withdrawal should be a part of discharge planning; clonidine hydrochloride has been used successfully in this setting, but should be carefully monitored.

All patients who are hospitalized for pain should have an **incentive spirometer** at the bedside. Ensure that the patient has been instructed on its usage and can demonstrate it appropriately.

Alternative methods of pain control (behavior modification, relaxation, visualization, self-hypnosis, and transcutaneous electrical nerve stimulation) are helpful adjuvants in the outpatient and inpatient setting but should not replace standard therapy. Children should have access to a psychologist who is experienced in the management of sickle cell pain.

Drug addiction is extremely rare and should not be a primary concern. The goal should be to provide patients with adequate relief by understanding the pharmacology of the medications, drug tolerance, and physical dependence. Drug tolerance is common, and withdrawal symptoms after hospitalization are probably underreported by the patients. All patients should start a narcotic taper while in the hospital and complete this as an outpatient. On average, patients admitted for the management of VOE require 3 to 7 days of inpatient care.

Acute chest syndrome/ pneumonia

Acute chest syndrome (ACS) is defined as the development of a new pulmonary infiltrate in the presence of fever or respiratory symptoms. As chest radiograph changes may be delayed, the diagnosis may not be apparent at presentation. Approximately 50% of children with sickle cell disease will have acute chest syndrome. ACS is frequently caused by community-acquired pathogens such as chlamydia, mycoplasma, and other bacterial or viral organisms. In older children, adolescents, and young adults, ACS may be more commonly associated with vaso-occlusion, infarction, fat embolism, or in situ sickling. These episodes are characterized by chest pain, fever, hypoxia, and pulmonary infiltrates. Although ACS usually improves with medical management, it can present with or progress rapidly to respiratory failure (acute respiratory distress syndrome), requiring mechanical ventilation and emergent exchange transfusion.

Sixty percent of children who have pneumonia on X-ray will be missed by physical exam alone. In addition, many children with a negative chest film on admission will

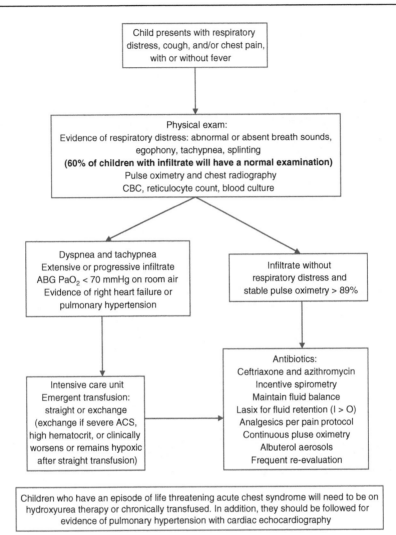

Figure 3.2 Sickle-cell disease with acute pulmonary infiltrate. (Abbreviations: CBC, complete blood count; ABG, arterial blood gas; ACS, acute chest syndrome).

develop findings after hydration. All children who have symptoms of pulmonary disease, such as fever, shortness of breath, tachypnea, chest pain, cough, wheezing, rales, or dullness to percussion, should have an assessment of oxygen saturation, a chest radiograph, receive parenteral antibiotics, and be admitted to the hospital (see Figure 3.2). Bronchodilators and incentive spirometry are helpful adjuncts in treatment and prevention of worsening ACS. If there is an infiltrate, the patient should be closely observed for hypoxia and progression of pulmonary infiltrates, with repeat chest radiographs. Overhydration can lead to pulmonary edema and exacerbate acute chest syndrome. Oversedation with narcotics can also lead to hypoventilation, increasing the risk for ACS. Narcotics should be used with caution in this setting.

Acute chest syndrome can develop in a matter of hours and is associated with a high rate of morbidity and mortality. Children should have oxygen saturation monitored and, if indicated, arterial blood gases also. Oxygen therapy should be used only for significant hypoxia (O_2 saturation $\leq$ 92%). Supplemental oxygen can decrease erythropoietin production and lead to more severe anemia. Pulmonary infections should be treated aggressively, and these children watched closely. If there is no improvement, and/or worsening anemia, a red blood cell transfusion (straight or exchange, dependent upon the severity of the hypoxia, anemia, and clinical status of the patient) may help to correct the anemia, decrease the percent Hgb S, and improve oxygen-carrying capacity to aid in reversing the pulmonary sickling and improve the clinical course. Transfusions are more effective when administered early in the course of ACS, rather than as a life-saving measure in a critically ill child.

There is a distinct difference between the etiology of acute chest syndrome in children and that of adolescents and adults. In children, the incidence of acute chest syndrome is seasonal, lower in the summer months with increasing rates in the winter when viral infections are prevalent. In adults and adolescents, ACS is frequently a complication of an episode of vaso-occlusion (without fever) due to pulmonary fat embolism. This event will progress to include chest pain, fever, and a pulmonary infiltrate (usually basilar with pleural effusion). Adults and adolescents more frequently need transfusions and less frequently have a viral or bacterial infection associated with their episode of acute chest syndrome. Individuals with Hgb SC disease have relatively more fat in their marrow and resultantly can have more severe pulmonary fat emboli when their course is complicated by acute chest syndrome.

Stroke and other central nervous system events are more common in children with ACS in the 2 week period after the event.

Laboratory evaluation of acute chest syndrome

- CBC with differential and reticulocyte count.
- Type and hold for possible blood transfusion (phenotypically matched, sickledex negative).
- Chest radiograph, as often as clinically indicated to monitor progression of disease.
- Continuous pulse oximetry and baseline arterial blood gas (on room air if possible).
- Blood culture for fever.

Management

All patients with evidence of acute pulmonary pathology should be admitted to the hospital. If fever is present or if an infectious process is suspected, antibiotic therapy should be started immediately. See *Fever and Infection* section, and Figures 3.1 and 3.2.

- Oxygen

Hypoxemic patients (P_aO_2 70 to 80 mmHg, O_2 saturation $\leq$92%): 2 L/min per nasal cannula.

Reevaluate arterial blood gas on oxygen.

- Antibiotics

Initiate broad spectrum antibiotic: **ceftriaxone** 50 mg/kg/d IV every 24 hours after blood cultures obtained (maximum 2 g/dose).

Due to the frequency of atypical organisms (e.g., chlamydia and mycoplasma), a macrolide or quinolone antibiotic should be included: **azithromycin** 10 mg/kg on day 1, followed by 5 mg/kg on days 2 to 5 (maximum 500 mg on day 1, 250 mg on days 2 to 5).

• Analgesics

As indicated for vaso-occlusive pain management, administration must be monitored to provide the maximum pain control and prevent hypoventilation or atelectasis from splinting or narcotization.

• Hydration

PO and IV hydration (D5W 1/2 NS) at a maximum of 1.25× maintenance. Caution should be used in patients with potential acute chest syndrome to avoid fluid overload. Monitor Is & Os, daily weight.

• Other supportive measures

Continuous pulse oximetry.

Incentive spirometry, 10 times an hour, every hour while awake (prevention of hypoventilation and atelectasis).

Albuterol aerosols q4 hours (airway hyperreactivity common in ACS).

• Physical therapy

Warm packs.

Ambulation as tolerated, sitting up in bed.

• Transfusion

Straight transfusion.

Exchange transfusion (for patients with hematocrit > 30% or moderate-to-severe ACS to more efficiently reduce Hgb S%).

Transfusion decreases the proportion of sickling red cells and increases blood oxygen affinity. The main indication is worsening respiratory function, as documented by hypoxemia (p_aO_2 <70 mmHg on room air), worsening chest pain, evolving clinical examination, or worsening infiltrates on chest radiography. For patients with chronic hypoxemia, a drop of >10% from baseline is a reasonable level at which to transfuse. Delays in instituting transfusion therapy, particularly in rapidly deteriorating patients, should be avoided.

Priapism

Forty percent of men who are homozygous for Hgb S report having priapism in their adolescence and early adulthood. Priapism has a second peak at 21 to 29 years. Priapism is defined as a **painful** erection that lasts for more than 30 minutes. It frequently results in interference with the urinary stream. Priapism can be precipitated by prolonged intercourse or masturbation, frequently occurs at night, and can be differentiated from a nocturnal erection by its duration and pain. Children will occasionally complain of dysuria as the first complaint of priapism. Prognosis is poorer in adolescents and adults who have recurrent prolonged priapism, and if aggressive treatment has not been successful, impotence may result. Children who have priapism generally have a better prognosis than adolescents and adults and usually do not have prolonged episodes requiring aggressive therapy. Priapism can occur with vaso-occlusive episodes as well as with fever and sepsis.

Priapism can last for hours, days, or weeks with moderate-to-severe pain, or it can occur as a pattern of painful erections that recur over a period of days to several weeks (stuttering priapism). Chronic nonpainful priapism can also occur.

Since priapism can lead to impotence, early medical management is indicated. A urologist familiar with priapism in sickle cell disease should be consulted. Treatment includes hydration, pain management, intracavernous injection of alpha-adrenergic agents, exchange transfusion, and shunting surgery. Oral alpha-adrenergics (e.g., pseudoephedrine hydrochloride 30 mg BID) have been used successfully to treat stuttering priapism. Chronic transfusion therapy has been used in patients with recurrent priapism (maintenance of Hgb S below 30% to 40%), although no controlled trials have been performed proving the efficacy of this therapy.

Stroke (cerebrovascular accident)

Stroke is a common event in children homozygous for Hgb S. Between 10% and 15% of children with sickle cell disease suffer from overt strokes. In children, strokes are more frequently the result of cerebral vascular stenosis and infarction. The mean age of occurrence of clinically evident stroke is 7 to 8 years with the highest risk occurring between 2 and 9 years. Hemorrhage and infarct may occur together.

Strokes in children who have sickle cell disease involve stenosis and occlusion of the major anterior arteries of the brain, including the carotids. The presenting symptoms of stroke can be dramatic and acute, such as coma, seizure, hemiparesis, hemianesthesia, visual field deficits, aphasia, or cranial nerve palsies. Subtle limb weakness (without pain) is often mistaken for an acute vaso-occlusive episode but can be due to stroke. By definition, the symptoms must persist for at least 24 hours to be classified as a stroke. The presentation of severe headache and vomiting with no other neurological findings can be symptoms of an intracranial hemorrhage.

Initially, a CT scan without contrast will be normal for up to 6 hours after a stroke but will rule out intracerebral hemorrhage, abscess, tumor, or other pathology that would explain the neurological symptoms. Magnetic resonance imaging (MRI) and magnetic resonance angiography (MRA) are much more sensitive methods to determine intracranial infarct but can remain normal for 2 to 4 hours after an event. All catastrophic neurological events should first be evaluated with CT since it is generally more available and will rule out acute pathology.

With clinical concern prior to definitive diagnosis by MRI/MRA imaging, children are exchange transfused to achieve a concentration of Hgb S of less than 30%. Blood pressure should be continually monitored during an exchange transfusion realizing that, relative to the normal population, children with sickle cell disease are hypotensive. The diagnosis of stroke in children should initially be made based on clinical findings and treated emergently. Children should be monitored until they are stable and the hemoglobin electrophoresis is documented. Those who have had a stroke require chronic transfusion therapy for an undetermined length of time.

Children with sickle cell disease have more frequent and more severe **headaches** than other children; these may be manifestations of cerebral hypoxia and vasodilation. Children who have severe headaches accompanied by vomiting need extensive evaluation with imaging as well as neurologic and neuropsychological testing.

Transcranial Doppler (TCD) has been shown to predict increased risk of stroke in children who have increased flow velocity in major cerebral arteries. Unsuspected cerebral vascular damage was detected by CT and MRI in 25% to 30% of children in the Cooperative Study of Sickle Cell Disease. No clinical factors, with the exception of transcranial Doppler, predicted the occurrence of stroke. In this study, there was a correlation between first stroke and transient ischemic attack, acute chest syndrome, elevated systolic blood pressure, and severe anemia. All children who can cooperate with transcranial Doppler (usually by 2 years of age) should have an annual evaluation if the study is available locally. Normal middle cerebral artery velocity in children with sickle cell disease is approximately 120 cm/s. Children who have velocities of 170 to 199 cm/s are considered at high risk and those with velocities $\geq$200 cm/s are at highest risk. The STOP trial (Stroke Prevention Trial in Sickle Cell Anemia) showed that transfusion greatly reduces the risk of first stroke in children who have abnormally high TCD velocity ($\geq$200 cm/s).

Prophylactic chronic transfusion should be strongly considered if there are two studies at least 2 weeks apart with velocities ≥200 cm/s. Compliance issues and risks of chronic transfusions must also be considered when deciding on this therapy.

Transient ischemic attacks are defined as focal neurological deficits with a vascular distribution persisting for less than 24 hours, although they typically last less than an hour. Patients with transient ischemic attacks are treated in a similar manner to those who have an infarct. The diagnosis is made in retrospect when the follow-up MRI is negative for a persistent lesion that would explain the neurological symptoms.

Intracerebral hemorrhage or **subarachnoid hemorrhage** may present without focal neurologic symptoms. Exchange transfusion should be carried out immediately. Arteriography is used to identify the arterial bleed and the patient may need emergent surgical intervention. Mortality is very high during the acute event (∼50%).

Acute anemia

There are two common causes of acute life-threatening anemia in sickle cell disease: splenic sequestration and aplastic crisis.

Splenic sequestration

Infants and young children who have Hgb SS and $S\beta^0$ thalassemia and older children (over 10 years) who have Hgb SC or $S\beta^+$ thalassemia syndromes can have intrasplenic pooling of large amounts of blood and platelets. This can lead to anemia, thrombocytopenia, hypovolemia, cardiovascular collapse, and sudden death within hours of the onset of sequestration. The syndrome has been reported in infants as young as 2 months of age. Classically, however, it occurs in children with Hgb SS after the disappearance of Hgb F from approximately

6 months to 3 years of age when the spleen becomes fibrotic due to multiple infarctions. These crises can occur in older children who have Hgb SC or $S\beta^+$ thalassemia but are usually not as severe; still, fatal events have been recorded for these children. The incidence is between 10% and 30% and the recurrence rate is 50%. Mild events can indicate the possibility of life-threatening sequestration events. Chronic sequestration can also be a sequelae with chronic anemia and thrombocytopenia.

The clinical presentation is usually rapid in onset; the child will typically have sudden weakness, pallor of the lips and mucous membranes, breathlessness, rapid pulse, faintness, and abdominal fullness. Evaluation of the CBC will frequently show a precipitous drop from the baseline hemoglobin.

The treatment for splenic sequestration is transfusion to restore circulating blood volume, usually with phenotypically matched blood (unless there is a life-threatening situation). As the shock is reversed and the transfused blood decreases the percentage of Hgb S, the splenomegaly regresses and much of the blood is remobilized with a rapid rise in the child's hemoglobin.

Splenectomy should be strongly considered in all children who have a splenic sequestration crisis. Transfusions can prevent recurrence until surgery can be arranged. Some children who have Hgb SS and older children who have other S hemoglobinopathies can have massive splenomegaly with **hypersplenism** after an episode of splenic sequestration. If hypersplenism (with resultant anemia, neutropenia, or thrombocytopenia) is persistent and severe, splenectomy is indicated.

Prior to splenectomy, younger children should have an evaluation of splenic function with a **pit count** and a spleen scan. In normally eusplenic persons, fewer than 1% of the circulating red cells are pitted; values of 2% to 12% may represent decreased splenic function. If they still have a functional spleen, usually under 2 years of age, a partial splenectomy can be performed. Children should have appropriate immunizations, including pneumococcal and meningococcal vaccinations, prior to splenectomy. **Penicillin** prophylaxis is continued indefinitely in all children who have been splenectomized.

Aplastic crisis

Severe anemia can develop over several days due to shortened red cell survival without compensatory reticulocytosis. Reticulocytopenia can last 7 to 10 days. The primary cause of transient red cell aplasia is parvovirus B19, though it can follow other viral infections as well. Parvovirus B19, the most common cause of aplasia in children with hemoglobinopathies, can also cause neutropenia. While many patients recover spontaneously, the anemia can be profound. Red cell transfusion is indicated for those who become symptomatic from anemia or if the hemoglobin falls 2 g/dL or more from baseline. Symptoms occurring with aplastic crisis include nausea and vomiting, myalgias, and arthralgias. Splenic and hepatic sequestration have also been reported with aplastic crises. If the ability to follow-up is of concern, the child should be hospitalized for observation. The patient should be isolated from other patients with chronic hemolytic anemias (sickle cell disease or thalassemia) or red cell aplasia and should not have pregnant caregivers. If the child is mildly anemic and asymptomatic, outpatient monitoring is reasonable.

Avascular necrosis

Bone pain is common in sickle cell disease. Marrow infarcts can cause pain that can last for weeks. Avascular necrosis (osteonecrosis) causes pain that can sometimes be confused with a bone infarct. Symptoms of avascular necrosis, such as limping, can sometimes be confused with stroke. Limping with weakness but without pain is stroke not avascular necrosis.

Avascular necrosis is common in all age groups but is more frequently diagnosed in the adolescent and usually involves the humeral and femoral heads. It is more common in individuals who have Hgb $S\beta^0$ thalassemia and Hgb SS with alpha-thalassemia. It is also seen, though with a lower frequency, in those who have Hgb $S\beta^+$ thalassemia. Individuals who have Hgb SS are more frequently affected than those with Hgb SC.

Avascular necrosis is a result of an infarct in the cancellous trabeculae in the head of either the femur or the humerus. The process of necrosis and repair can be progressive, leading to collapse of the head or arrest with varying degrees of disability and sclerosis. Below is a method of describing the progression of avascular necrosis:

Stage 0: no evidence of disease

Stage 1: X-ray normal, bone scan abnormal, MRI abnormal

Stage 2: X-ray: sclerosis and cystic changes without collapse

Stage 3: Subchondral collapse (crescent sign) without collapse

Stage 4: Collapse and flattening of the femoral head without acetabular involvement, normal joint space

Stage 5: Joint narrowing and/or acetabular involvement

Stage 6: Increased joint narrowing and/or acetabular involvement

Treatment for avascular necrosis of the femur includes bed rest with crutch walking for 6 weeks, nonsteroidal anti-inflammatory drugs (NSAIDs), and core decompression surgery for stages 1 or 2. Extensive physical therapy has been found to be beneficial but is often difficult to perform. Decompression surgery is relatively simple; a core is removed from the head of the femur. The coring begins approximately 2 cm below the trochanteric ridge extending through the neck and into the head of the femur. Acutely this procedure provides relief of pain and is thought to arrest the progression of avascular necrosis; however, this has not been confirmed in a prospective trial. Higher stage avascular necrosis requires joint replacement.

Retinopathy/Hyphema

The eye is particularly sensitive to hypoxia. Vaso-occlusion of retinal vessels and hypoxia of the retina cause permanent retinal damage. Blood in the anterior chamber of the eye (hyphema) becomes rapidly deoxygenated and permanently sickled, obstructing the outflow from the aqueous humor. The accumulation of aqueous humor in the anterior chamber increases intraocular pressure leading to decreased blood flow to the retina until the perfusion pressure of the globe is reached. This leads to sudden vascular stasis and blindness. The events occurring in hyphema can also occur in children who have sickle cell trait.

Retinal vascular occlusion initially occurs in peripheral retinal vessels without significant sequelae. It eventually leads to neovascularization from the retina into the vitreous (sea fans). These abnormal vessels are fragile and can bleed into the vitreous causing "floaters" or blindness if the hemorrhage is sufficient. If bleeds do not obscure vision and are unnoticed, they can cause collapse of the vitreous, traction on the retina, and eventually cause retinal detachment. Retinal disease of the eye is common in sickle cell disease. It

occurs most commonly in individuals who have Hgb SC.

Treatment of sickle cell retinopathy requires recognition. The damaged peripheral vessels are not generally appreciated by direct ophthalmic examination and require the use of indirect binocular stereoscopic ophthalmoscopy. Sea fanning, vitreous hemorrhage, and retinal detachment can be observed by direct ophthalmoscopy. Annual ophthalmic evaluations should begin at age 10 for all children with sickle cell disease. Treatment of early neovascularization requires laser photocoagulation. Surgical approaches are required for advanced lesions.

Hyphema is a medical emergency in sickle cell disease. It requires immediate ophthalmic evaluation and transfusion (exchange or straight) to reduce sickling and improve oxygenation. If a conservative approach is not successful, anterior chamber paracentesis is performed to relieve intraocular pressure and remove the hyphema.

Hyperbilirubinemia/Gallstones

Bilirubin gallstones can eventually be detected in most patients with chronic hemolytic anemia. In sickle cell disease, gallstones occur in children as young as 3 to 4 years of age, and are eventually found in approximately 70% of patients. It may be difficult to differentiate between gallbladder disease and abdominal vaso-occlusive crisis in patients with recurrent abdominal pain. Cholecystectomy may be necessary for patients with fat intolerance, presence of gallstones, and recurrent abdominal pain.

Hepatomegaly and liver dysfunction may be caused by a combination of intrahepatic trapping of sickled cells, transfusion-acquired infection, or transfusional hemosiderosis. The combination of hemolysis, liver dysfunction, and renal tubular defects can result in very high bilirubin levels. Benign cholestasis of sickle cell disease results in severe asymptomatic hyperbilirubinemia without fever, pain, leukocytosis, or hepatic failure.

Perioperative management of sickle cell patients

Following are guidelines for the management of sickle cell patients who have surgical procedures or require anesthesia for other purposes. General anesthesia results in atelectasis and hypoxia, which is poorly tolerated by the patient with sickle cell disease; therefore, special precautions must be taken perioperatively to decrease morbidity and mortality associated with even minor surgical procedures. Other risk factors include the presence of chronic organ damage in some patients, the effects of asplenia, and the propensity for sickling and obstruction of microvasculature with even mild hypoxia. The guidelines suggested below are extrapolated from a multicenter randomized trial of transfusion (exchange vs straight) in the perioperative period.

Preoperative care
1. Admission to the hospital the afternoon prior to scheduled surgery.
2. Hydration at $1.25\times$ maintenance (IV + PO) the evening and night prior to surgery.
3. Pulse oximetry on room air (spot checks).
4. Incentive spirometry at least 10 times per hour while awake.
5. Lab work: CBC with differential and reticulocyte count, urinalysis, type and cross, chemistry panel.
6. Transfusion: All sickle cell patients should have a **red cell phenotype** study obtained prior to any transfusion. Sickle cell patients should receive phenotypically matched blood to decrease the risk of alloimmunization. In addition, all blood should be sickledex negative and leukodepleted. The following transfusion guidelines are recommended. See also Chapter 5.

    a. Patients with Hgb SS or $S\beta^0$ disease who are undergoing any procedure other than myringotomy tube placement should have a simple transfusion to achieve a hemoglobin of 10 to 12 g/dL. Do not exceed 12 g/dL due to the risk of stasis/sludging.

    b. Patients with Hgb SC disease or $S\beta^+$ who have baseline hemoglobin below 10 g/dL may need transfusions to achieve a hemoglobin of 10 to 12 g/dL. However, do not transfuse these patients prior to consulting the hematologist. Many factors may affect this decision including a history of significant complications of their sickle cell disease (i.e., pneumonia, vaso-occlusive episodes, priapism, and aseptic necrosis).

    c. Consult the hematologist if there is confusion regarding individual patients.

7. Patients with central venous catheters or those undergoing dental procedures should receive antibiotic prophylaxis prior to surgery.

Postoperative care
1. Adequate pain management to prevent splinting and atelectasis, with care to prevent narcosis.
2. Pulse oximetry for at least the first 12 to 24 hours postoperatively.
3. Incentive spirometry at least 10 times per hour while awake. Be aggressive!
4. Ambulation as early as possible, taking into account the specific surgical procedure.
5. Lab work: CBC with reticulocyte count daily.

6. Follow-up in clinic approximately 1 week post-hospital discharge or sooner if there are ongoing problems.

Transfusion therapy

Red blood cell transfusion increases oxygen-carrying capacity and improves microvascular perfusion by decreasing the proportion of sickle red cells (Hgb S%). Transfusions are given to patients with sickle cell disease to stabilize or reverse an acute medical complication, or as part of chronic therapy in certain situations to prevent future complications.

Indications
Acute illnesses
Splenic sequestration
Transient red cell aplasia
Hyperhemolysis (infection, ACS)

Patients should be transfused if there is evidence of cardiovascular compromise (heart failure, dyspnea, hypertension, or marked fatigue). Generally, transfusion is indicated if the hemoglobin falls below 5 g/dL or drops greater than 2 g/dL from the steady state.

Sudden severe illness
Acute chest syndrome
Stroke
Sepsis
Acute multiorgan failure

These life-threatening illnesses are often accompanied by a falling hemoglobin. Transfusion therapy has become standard medical practice in the management of these illnesses. When ACS is associated with hypoxia and a falling hemoglobin, transfusion is indicated. Many patients can be treated with straight transfusion, though in severe cases, exchange transfusion or red cell pheresis is recommended. Studies suggest early transfusion may prevent progression of acute pulmonary disease.

The efficacy of transfusion in the management of acute stroke has not been well studied, though anecdotal reports indicate that early exchange transfusion may limit neuronal damage by improving local oxygenation and perfusion. Chronic transfusion therapy reduces the rate of recurrence and is indicated in all patients after a first stroke.

Perioperative transfusion
Patients with sickle cell anemia undergoing major surgery should be prepared in advance by transfusion to a hemoglobin of approximately 10 g/dL and a decrease in Hgb S% to approximately 60%. While standard practice guidelines have not been developed for Hgb SS patients undergoing minor procedures or those with Hgb SC, it is generally acceptable to not transfuse these patients, assuming they are medically stable.

Chronic transfusion therapy
Chronic transfusions are indicated in several conditions in which the potential medical complications warrant the risks of alloimmunization, infection, and transfusional iron overload. Transfusions are given every 3 to 4 weeks, with a goal to maintain the Hgb S% at 30% to 50%. While straight transfusions are acceptable, red cell pheresis or exchange transfusions may be preferred to decrease the rate of iron overload.

Indications
1. Primary stroke prevention
2. Pulmonary hypertension/chronic lung disease
3. Frequent ACS
4. Chronic debilitating pain

Other indications for transfusions:

Transfusions are sometimes suggested for a number of conditions in which efficacy is unproven, but may be considered under severe circumstances. Such circumstances include:

Acute priapism

Pregnancy (frequent complications)

"Silent" cerebral infarcts

Leg ulcers

Hydroxyurea therapy

Hydroxyurea (HU) was originally utilized as an antineoplastic agent, but due to its effects on increasing fetal hemoglobin (Hgb F), it has gained favor in the treatment of patients with sickle cell disease. Hydroxyurea's mechanism of action is not clearly understood; however, it is thought that inhibition of ribonucleotide reductase leads to downstream cytotoxicity of erythroid progenitors leading to upregulation of fetal hemoglobin production. In addition, hydroxyurea's cytotoxic effects lead to leukopenia and neutropenia, beneficial in sickle cell disease secondary to the viscous properties of these cells during vaso-occlusion.

Long-term adult studies have shown no significant complications of HU usage and it is being used more commonly in pediatric patients with sickle cell disease. Current recommendations for HU usage include the following:

• Frequent episodes of VOE including dactylitis

• Acute chest syndrome

• Chronic hypoxia

• Low hemoglobin and Hgb F

• Signs of increased hemolysis (increased LDH and total bilirubin)

• Abnormal TCD or history of stroke with refusal for chronic transfusion therapy

As experience grows with HU therapy, practitioners are recommending HU as prophylaxis in more patients. Some would argue that all patients with hemoglobin SS and $S\beta^0$ thalassemia should be on HU therapy; this may become the standard of care in the near future.

HU therapy begins at 20 mg/kg/d and should be titrated based on beneficial increment in Hgb F% and resultant increase in hemoglobin and MCV. Potential toxicities with HU therapy that should be monitored closely include neutropenia, leukopenia, and anemia. Elevation in ALT and thrombocytopenia can also occur, though less commonly.

Hematopoietic stem cell transplantion in sickle cell disease

Hematopoietic stem cell transplantion is curative for patients with sickle cell disease and should be considered in young patients with hemoglobin SS and $S\beta^0$ thalassemia and a matched sibling donor.

Patients with severe manifestations of sickle cell disease including multiple pain episodes, recurrent ACS, stroke, and end-organ damage should be considered for unrelated bone marrow or umbilical cord blood transplantation when a matched sibling donor is not available.

Case study for review

You are a primary care physician taking care of a 2-year-old with known sickle cell disease (Hgb SS). You are counseling the family on particular risks for the patient at this age.

1. What are some of the main areas of discussion?

In evaluating the patient as a whole, one must first discuss growth and development and the risks of low hemoglobin on brain development. Assuming the patient has had previous laboratory studies, past hemoglobin values can help objectively guide this discussion as phenotypic disease is related to level of anemia and concomitant reticulocytosis, amount of leukocytosis, as well as evidence of hemolysis (total bilirubin and LDH levels). In this discussion, newer treatment modalities including hydroxyurea therapy and the potential for hematopoietic stem cell transplantation should be discussed.

Fortunately, this child has had a relatively benign course to date.

2. What are some of the potential acute risks that should again be discussed with the family?

The major risks to the child include severe infection, pain including dactylitis, and splenic sequestration. These risks should all be discussed in detail with the family.

In terms of severe infection, the family should be aware that they should monitor the child closely if the child appears ill and check the temperature before administering antipyretics, even if given for pain alone. In addition, they should be aware that if the child appears ill, they should immediately call the on-call physician and will likely require immediate evaluation including blood work, chest radiography, parenteral antibiotics, and hospital admission and observation. You should again reinforce the need for the child to be on penicillin prophylaxis. Finally, one should review the child's vaccinations to ensure they are up to date, especially for encapsulated bacteria including *S. pneumoniae*, *H. influenzae*, and *N. meningitidis*.

Regarding episodes of pain, although it is reassuring the child has had a relatively unremarkable course to date, VOE can start at any age. At 2 years of age, the child is still at risk for developing episodes of dactylitis. The family should be advised on the signs and symptoms to monitor for pain in a young child which may present as irritability, refusal to walk, decreased appetite, as well as localized swelling and/or tenderness. A pain plan should be established with the family which should include the availability of oral medications at home (e.g., acetaminophen, ibuprofen, Tylenol with codeine, and/or Lortab elixir) as well as adjuvant strategies such as warm bath and heating pads.

Finally, the practitioner should discuss other potential acute complications such as splenic sequestration. If the child has a palpable spleen, the family should be advised on the current size and to monitor for changes in size if the patient appears to be pale or weak. In addition, if the child does appear to have these symptoms without a change in the size of the spleen or does not have a palpable spleen, the family should be advised that these symptoms should again lead to prompt evaluation as they could be signs of splenic sequestration or an aplastic crisis.

Suggested Reading

Adams RJ, McKie VC, Hsu L, et al. Prevention of a first stroke by transfusion in children with sickle cell anemia and abnormal results on transcranial Doppler ultrasonography. N Engl J Med 339:5–11, 1998.

Ballas SK. Current issues in sickle cell pain and its management. Hematology Am Soc Hematol Educ Program 97–105, 2007.

Claster S, Vichinsky EP. Managing sickle cell disease. BMJ 327:1151–1155, 2003.

Rees DC, Olujohungbe AD, Parker NE, et al. Guidelines for the management of the acute painful crisis in sickle cell disease. Br J Haematol 120:744–752, 2003.

Vichinsky EP, Neumayr LD, Earles AN, et al. Causes and outcomes of the acute chest syndrome in sickle cell disease. National Acute Chest Syndrome Group. N Engl J Med 342:1855–1865, 2000.

Ware RE. How I use hydroxyurea to treat young patients with sickle cell anemia. Blood 115:5300–5311, 2010.

4 Thalassemia

The thalassemias are a diverse group of genetic diseases characterized by absent or decreased production of normal hemoglobin, resulting in a microcytic anemia. The alpha-thalassemias are concentrated in Southeast Asia, Malaysia, and southern China. The beta-thalassemias are seen primarily in the Mediterranean, Africa, and in Southeast Asia. Due to global migration patterns, there is an increase in the incidence of thalassemia in North America, primarily because of immigration from Southeast Asia. Like with sickle cell anemia, development of thalassemia is directly related to evolutionary pressure secondary to malaria.

Normally, $\geq 95\%$ of adult hemoglobin found on electrophoresis is Hgb A $(\alpha_2\beta_2)$. Two minor hemoglobins occur: 2% to 3.5% is Hgb A2 $(\alpha_2\delta_2)$ and $\leq 2\%$ is Hgb F $(\alpha_2\gamma_2)$. A mutation affecting globin chain production or deletion of one of the globin chains leads to a decreased production of that chain and an abnormal globin ratio. The globin that is produced in normal amounts is in excess and forms aggregates or inclusions within the red cells. These aggregates become oxidized and damage the cell membrane leading to ineffective erythropoiesis, hemolysis, or both. The quantity and properties of these globin chain aggregates determine the phenotypic characteristics of the thalassemia.

An excess of alpha-globin chains (beta-thalassemia) leads to the formation of alpha-globin tetramers that accumulate in the erythroblast. These aggregates are very insoluble and precipitation of these aggregates interferes with erythropoiesis, cell maturation, and cell membrane function leading to ineffective erythropoiesis and anemia.

An excess of beta-globin chains (alpha-thalassemia) leads to tetramers of beta-globin, Hgb H. These tetramers are more stable and soluble, but as the red cell ages in the circulation and, under conditions of oxidant stress, Hgb H precipitates and interferes with cell membrane function leading to an increase in hemolysis.

Alpha-thalassemia

The alpha-thalassemias are caused by a decrease in the production of alpha-globin due to a deletion or mutation of one or more of the four alpha-globin genes located on chromosome 16. Alpha-gene mapping can be obtained to determine the specific mutation. The alpha-thalassemias are categorized as: silent carrier, alpha-thalassemia trait, hemoglobin H disease, hemoglobin H-constant spring, and alpha-thalassemia major. Frequently, the diagnosis of

Handbook of Pediatric Hematology and Oncology: Children's Hospital & Research Center Oakland, Second Edition. Caroline A. Hastings, Joseph C. Torkildson, and Anurag K. Agrawal.
© 2012 John Wiley & Sons, Ltd. Published 2012 by John Wiley & Sons, Ltd.

alpha-thalassemia trait in a parent is discovered after the birth of an affected child.

Silent carrier status is characterized by three functional genes for α-globin: $(-\alpha/\alpha\alpha)$. Outside the newborn period, it is not possible to make this diagnosis by conventional methods. There is overlap between the red blood cell indices of these individuals and normals, although the MCV may be slightly lower. This state is deduced when a "normal" individual has a child with Hgb H disease or with microcytic anemia consistent with alpha-thalassemia trait. An unusual case of the silent carrier state is the individual who carries the hemoglobin constant spring mutation ($\alpha_{cs}\alpha/\alpha\alpha$ or $\alpha\alpha_{cs}/\alpha\alpha$). This is an elongated α-globin due to a termination codon mutation. Individuals who have this mutation have normal red blood cell indices, but can have children who have Hgb H-constant spring if the other parent has alpha-thalassemia trait ($\alpha\alpha/-$). Generally, these children are more affected clinically than other children who have Hgb H.

Individuals who have **alpha-thalassemia trait** ($-\alpha/-\alpha$) or ($\alpha\alpha/-$) are identified by microcytosis, erythrocytosis, hypochromia, and mild anemia. The diagnosis is made by genetic studies, ruling out both iron-deficiency anemia and beta-thalassemia trait. In the neonatal period, when hemoglobin Bart's (γ_4) is present ($\sim5\%$ on newborn screen), the diagnosis can be suspected. In children, there are no markers such as elevated Hgb A_2 and Hgb F (as seen in beta-thalassemia trait) to make the diagnosis. The diagnosis is one of exclusion and is often mistaken for iron-deficiency anemia secondary to the microcytosis. Clues for the diagnosis include a normal RDW and an increase in red blood cells for the level of hemoglobin. During pregnancy, the microcytic anemia can be mistaken for anemia of pregnancy, and may be a clue for a family history of alpha-thalassemia trait.

Hemoglobin H ($-/-\alpha$) should be considered in the case of a neonate in whom all of the red blood cells are very hypochromic. Neonates who have Hgb H will also have a high percentage of Hgb Bart's on their newborn screen ($\sim20\%$). In children, this hemoglobinopathy is characterized by moderate anemia with a hemoglobin in the 8 to 10 g/dL range, hypochromia, microcytosis, red cell fragmentation, and a fast migrating hemoglobin (Hgb H) on electrophoresis.

Hemoglobin H does not function as a normal hemoglobin, and has a high oxygen affinity, so the measured hemoglobin in these children is misleading. Individuals who have Hgb H generally have a persistent stable state of anemia that may be accentuated by increased hemolysis during viral infections and by exposure to oxidant medications, chemicals, and foods such as sulfa-drugs, benzene, and Fava beans, similar to individuals who have G6PD deficiency. As the red cells mature, they lose their ability to withstand oxidant stress and Hgb H precipitates, leading to hemolysis. Therapy for individuals who have Hgb H disease includes folate, avoidance of oxidant drugs and foods, genetic counseling, education, and frequent medical care. Uncommon occurrences in a child with Hgb H would be severe anemia, cholelithiasis, skin ulceration, and splenomegaly requiring splenectomy. Unlike individuals who have beta-thalassemia, hemosiderosis is rare in Hgb H disease.

Children with **hemoglobin H-constant spring** ($-/\alpha_{cs}\alpha$ or $\alpha_{cs}-/\alpha-$) have a more severe course than children who have Hgb H. They have a more severe anemia, with a steady-state hemoglobin ranging between 7 and 8 g/dL. They more frequently have splenomegaly and severe anemia with febrile illnesses and viral infections, often requiring transfusion. If anemia is chronically severe and the child has splenomegaly, a splenectomy may be performed. If splenectomy is anticipated, a complication can be severe postsplenectomy thrombocytosis with hypercoagulability leading to thrombosis of the splenic vein or hepatic veins. This complication has also been reported as recurrent pulmonary emboli and clotting diathesis. Children who are scheduled to have surgery are treated with low-molecular-weight heparin, followed by low-dose aspirin, continued indefinitely.

The most severe form of alpha-thalassemia is **alpha-thalassemia major** $(-/-)$. This diagnosis is frequently made in the last months of pregnancy when fetal ultrasound indicates a hydropic fetus. The mother frequently exhibits toxemia and can develop severe postpartum hemorrhage. These infants are usually stillborn. There can be other congenital anomalies, though none are pathognomonic for alpha-thalassemia major. Because of in utero hypoxia, the hemoglobins found in these infants are Hgb Portland $(\zeta_2\gamma_2)$, Hgb H (β_4), and Hgb Bart's (γ_4), and no Hgb A or A_2. These babies can have other complications associated with hydrops such as heart failure and pulmonary edema.

If the diagnosis is made early, intrauterine transfusions can be performed. There are reports of survival with chronic transfusion in these infants, now more recently replaced by curative hematopoietic stem cell transplantation. Undoubtedly, more of these infants could be saved if the diagnosis was anticipated by prenatal diagnosis and the treatment provided.

Beta-thalassemia

Beta-thalassemia is caused by mutations in the beta-globin gene. Although there have been hundreds of mutations identified within the beta-globin gene locus, about 20 different alleles make up about 80% of the mutations found worldwide. Within each geographic population, there are unique mutations. Individuals with beta-thalassemia major are usually homozygous for one of the common mutations (as well as having one of the geographically unique mutations) that lead to the absence of beta-chain production.

The **beta-thalassemia syndromes** are much more diverse than the alpha-thalassemia syndromes due to the diversity of the mutations that produce the defects in the beta-globin gene. Unlike the deletions that constitute most of the alpha-thalassemia syndromes, beta-thalassemias are caused by mutations on chromosome 11 that affect all aspects of beta-globin production: transcription, translation, and the stability of the beta-globin product. Most hematologists feel there are three general categories of beta-thalassemia: beta-thalassemia trait, beta-thalassemia intermedia, and beta-thalassemia major. However, with the lack of genotypic differentiation, there remains phenotypic overlap between these three general categories.

Splice site mutations also occur and are of clinical consequence when combined with a thalassemia mutation. Three splice site mutations occur in exon 1 of the beta-globin gene. These mutations result in three different abnormal hemoglobins: Malay, E, and Knossos. **Hemoglobin E** is a very common abnormal hemoglobin in the Southeast Asian population and when paired with a β_0-thalassemia, mutation can produce severe transfusion-dependent thalassemia. Hemoglobin E is described in the section on newborn screening.

Individuals who have **beta-thalassemia trait** have microcytosis and hypochromia; there may be targeting and elliptocytosis, though some individuals have an almost normal smear. These hematologic features can be accentuated in women with trait who are pregnant and individuals who are folate or iron deficient. If iron deficiency is concurrent with beta-thalassemia trait, there may be a normal Hgb A_2. Iron deficiency causes decreased hemoglobin production and folate or vitamin B_{12} deficiency can lead to megaloblastic anemia with increased Hgb A_2. Both of these deficiencies need to be treated prior to evaluation for thalassemia trait. In iron-, B_{12}-, and folate-replete individuals, the Hgb A_2 can be as high as 3.5% to 8% and the Hgb F as high as 2% to 5%. Generally, beta-thalassemia trait is milder in African-Americans (who frequently have a promoter gene mutation) but has a similar presentation in individuals of Chinese, Southeast Asian, Greek, Italian, and Middle Eastern heritage.

Infants born in most states in the United States are screened for hemoglobinopathies. In states without newborn screening for hemoglobinopathies and in recent immigrants to this country, affected children are frequently found later than the newborn period, and the evaluation of their microcytic anemia includes differentiation between iron deficiency and beta-thalassemia trait. The red blood cell indices can be helpful in this differentiation as the hemoglobin concentration and the red cell count will generally be lower in iron deficiency. The distinguishing finding in beta-thalassemia is a hemoglobin electrophoresis with an elevated Hgb A_2 and F. Both will be increased in beta-thalassemia trait without iron deficiency, and will be normal or decreased in alpha-thalassemia and isolated iron-deficiency anemia. There are several formulas to help in office screening, but they are also based on the assumption that the child is not iron deficient. Usually, iron deficiency can be ruled out using free erythrocyte protoporphyrin, transferrin saturation, or ferritin as a screening test in children who have a hypochromic microcytic anemia. The least expensive test is a trial of iron and a repeat hemogram after a month. A lead level should be obtained if there is an index of suspicion for lead toxicity.

Problems can still arise if both alpha- and beta-thalassemia coexist since the changes in Hgb A_2 and F will not be apparent as noted above. Family studies and DNA analysis can be used to make a definitive diagnosis.

Children who are diagnosed with **thalassemia intermedia** have a homozygous or heterozygous beta-globin mutation that causes a greater decrease in beta-chain production than seen in thalassemia minor, but not to the degree for which chronic transfusion therapy is required. The phenotype can also occur in children who have a mutation that increases production of α-globin, in children who have coinherited alpha- and beta-thalassemia, and in other rarer mutations. Children who have thalassemia intermedia are able to maintain a hemoglobin of 7 g/dL or slightly higher with a greatly expanded erythron and may manifest bony deformities, pathological fractures, and growth retardation. Children who have thalassemia intermedia can also have delayed pubescence, exercise intolerance, leg ulcers, inflammatory arthritis, and extramedullary hematopoiesis causing spinal cord compression—a medical emergency requiring radiation therapy and transfusion. They can also have iron overload due to increased absorption of iron from the gastrointestinal tract and intermittent transfusion. They are at risk for the cardiac and endocrine complications of hemosiderosis, but usually at an older age than chronically transfused children. Chelation therapy is indicated for increasing ferritin and elevated liver iron.

Children who cannot maintain a hemoglobin between 6 and 7 g/dL should have an alternative diagnosis considered. If thalassemia is the cause of the anemia, transfusion and/or splenectomy should be considered. Frequently, adolescents and adults are unable to tolerate the degree of anemia that is seen in thalassemia intermedia. Hypersplenism, splenic pain, congestive heart failure, severe exercise intolerance, thrombocytopenia, and leukopenia should be considered indications for transfusion and splenectomy.

Appropriate clinical management of thalassemia intermedia patients may be more difficult than patients with thalassemia major requiring chronic transfusion due to phenotypic heterogeneity. Patients with clinically mild disease still may have serious long-term complications as described above due to ineffective erythropoiesis as well as chronic hemolysis, leading to pulmonary hypertension with resultant congestive heart failure and thrombosis in addition to cholelithiasis. Currently, transfusion therapy is limited to patients with symptomatic anemia or in children with delayed growth and development and is generally tailored to the individual patient. Hydroxyurea has been utilized as in sickle cell anemia, increasing Hgb F and obviating some of the need for transfusion. Splenectomy has been utilized but now is thought to be at least partly responsible for the development of pulmonary hypertension and thrombosis secondary to chronic hemolysis. Some argue that transfusion therapy is underutilized in thalassemia intermedia and improved risk stratification is needed.

Thalassemia major was first described by a Detroit pediatrician, Thomas Cooley, in 1925. The clinical picture he described is prevalent today in countries without the necessary resources to provide patients with chronic transfusions and iron chelation therapy. Children who have untreated thalassemia major have ineffective erythropoiesis, decreased red cell deformability, and enhanced clearance of defective red cells by macrophages. The result is a very hypermetabolic bone marrow with thrombocytosis, leukocytosis, and microcytic anemia in the young child prior to the enlargement of their spleen. At presentation, they have almost 100% Hgb F (these cells have a longer life span due to a balanced globin ratio as γ, rather than β, globin is present in Hgb F). These children have little or no Hgb A_2 and a low reticulocyte count. The diagnosis can be made with certainty by demonstrating thalassemia trait in both parents, by globin biosynthetic ratios, or by beta-gene screening. Beta-gene screening identifies the most common and some uncommon mutations, but not all mutations. An electrophoresis showing only Hgb F, a complete blood count, and a peripheral blood smear will generally be diagnostic. In most states, these children will be discovered by newborn screening or occasionally by the obstetrician who makes a diagnosis of thalassemia trait in the mother and obtains a family history of thalassemia or anemia in both parents prior to the birth of the baby.

Children who have untreated thalassemia die in the first decade of life from anemia, septicemia, and pathologic fractures. When palliative transfusions are introduced, children live into their late teens eventually succumbing to heart failure due to iron overload.

With the introduction of frequent chronic transfusion therapy with regular iron chelation, children are now surviving into adulthood, adding to the complexity of the disease. The longevity of patients who are compliant with their chelation therapy, or in those who have received bone marrow transplantation, is not yet known.

Neonatal screening for hemoglobinopathies

Newborn screening identifies patients with beta-thalassemia major, hemoglobin H, and sickle cell disease. Patients with beta-thalassemia major and sickle cell disease will be asymptomatic at birth due to high fetal hemoglobin levels but will become symptomatic over the next 2 to 3 months as normal production of Hgb F wanes. Patients

Table 4.1 Classification of the alpha-thalassemias.

Diagnosis	Genetic finding	Symptoms	Barts (%)
Silent carrier	$\alpha-/\alpha\alpha$	Hematologically normal	1–3
α-thalassemia trait	$\alpha-/\alpha-$ or $\alpha\alpha/--$	Mild anemia with microcytosis and hypochromia	3–6
Hemoglobin H disease OR Hemoglobin H-constant spring	$\alpha-/--$ $\alpha\alpha_{CS}/--$ or $\alpha-/\alpha_{CS}-$	Moderately severe hemolytic anemia Icterus and splenomegaly	5–20
α-thalassemia major	$--/--$	Severe anemia not compatible with life; hydrops fetalis without intrauterine transfusion	100

with significant Bart's hemoglobin (see Table 4.1) should be considered to have hemoglobin H and require alpha-gene screening to detect the possibility of Hgb H-constant spring.

The presence of Hgb F only on the newborn screening will be interpreted as beta-thalassemia major (see Table 4.2). This diagnosis must be confirmed with parental electrophoresis and repeat testing of the infant at 2 to 3 months after fetal hemoglobin wanes with concomitant increase in

hemoglobin A and A2 in the normal patient. The pattern FA is normal and should not be interpreted as beta-thalassemia trait. This is a diagnosis made by the practitioner when microcytic anemia is seen during routine childhood screening and an investigation for thalassemia confirms the diagnosis.

Hgb FE will be presumed to be Hgb E-beta-thalassemia until that diagnosis is investigated and confirmed, or ruled out by repeat electrophoresis and family studies. Hemoglobin E is the most common abnormal

Table 4.2 Interpretation of common newborn screening results.*

Result	Diagnostic possibilities	Action required
FA	Normal	None
	β-thalassemia trait	Genetic counseling
F	β-thalassemia major	Referral to hematologist
FAS	Sickle cell trait	Genetic counseling
FS	Sickle cell disease (Hgb SS)	Repeat testing at 2–3 months
	Hgb S/β_0-thalassemia	Family studies Referral to hematologist
FSA	Hgb S/β_+-thalassemia	Referral to hematologist
FSC	Sickle cell disease (Hgb SC)	Referral to hematologist
FAC	Hemoglobin C trait	Genetic counseling
FE	Hgb E/β-thalassemia	Repeat testing at 2–3 months
	Hgb EE	Family studies
FAE	Hgb E trait	Genetic counseling

*Order of results is listed from highest to lowest frequency (i.e., in FA, higher percentage of Hgb F than Hgb A).

hemoglobin discovered in the state of California on newborn screening. It is common in Laos, Cambodia, and Thailand. Hemoglobin E results from a mutation in an exon (exon 1, codon 26: GAG to AAG) that creates an alternate splice site competing with the normal splice site. This results in abnormal hemoglobin production and mild microcytic anemia (Hgb ≥ 10 g/dL) in the homozygous state. Electrophoresis reveals about 90% Hgb E with varying amounts of Hgb F. The heterozygote has a hemoglobin of about 12 g/dL with microcytosis and an electrophoretic pattern consistent with Hgb E plus Hgb A. When combined with other more severe beta-thalassemias, Hgb E-beta-thalassemia can produce an anemia that is profound requiring chronic transfusion therapy. All children who have Hgb E and Hgb F on their state screen require scrutiny for the emergence of a severe thalassemia syndrome. Individuals who are homozygous for Hgb E should not have a significant anemia and do not require special care. Like patients with alpha-thalassemia, they should not be treated with iron for their microcytic anemia unless they are proven to have concomitant iron deficiency.

Case study for review

You are seeing an infant that has been following in your clinic since the newborn period. The baby was born full-term without any significant issues. You are now seeing the baby back at 4 months for the well-child check and their secondary vaccinations. The parents note that the baby has been more listless, not eating as well, and looking paler. There are no recent infections or fevers.

1. Assuming this baby is anemic, what would your differential diagnosis be at this point?

Causes of anemia are quite broad at this point. Complete blood count with differential,

MCV, and reticulocyte count would be helpful to narrow the differential. Iron deficiency is unlikely before 6 months of age due to maternal iron stores unless the baby was born prematurely (and would have been routinely put on iron therapy) or if the mother had severe anemia during pregnancy or if there was acute or occult blood loss. Viral suppression or aplasia from infections such as parvovirus is possible, but less likely without any history of recent infection or fever. Beta-thalassemia as well as sickle cell anemia should be high in the differential as fetal hemoglobin lives 60 to 90 days and therefore by 4 months of age the infant will be producing little fetal hemoglobin ($\alpha_2\gamma_2$) and should have moved to almost solely hemoglobin A ($\alpha_2\beta_2$) unless there is a problem with the β-globin chain. Additional possibilities include a hemolytic anemia, transient erythroblastopenia of childhood (though rarely seen at this young of an age), infant leukemia, and folate and vitamin B_{12} deficiency if the baby is being fed goat's milk or the mother is vegan, respectively.

2. What additional piece of information may be helpful in this young child?

In addition to asking about a family history of sickle cell anemia and thalassemias, the provider should look for the results of newborn screen which could be very helpful in this case. If the patient has a newborn screen that is FA, sickle cell anemia and β-thalassemia major can be ruled out. More concerning newborn screening results would include F (β-thalassemia major), FS (Hgb SS disease or Hgb S/β^0-thalassemia), and FSA (Hgb S/β^+-thalassemia). β^0- and β^+-thalassemia are differentiated based on the presence (β^+) or absence (β^0) of hemoglobin A, although phenotypically the patient can have an extremely variable clinical presentation, in part due to the persistence of fetal hemoglobin. If the patient had sickle cell trait, their newborn screen result would be FAS as the percentage of hemoglobin A should be greater than the percentage of hemoglobin S. If necessary, results can be confirmed at 4 to 6 months of age after fetal hemoglobin levels should be significantly decreased or, if possible, the parents can be tested. In this case, the newborn screen results are F only.

3. How might repeat hemoglobin electrophoresis be different at this age?

The patient that has no hemoglobin A will be on the extreme end of the clinical spectrum with definitive β-thalassemia major. For those patients with some β-globin production, the clinical severity of disease at this point cannot be determined on a molecular level. Patients who are solely fetal hemoglobin ($\alpha_2\gamma_2$) on newborn screen will likely continue to make some amount of fetal hemoglobin in addition to hemoglobin A2 ($\alpha_2\delta_2$). Their repeat hemoglobin electrophoresis will represent this with variable amounts of hemoglobin A2 and F and no hemoglobin A.

4. What would you expect the parents' hemoglobin electrophoresis to show?

The parents likely both have β-thalassemia trait. If they were tested as newborns, they would be FA. As adults, after fetal hemoglobin production has decreased, they would have increased amounts of both A2 ($>3.5\%$) and F ($>2\%$) in addition to hemoglobin A.

5. What other clinical signs might be apparent in the infant?

One would expect to see increasing signs of extramedullary hematopoiesis with increasing age and decreasing fetal hemoglobin production. Some of the early signs could be frontal bossing as well as maxillary and mandibular prominence. The infant may have failure to thrive as well as the development of hepatosplenomegaly.

Suggested Reading

Aessopos A, Kati M, Meletis J. Thalassemia intermedia today: should patients regularly receive transfusions? Transfusion 47:792–800, 2007.

Olivieri NF. The beta-thalassemias. N Engl J Med 341:99–109, 1999.

Singer ST, Kim HY, Olivieri NF, et al. Hemoglobin H-constant spring in North America: an alpha-thalassemia with frequent complications. Am J Hematol 84:759–761, 2009.

Taher AT, Musallam KM, Karimi M, et al. Overview on practices in thalassemia intermedia management aiming for lowering complication rates across a region of endemicity: the OPTIMAL CARE study. Blood 115: 1886–1892, 2010.

5 Transfusion Medicine

Transfusion of blood products continues to be an important and necessary part of therapy in children with hematologic and oncologic diagnoses. Many complications can result from transfusion, both infectious and noninfectious. With continued improvements in donor screening, and better testing techniques, infections from known entities have become a rarity. However, as long as blood component therapy is derived from human blood donation, the risk will persist. Donor selection criteria are designed to screen out potential donors with increased risk of infection with HIV-1/2, HTLV-I/II, and hepatitis B and C, as well as other infectious pathogens. Despite rigorous screening and testing for these infections, the risk of transmitting these viruses is not totally eliminated.

Clerical errors and misidentification are major risks for transfusion and can result in serious consequences, including death. It is essential that all blood samples drawn for a type and cross-match be clearly labeled with the patient's identification. Before administration of the blood product, the order should be checked, patient identification reviewed (patient's identification band), and blood type verified. Many institutions have moved toward testing two separate blood type specimens for nonemergent transfusion in previously untransfused patients to eliminate the risk of clerical error.

Directed donation from first-degree relatives (especially maternal) should be discouraged for patients who may be candidates for an allogeneic bone marrow transplant due to the possibility of antigen sensitization. If it cannot be avoided, the blood should be irradiated to prevent graft-versus-host disease (GVHD). Studies have shown that blood from directed donation is not safer than the general donation pool due to current sophisticated screening and testing methods.

These risks must be carefully considered and weighed against expected benefit each time a transfusion is contemplated. Informed consent should be obtained prior to every nonemergent transfusion. In California, the Gann Act must be renewed on a yearly basis for those patients undergoing frequent transfusion due to an underlying hematologic or oncologic condition.

Packed red blood cell transfusion

Transfusion decisions are made on the basis of clinical context, rather than the level of hemoglobin alone (see Figure 5.1). Prior to transfusion, it is necessary to assess the

Handbook of Pediatric Hematology and Oncology: Children's Hospital & Research Center Oakland, Second Edition. Caroline A. Hastings, Joseph C. Torkildson, and Anurag K. Agrawal.
© 2012 John Wiley & Sons, Ltd. Published 2012 by John Wiley & Sons, Ltd.

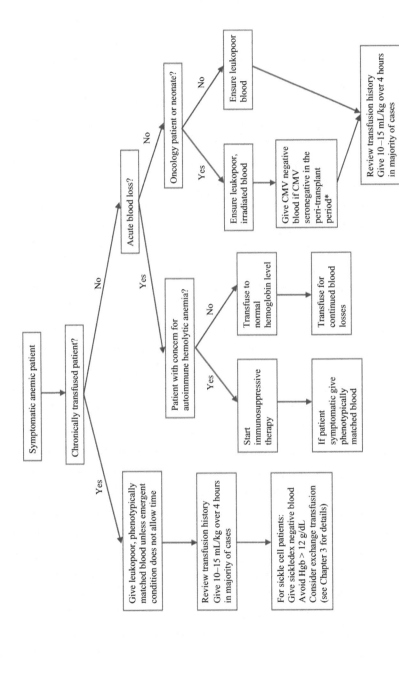

Figure 5.1 Blood transfusion guidelines. (*Refer to institutional guidelines as transfusion of CMV seronegative PRBCs is controversial.)

mechanism responsible for anemia (bone marrow infiltration, ineffective erythropoiesis of chronic disease, occult or obvious blood loss, transfusion or drug-related suppression of normal hematopoiesis, and nutritional deficiency), the severity of the signs and symptoms, and the likelihood of resumption of normal hematopoiesis.

Whole blood is rarely, if ever, utilized in standard practice, though may occasionally be utilized for massive transfusion after military trauma. Packed red blood cells (PRBCs) are depleted of the majority of platelets and white blood cells and need to be ABO and RhD compatible, at the minimum. Phenotypically, and now more recently genotypically, matched blood for minor antigens should be utilized for patients undergoing chronic transfusion (e.g., sickle cell disease). One unit of PRBCs is approximately 250 to 350 mL with a hematocrit of 55% to 60% when prepared with adsol. Based on the hematocrit of the stored PRBCs, one can calculate the presumed rate of rise from blood transfusion. For adsol-preserved units, the transfusion factor is approximately 5 (assuming no hemolysis of transfused blood or blood loss). The estimated hemoglobin (Hgb) increase can be derived utilizing this transfusion factor:

$$\text{Estimated hemoglobin rise (g/dL)} = \frac{\text{Volume of PRBC transfusion (mL/kg)}}{\text{Transfusion factor}}$$

For example, for a transfusion of 15 mL/kg, the estimated hemoglobin increase should be 3 g/dL. Of note, waiting a certain period of time for a posttransfusion "reequilibration" prior to rechecking the hemoglobin is not necessary.

Removal of the vast majority of remaining white blood cells, or **leukoreduction**, is an important step in reducing transfusion-related risks including risk of infection, febrile nonhemolytic transfusion reactions (FNHTRs), and alloimmunization from PRBC transfusion. Although not universal as yet in the United States, leukoreduction is becoming standard of care and is universal in Canada and much of Europe.

Irradiation of blood products should be utilized for all patients who are immuno compromised in order to prevent transfusion-associated graft-versus-host disease (TA-GVHD). This should include all oncology patients as well as neonates.

Cytomegalovirus (CMV)-negative blood should be considered in patients in the peritransplant period who are noted to be CMV seronegative in addition to neonates born to CMV-negative mothers and patients with immunodeficiencies. Institutional guidelines vary and should be consulted in determining the need for CMV-negative blood secondary to the limited supply of this product.

Finally, **washing** of PRBCs is rarely indicated and decreases the red cell mass by approximately 20%. Washing is indicated for severe allergic transfusion reactions, hyperkalemia, large-volume transfusions, and selective IgA deficiency.

Indications for PRBC transfusion

Neonates

Guidelines for transfusion in neonates and infants vary widely in the literature. Clinical correlation is required in addition to the following basic guidelines:

• Transfusion of leukopoor, irradiated blood in premature infants and low-birth weight neonates (CMV-negative if CMV status of mother is negative or unknown)
• High oxygen requirement or severe cardiac disease, keep Hgb 11 to 15 g/dL
• Mild-to-moderate respiratory distress or perioperative care, keep Hgb 10 g/dL

- Stable infants who become symptomatic from anemia, keep Hgb > 7 to 8 g/dL (based on degree of symptoms)

Acute blood loss and nonimmune hemolytic anemia

Unlike chronic conditions that result in a slow drop in hemoglobin and time for compensation, patients with acute blood loss or nonimmune hemolytic anemia may be symptomatic at much higher hemoglobin levels and should be transfused accordingly. In situations of continuing blood loss, patients should be transfused to achieve an expected hemoglobin level in addition to receiving blood to compensate for ongoing losses. In an emergent situation, transfusion consent is not required, and if there is no time for a cross-match, O-negative blood should be given.

Severe chronic anemia

In pediatric patients, iron-deficiency anemia is the most likely cause of severe chronic anemia (i.e., Hgb < 5 g/dL), in addition to viral suppression, transient erythroblastopenia of childhood, aplastic anemia, and newly diagnosed leukemia. Pediatric patients can present with an extremely low hemoglobin (e.g., 2 to 3 g/dL) and yet be relatively well compensated. Patients should be assessed closely for subtle signs of congestive heart failure (cardiomegaly on chest radiograph, increased diastolic blood pressures, hepatomegaly, oliguria, and periorbital edema) prior to transfusion. Slow transfusion (e.g., 1 mL/kg/h) has been recommended in the past, although studies have shown that 2 to 3 mL/kg/h is safe in patients with normal underlying cardiopulmonary function. Those with signs of cardiopulmonary dysfunction should be transfused slowly with judicious usage of diuretics, and exchange transfusion should be considered in those with heart failure.

Oncology patients

In general, a hemoglobin of 7 g/dL is used as the threshold for transfusion in pediatric oncology patients. This may be altered in cases where the patient is asymptomatic with imminent recovery of red blood cells (often heralded by increase in platelet count). Infants with effects on growth and development due to anemia should be maintained at higher hemoglobins; similarly, adolescents may complain of headache and fatigue and be less symptomatic with hemoglobins in the 8 to 10 g/dL range. Those with cardiopulmonary dysfunction and those requiring procedural sedation with anticipated blood loss should be kept in the 8 to 10 g/dL range as well.

Autoimmune hemolytic anemia

In patients with an autoimmune hemolytic anemia, immunosuppressive therapy is usually sufficient to abate the underlying process. In those patients who are symptomatic with a continuing drop in hemoglobin and/or resultant significant cardiopulmonary dysfunction, phenotypically matched blood may be given with close observation knowing that hemolysis is likely to continue and may even be augmented.

Chronically transfused patients

Patients with β-thalassemia major as well as some with β-thalassemia intermedia, Hgb SS, and Hgb S/β^0-thalassemia require chronic transfusion therapy, as outlined in previous chapters. These patients should have a red cell phenotype prior to initiating transfusions and based on institutional practice will usually receive phenotypically matched blood to a small panel of antigens (at our institution, other Rh antigens including C/c and E/e as well as Kell). If the patient develops antibodies to other minor red cell antigens (e.g., MNS, Duffy [Fy^a/Fy^b], Kidd [Jk^a/Jk^b], and Lewis [Le^a/Le^b]), more extensive phenotype matching is performed in order to decrease the continued risk for alloimmunization. Genotyping for a wider range of antigens is becoming more universally available and will likely become the future standard of care. Sickle cell patients in addition should receive sickledex-negative blood as blood donors are not screened for sickle cell trait. Transfusion is given on a regular basis (i.e., every 3 to 4 weeks) in order to suppress ineffective erythropoiesis.

Dosing of PRBC transfusion

The desired incremental increase in hemoglobin should be considered when determining the amount of blood to be transfused. In general, 10 to 20 mL/kg over 4 hours is given in order to increase the hemoglobin by 2 to 4 g/dL. Care should be taken to not waste blood; therefore, orders should be rounded to the nearest unit or half unit, as feasible. Remaining blood may be sterilely aliquoted and used later in the same patient in order to decrease exposure to multiple donors. Slow transfusion should be given in patients with signs of volume overload or cardiopulmonary dysfunction. Patients with frank heart failure should be exchange transfused. Care should be taken to not increase the hemoglobin above 12 g/dL in patients with sickle cell disease secondary to hyperviscosity and increased risk of CNS events. Similarly, in leukemic patients with hyperleukocytosis at diagnosis (white blood cell count > 100×10^9/L), the hemoglobin should preferably be kept below 10 g/dL and transfusion avoided if possible due to the same risks of increasing viscosity and the propensity for leukostasis.

Exchange transfusion

Exchange transfusion or erythrocytopheresis may be indicated in the severely anemic patient with congestive heart failure, acute sickle cell events, hyperbilirubinemia, or in an anemic patient treated with severe fluid restriction (increased ICP). In sickle cell disease, exchange transfusion quickly reduces the concentration of sickle cells without increasing the hematocrit or whole blood viscosity. In addition, red cell exchange transfusion reduces iron accumulation since an equal volume of red cells and iron are removed as infused. Therefore, for sickle cell disease, erythrocytopheresis is preferred over straight transfusion in patients requiring chronic transfusion in addition to those patients with acute events. Automated erythrocytopheresis can be done rapidly and safely in most situations. Limitations of this technique include increased red cell utilization, venous access, and increased cost.

Platelets

Platelet transfusions are indicated for thrombocytopenic patients with bleeding due to severely decreased platelet production or for patients with bleeding secondary to functionally abnormal platelets. Transfusion is not indicated for those with rapid destruction (e.g., immune thrombocytopenic purpura and neonatal alloimmune thrombocytopenia) unless there is life-threatening hemorrhage; however, transfusion may be useful in the bleeding patient with rapid consumption (e.g., disseminated intravascular coagulation [DIC]) or dilutional thrombocytopenia (massive transfusion or exchange). Platelets are frequently needed in the patient receiving chemotherapy or one thrombocytopenic secondary to a marrow infiltrative process.

Indications for platelet transfusion

1. Premature or sick infants
   a. Stable infant with platelet count <50×10^9/L

b. Distressed infant with platelet count $<100 \times 10^9$/L

2. Children

   a. Platelet count $<10 \times 10^9$/L; higher if febrile, septic, or with active bleeding

   b. Platelet count <20 to 50×10^9/L with a minor invasive procedure such as:

      i. Lumbar puncture

      ii. ECMO or CV bypass

      iii. Other minor procedures such as central line placement

   c. Invasive procedure in a patient with a qualitative platelet defect

   d. More invasive procedures will require discussion with the surgical team regarding platelet transfusion threshold, although recommendations are generally not evidence based

3. Patients undergoing therapy for malignancy

   a. Platelet count $<10 \times 10^9$/L; higher if febrile, septic, or with active bleeding

   b. Induction chemotherapy:

      i. ALL $<10 \times 10^9$/L

      ii. AML <10 to 20×10^9/L

   c. Children undergoing intensive therapy with active mucositis should have their platelet count maintained at 30 to 50×10^9/L (i.e., Head Start protocol for brain tumors)

   d. Lumbar puncture with platelet count <20 to 50×10^9/L; potentially <50 to 100×10^9/L with diagnostic lumbar puncture

   e. Bleeding patient with normal coagulation studies, platelets $<50 \times 10^9$/L; with abnormal coagulation studies, platelet count $<100 \times 10^9$/L

   f. Patient requiring a moderately invasive surgical procedure, with a platelet count <50 to 100×10^9/L (requiring discussion with surgical team secondary to lack of evidence-based guidelines). Most surgeons would like platelet count to remain >50 to 75×10^9/L for 48 to 72 hours after the surgical procedure

   g. Intramuscular injection (i.e., PEG-asparaginase) with platelet count $<20 \times 10^9$/L

Dosing of platelet transfusion

One unit of random platelets ($\sim$40 mL) per 10 kg will increase the platelet count by 40 to 50×10^9/L if there is no active consumptive process (e.g., fever, immune thrombocytopenic purpura, sepsis, alloimmunization, or DIC) or sequestration. This is equivalent to an increment in platelet count of 10×10^9/L per mL/kg of transfused platelets (i.e., in a 10 kg child, 10 mL/kg or 100 mL of transfused plates should raise the platelet count by 100×10^9/L). The platelet count should be checked 1 to 2 hours after infusion to identify refractory patients. A patient is refractory if 1 hour after transfusion the platelet increment is less than 5 to 10×10^9/L per unit transfused for two separate transfusions.

A patient may have platelet refractoriness secondary to alloantibodies (immune mediated). Nonimmune causes of platelet refractoriness are common and include splenomegaly, fever, infection, DIC, and use of amphotericin B.

For refractory patients, a trial of cross-matched platelets should be given. Other possibilities for treatment should this fail include leukocyte-depleted, human leukocyte antigen (HLA)-matched platelets, intravenous immunoglobulin (IVIG) with HLA-matched platelets, or massive transfusion with random donor platelets (to overwhelm the antibody).

Most institutions now utilize pheresed platelets that are harvested from a single donor and generally contain greater than 30×10^9/L of platelets, equivalent to approximately 6 to 8 units of random platelets. The volume is usually 250 to 350 mL. Secondary to the apheresis, these platelet products are considered to be leukoreduced. In addition, although controversial, most believe that apheresis is sufficient to reduce the risk of CMV transmission. Plasma ABO compatibility should generally be utilized, especially with increasing volume of transfusion. Type-specific platelets can be given in cases of refractoriness and should be given to patients in the peritransplant period to eliminate the production of any potential red blood cell antibodies. As with PRBC transfusion, platelet irradiation is required in oncology patients, premature or low birth weight newborns, and patients with immunodeficiencies.

Dosage of platelet transfusion is generally 10 to 15 mL/kg and can be given over 30 minutes to 1 hour. Due to the expected increase in platelet count and short lifespan of platelets, 1 unit of pheresed platelets is usually sufficient for transfusion in patients over 30 kg. As with PRBCs, pheresed platelet units should be rounded to the nearest half and full units as feasible to decrease waste and may be sterilely aliquoted as needed.

Fresh frozen plasma

Fresh frozen plasma (FFP) is a source of plasma proteins, including nonlabile clotting factors, such as fibrinogen. It is used for the treatment of stable clotting factor deficiencies in which no concentrate is available (not for factor VIII or IX). By definition, each milliliter of undiluted plasma contains 1 international unit (IU) of each coagulation factor.

Plasma consists of the anticoagulated clear portion of blood separated by centrifugation. FFP is collected from single donors, with each unit being removed from a unit of whole blood and frozen within 6 to 8 hours of collection. FFP should not be used when the coagulopathy can be corrected more effectively with specific treatment such as vitamin K, cryoprecipitate, or factor concentrate. Due to the high concentration of plasma antibodies, FFP is often the cause in cases of transfusion-associated acute lung injury (TRALI) and therefore should be used judiciously. The direct antiglobulin test (DAT; Coombs test) may also be positive for this reason.

Indications for FFP
- Bleeding or invasive procedure with documented clotting factor deficiency and appropriate factor not available
- Treatment of protein C or S deficiency, factor XI deficiency (hemophilia C)
- Bleeding during massive transfusion, not from thrombocytopenia

Dosing of FFP
The usual dosage of FFP is 10 to 15 mL/kg over 1 hour, which is expected to increase the concentration of coagulation factors by 25% to 50%. Due to the presence of isohemagglutinins, FFP should be ABO matched. White blood cells are killed or made nonfunctional during the freezing process; therefore, leukoreduction and irradiation are unnecessary.

Cryoprecipitate

Cryoprecipitate is prepared by thawing FFP and recovering the cold precipitate. Each bag contains >80 U factor VIII coagulant activity and >150 mg fibrinogen in approximately 15 mL of plasma. In addition, cryoprecipitate contains factor XIII and von Willebrand factor. Bags must usually be pooled to achieve an adequate dose.

Indications for cryoprecipitate
- Bleeding or invasive procedure with factor VIII deficiency or von Willebrand disease and factor concentrate not available
- Bleeding or invasive procedure with hypofibrinogenemia or factor XIII deficiency

Dosing of cryoprecipitate

The usual dosage for cryoprecipitate is 1 unit/5 kg. Obtain a fibrinogen level at 30 minutes postinfusion. For hypofibrinogenemia with coagulopathy, the goal is to maintain fibrinogen >100 mg/dL Specific factor or coagulation protein levels need to be determined in addition to assessing clinical status to decide on frequency of transfusion. As with FFP, cryoprecipitate is preferably ABO compatible and leukoreduction and irradiation are not required.

Antithrombin III

Antithrombin III (ATIII) concentrate is available for use in patients with inherited or acquired ATIII deficiency (sepsis, thrombosis, and medication induced). It may also be needed in patients receiving heparin therapy who have a low ATIII level. Patients with thrombosis after asparaginase therapy should have an ATIII level checked and repletion as necessary. ATIII replacement should also be considered in patients with veno-occlusive disease (sinusoidal obstructive syndrome) after hematopoietic stem cell transplantation. Dosing of ATIII is based on the baseline and desired level.

Granulocyte transfusion

Patients with profound and prolonged neutropenia are at increased risk for serious life-threatening fungal and bacterial infections. The beneficial effect of granulocyte transfusion in this population, with known persistent infection, especially with Gram-negative organisms and fungus, is yet to be proven by randomized controlled trials, although observational studies are available. Donor mobilization with granulocyte colony-stimulating factor (G-CSF) has increased granulocyte yields, and therefore the therapeutic benefit of transfusion, as the dose of granulocytes is the most important factor in success of this treatment modality.

Granulocytes migrate toward, phagocytize, and kill bacteria. When given a granulocyte transfusion, the cells migrate to the foci of infection, though there is rarely a measurable increase in the peripheral granulocyte count. This is likely from sequestration at the site of infection, prior immunization to leukocyte antigens, or a consumptive process secondary to the infection. Side effects of granulocyte transfusion include the risk of CMV infection, TA-GVHD, respiratory distress with pulmonary infiltrates (TRALI, concurrent administration of amphotericin B, or secondary to granulocyte sequestration), and alloimmunization.

Preparation of granulocyte concentrates

Donor mobilization is recommended with G-CSF at 5 mcg/kg (maximum 300 mcg IV/SC) and dexamethasone 12 hours prior to col-lection. Granulocytes are then collected by apheresis and ideally should be transfused within 8 to 12 hours of collection. RBC contamination requires ABO compatibility. Due to risks of TA-GVHD and CMV infection, irradiation and CMV seronegativity are required (in those that are CMV-negative), respectively. Amphotericin B and concomitant granulocyte transfusion is potentially associated with severe pulmonary reactions, although the evidence is controversial; however, it is reasonable to space these therapies apart by at least 4 hours. HLA-matched granulocytes should be given in patients with known alloimmunization. Since granulocyte half-life is only 7 hours, daily collection and transfusion for several days are likely required for benefit.

Indications for granulocyte transfusion

With a lack of randomized controlled trials, there are no evidence-based guidelines for granulocyte transfusion. Limited data in neonates with sepsis has failed to show a significant benefit. After weighing the potential risks and benefits, as well as determining the daily availability of an eligible donor and collection site, granulocyte transfusion can be considered in severely neutropenic patients with a refractory or progressive bacterial or fungal infection on appropriate, aggressive therapy with neutropenia that is expected to continue for, at the least, several days.

Transfusion reactions

Approximately 4% of transfusions are associated with some form of adverse reaction, ranging from brief episodes of fever to life-threatening episodes of hemolysis and shock. Fortunately, the majority of reactions are short-term, specifically FNHTRs and allergic reactions, and easily managed. Life-threatening reactions are nearly always due to clerical error resulting in transfusion of an ABO incompatible unit. The challenge for the clinician is to promptly recognize potential serious complications that may present with common symptoms such as fever. For any transfusion reaction, a bedside check of all labels, forms, and patient identification should be done, in addition to notifying the blood bank. Transfusion reactions are summarized below and include FNHTRs, allergic reactions, immune-mediated hemolysis, TRALI, transfusion-associated circulatory overload (TACO), TA-GVHD, and acute infection.

Hemolytic transfusion reactions

Hemolytic transfusion reactions can either be acute or delayed. Acute hemolytic transfusion reactions (AHTRs) are usually due to clerical error resulting in the transfusion of an ABO incompatible unit. AHTRs classically present with fever, chills, nausea, and vomiting in addition to dyspnea, hypotension, shock, hemoglobinuria, and DIC. Bacterial contamination must be considered in the differential for an AHTR. **Delayed hemolytic transfusion reactions (DHTRs)** present 2 to 14 days after transfusion with milder symptoms including low-grade fever, jaundice, and a posttransfusion hemoglobin increment less than expected due to minor antigen incompatibility (alloimmunization) from prior transfusion.

Evaluation of a potential AHTR should include work-up of all recently transfused blood products (see Figure 5.2). A bedside check of labeling should occur followed by laboratory evaluation including repeat cross-matching and a DAT (Coombs test). The DAT may not always be positive if all the antibodies have been destroyed during the hemolytic crisis. Other labs that should be sent to rule out intravascular hemolysis include indirect bilirubin, LDH, plasma-free hemoglobin (and/or haptoglobin), and urinalysis for hemoglobinuria.

DHTRs lead to extravascular hemolysis and should be evaluated in a patient with clinical or laboratory symptoms after the first 24 hours. Labs to follow include a posttransfusion hemoglobin level and reticulocyte count, indirect bilirubin, LDH, and DAT.

If an AHTR is suspected, emergent management is vital. The transfusion should be immediately stopped and IV fluid resuscitation commenced. Inotropic support may be required for hypotension and shock. Renal perfusion and urine output should be followed closely and additional blood product support may be required. DHTRs usually do not require intervention although may rarely cause profound anemia.

FNHTRs were significantly more common prior to near universal leukoreduction

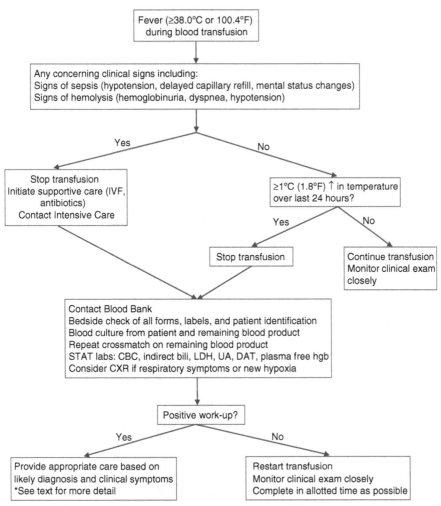

Figure 5.2 Approach to fever during blood transfusion. (Abbreviations: CBC, complete blood count; LDH, lactate dehydrogenase; UA, urinalysis; DAT, direct antiglobulin test, (Coombs); CXR, chest X-ray).

and occur due to pyrogenic cytokines released by leukocytes during blood component storage. FNHTR is defined as a temperature increase of 1 °C (1.8 °F) without any other attributable cause. More serious causes of fever including AHTR and bacterial contamination must be ruled out prior to the diagnosis of FNHTR being made. Transfusion must therefore be discontinued until an AHTR can be ruled out (see Figure 5.2). Fever due to FNHTR is usually self-limited and resolves with antipyretic usage and stopping the transfusion. Chills, rigors, and discomfort can occur, mimicking an AHTR. Transfusion can potentially be restarted after AHTR has been ruled out based on the clinical status of the patient and urgency of the transfusion.

Although patients with a history of FNHTR often receive premedication with acetaminophen with future transfusions, this practice is not evidence based. Antipyretics should be considered for the patient with multiple FNHTRs; if acetaminophen is not effective, a trial of washed blood components can be considered. Of note, transfusion can be given to the febrile patient if urgently necessary, as the criteria for workup (beyond a close and continued clinical assessment) is an increase of 1 °C in fever compared to the fever curve from the previous 24 hours.

Allergic transfusion reactions

Allergic reactions are typically type I hypersensitivity reactions to plasma in blood components. Allergic reactions are common, occurring in 1% to 5% of transfusions, and usually with mild symptoms such as urticaria, although anaphylaxis can occur. For the majority of allergic reactions, an antihistamine such as diphenhydramine is sufficient to alleviate symptoms and the transfusion can likely be completed in the allotted time. For more severe symptoms, the transfusion should be stopped. Steroids, an H2 blocker (e.g., ranitidine), epinephrine, volume expansion, β2 agonists (e.g., albuterol), and oxygen may be required. Patients with a severe allergic reaction should be tested for IgA deficiency. As with FNHTRs, premedication (with an antihistamine) remains controversial in patients with a history of a reaction. Patients with multiple episodes may benefit from premedication with an antihistamine and, if not effective, potentially corticosteroids. If allergic reactions continue, washed blood products should be utilized.

Transfusion related acute lung injury

TRALI is becoming increasingly recognized as an important cause of morbidity after transfusion with plasma-containing blood components. Signs and symptoms include hypoxia, chest infiltrates (without volume overload), dyspnea/tachypnea, fever, and hypotension. TRALI generally should occur within 6 hours of transfusion completion. A majority of patients with TRALI will recover in a 2- to 4-day period, although respiratory support, and in some cases mechanical ventilation, is often required.

Transfusion-associated circulatory overload

TACO also is becoming more widely recognized but is likely rare in the pediatric population. TACO occurs due to cardiogenic edema from too rapid or too large a volume of transfusion. Clinical signs such as dyspnea/tachypnea and hypoxia may be confused with TRALI. Differentiating features include hypertension rather than hypotension due to pulmonary overcirculation with a positive fluid balance. Chest radiograph should be more consistent with pulmonary edema/effusion rather than infiltrates. Aggressive diuresis should be utilized.

Transfusion-associated graft-versus-host disease

TA-GVHD can occur in immunocompromised patients who receive nonirradiated blood or platelet transfusion due to donor T-lymphocytes that cannot be rejected by the host. TA-GVHD has also been reported in immunologically normal patients with an HLA-compatible donor such as in homogeneous populations or in cases where the donor is a close relative (directed donation). Clinical symptoms are equivalent to those with transplant GVHD including fever, anorexia, vomiting/diarrhea, and skin rash. Hepatic dysfunction and pancytopenia can similarly manifest.

Bacterial infections

Blood components may be contaminated with bacteria at the time of collection or during processing. Infection rates are higher after platelet transfusion since platelets are stored at room temperature, although clinical signs and symptoms are often more severe after transfusion of contaminated PRBCs. Infection is associated with a rapid onset of symptoms and a high rate of morbidity and mortality, especially from Gram-negative organisms. The patient may present acutely septic with fever/chills, hypotension, tachycardia, and shock. If bacterial contamination is suspected, the transfusion should be stopped immediately. Aggressive supportive treatment including IV fluid resuscitation, initiation of broad-spectrum antibiotics, and potential therapy for renal failure, shock, and/or DIC should be started emergently.

Case study for review

You are following a 12-year-old, 60-kg boy admitted to the pediatric intensive care unit with septic shock. He is secondarily found to be anemic and thrombocytopenic with coagulopathy and hypofibrinogenemia in DIC.

After initial stabilization of the patient with IVF, antibiotics, mechanical ventilation, and pressors, the PICU team is determining their transfusion plan. Current hemoglobin is 7.0 g/dL, platelets are 34×10^9/L, PT is 27.2 seconds, PTT is 74.6 seconds, and fibrinogen is 76 mg/dL. There is no noted active bleeding. 1:1 mixing studies correct both the PT and PTT, implying a factor deficiency rather than an antibody. The patient does appear to have some amount of hemolysis with an elevated indirect bilirubin and LDH but has a negative direct Coombs test.

1. What blood products should be transfused?

2. What amount of PRBCs should be given?

3. Are there any special considerations for the type of blood product required?

4. What are some specific risks with this patient presentation?

First, the patient should be given PRBCs, pheresed platelets (if possible), and FFP. Cryoprecipitate may or may not be required dependent on the increase in fibrinogen with FFP. If the patient is clinically worsening (e.g., problems oxygenating, dropping blood pressures), consideration should be given to transfusing O-negative PRBCs while awaiting cross-matching.

Second, one can utilize the transfusion factor to estimate the increment in hemoglobin with transfusion. In this case, the transfusion factor will likely overestimate the bump as the patient is actively septic and therefore hemolyzing PRBCs and consuming platelets. Still, estimating will help determine a reasonable plan. Assuming the decision is made to give 15 mL/kg (3 units), one would expect at most an increase in hemoglobin of 3 g/dL:

Transfusion amount (mL/kg)/transfusion factor = Hgb increase (g/dL)

Therefore, in this case (15 mL/kg)/5 = 3 g/dL

In general, platelet and FFP transfusion will also be 10 to 15 mL/kg. Platelet transfusion should initially be a maximum of one pheresed unit (approximately 250 to 350 mL). Posttransfusion hemoglobin, platelets, and coagulation studies can help determine the need for additional transfusion as well as the likely frequency of necessary transfusion (directly dependent on the clinical status of the patient). Time for "equilibration" after the completion of transfusion is unnecessary.

Third, in this case, no significant special arrangements need to initially be made in regards to the transfusions. The patient does not need sickledex-negative blood unless they have concomitant sickle cell disease. Also, phenotypically matched blood is unnecessary. As the patient does not have a known underlying reason to be immunocompromised, irradiated blood and platelets are not required. Similarly, CMV-negative blood is unnecessary.

Finally, specific risks exist for this patient and must be considered during transfusion. Due to the likelihood of continued transfusions as well as the presence of sepsis, the patient may develop volume overload and potentially TACO; therefore, the judicious use of diuretics with transfusion should be considered. In addition, a significant volume of PRBC transfusion can have a dilutional effect on platelets and coagulation factors, thus increasing transfusion requirements for these blood products. The patient is also at risk for hyperkalemia with increasing PRBC transfusion. If hyperkalemia begins to occur, washed PRBCs should be given. Massive PRBC or whole blood transfusion has been shown to induce transfusion-associated microchimerism. Microchimerism is the presence of donor lymphocytes in the recipient's circulation. The significance of transfusion-associated microchimerism is unknown. Patients receiving large amounts of plasma are at risk for developing TRALI that must be considered with worsening respiratory symptoms.

Suggested Reading

Eder AF, Chambers LA. Noninfectious complications of blood transfusion. Arch Pathol Lab Med 131:708–718, 2007.

Fasano R, Luban NL. Blood component therapy. Pediatr Clin N Am 55:421–445, 2008.

Klein HG, Spahn DR, Carson JL. Red blood cell transfusion in clinical practice. Lancet 370:415–426, 2007.

Roseff SD, Luban NL, Manno CS. Guidelines for assessing appropriateness of pediatric transfusion. Transfusion 42:1398–1413, 2002.

Stroncek DF, Rebulla P. Platelet transfusions. Lancet 370:427–438, 2007.

6 Chelation Therapy

Transfusional iron overload

Iron overload may occur in any patient receiving intermittent transfusions for acute illness (e.g., sickle cell disease), chronic transfusion therapy (thalassemia, sickle cell disease, red cell aplasia, bone marrow failure syndromes), or in those having received an intensive period of frequent transfusion (myelosuppressive chemotherapy/radiation for treatment of malignancy and after hematopoietic stem cell transplant). Each milliliter of blood contains 1 mg of iron and normal iron stores are approximately 3 g, with 2 g in the blood and 1 g in the liver. Therefore, patients receiving frequent transfusion likely will have received a large amount of transfused iron and should be monitored for evidence of iron accumulation.

There is no simple test for quantifying total iron burden. Serial serum ferritin levels are helpful in determining hepatic iron stores, but values are altered in states of inflammation. Liver biopsy remains the gold standard for quantification of total body iron but is an invasive procedure. Liver iron levels ≥ 7 mg/g dry weight liver are indicative of iron overload. The superconducting quantum interference device (SQUID) is accepted as a noninvasive method to quantitate total body iron, but its limited availability does not allow for routine use. Currently, R2 MRI (proton magnetic resonance imaging) is becoming more widely utilized as an accurate and noninvasive measure of organ iron content, and T2* MRI is becoming the new standard for measuring cardiac iron stores. Further study is required for these new techniques to become uniformly calibrated methods.

Institution of chelation therapy relative to transfusion frequency is based on institutional practice. Patients that will require chronic transfusion therapy should be chelated before their liver iron reaches a high level, measured by liver biopsy, MRI quantification, or based on the number of transfusions received (i.e., chelation initiated after receiving 10 to 20 transfusions, or approximately 3 to 6 g of transfusional iron in a 30 kg patient). Thalassemia patients tend to have a higher iron burden than sickle cell patients as the chronic inflammatory state in sickle cell disease limits gastrointestinal iron absorption. Thalassemia patients should be counseled to be on a low-iron diet.

Patients receiving intermittent transfusion or those receiving frequent transfusion therapy in a short period of time (e.g., with intensive leukemia therapies) may have a more insidious development of iron overload. Patients with leukemia should have serum ferritin levels checked at the end of therapy. Those with ferritin levels > 1000 ng/mL

Handbook of Pediatric Hematology and Oncology: Children's Hospital & Research Center Oakland, Second Edition. Caroline A. Hastings, Joseph C. Torkildson, and Anurag K. Agrawal.
© 2012 John Wiley & Sons, Ltd. Published 2012 by John Wiley & Sons, Ltd.

should have serial checks every 3 months; if ferritin remains above this threshold after 6 to 12 months, the patient should undergo liver biopsy or R2 MRI for more accurate iron quantification. These patients, especially male adolescents, may benefit from monthly phlebotomy which can be discontinued when the ferritin and liver iron concentration reach normal levels (i.e., 1.6 mg/g dry liver weight). Younger children and menstruating females have been shown to have reversible iron overload in most such cases.

Current treatment strategies for iron overload and potential side effects of iron chelators are summarized in Table 6.1. Desferoxamine (Desferal) has the longest treatment record but requires parenteral administration and has been widely replaced by deferasirox (Exjade) due to the convenience of oral intake and therefore presumed increased compliance. Exjade may not be effective in all patients, which must be weighed against the risks of noncompliance with Desferal. Deferiprone (Ferriprox or Kelfer) was approved by the Food and Drug Administration (FDA) in October 2011. Usage of two agents concomitantly is currently undergoing clinical trials and may have particular benefit in chelation of cardiac iron.

Concomitant administration of ascorbic acid (vitamin C) increases the excretion of iron when given with chelation. Iron chelators should not be administered when there is concern for a bacterial infection. By mobilizing free iron, chelators promote bacterial growth, in particular *Yersinia enterocolitica*. For febrile patients on chelator therapy, chelation should be stopped until blood cultures are definitively negative. Broad-spectrum antibiotic prophylaxis should be initiated and include coverage for this unusual organism.

Table 6.1 Iron chelators.

Name	Desferoxamine (Desferal)	Deferasirox (Exjade)	Deferiprone (Ferriprox/Kelfer/L1)
Dose (mg/kg/d)	25–50	20–40	75–100
Administration	SC/IV, given as continuous infusion over 8–24 hours, 5–7 d/wk	PO, daily	PO, TID
Side effects	Irritation at infusion site, ototoxicity (tinnitus, transient hearing loss), ocular disturbance (decreased night vision), allergic reactions, growth failure, skeletal disturbance, pulmonary hypersensitivity	GI disturbance, rash, renal and hepatic impairment, GI hemorrhage	Agranulocytosis, neutropenia, GI disturbance, transaminitis, arthropathy, progression of hepatic fibrosis
Potential therapeutic issues	Highly effective but compliance may be an issue due to route of administration	Long-term data lacking; may not be effective in all patients	Recently approved for use by the FDA; long-term data lacking

Abbreviations: SC, subcutaneous; IV, intravenous; GI, gastrointestinal; FDA, Food and Drug Administration.

Lead toxicity

Lead poisoning is an environmental disease that has undergone a major evolution in the past few decades. Recognition of the devastating neurologic effects of high lead levels and knowledge of the causes have led to universal efforts to decrease environmental lead contamination, with a resultant decrease in measured blood lead levels in children over the past 2 to 3 decades. Sources of lead have included gasoline additives, food can soldering, lead-based paints, ceramic glazes, certain toys, drinking water systems (lead pipes), and folk remedies. The use of these products has been markedly reduced as the result of federal guidelines and the development of cost-effective alternatives. Lead in gasoline and paint is at extremely low levels and has been eliminated altogether from food can soldering. Housing built prior to 1960 is likely to have been painted with high-content lead-based paint, and since lead isotopes are very stable, environmental exposure presents an ongoing risk. High risk populations have a greater likelihood of living in older housing, which has not had lead abatement. Risk factors for excessive lead exposure include poverty, age younger than 6 years, African-American ethnicity, and urban housing.

Lead may enter the body through direct ingestion, inhalation, or via skin absorption. The most common pathway among young children is through the mouth. Lead absorption is enhanced in the presence of other dietary mineral deficiencies, such as calcium and iron, due to competitive biochemical pathways. Pica behavior enhances the likelihood of direct ingestion. Toddlers in particular are at risk due to normal developmental behaviors such as putting objects and toys in the mouth and chewing on unusual surfaces (e.g., window sills).

Lead entering the intravascular space rapidly attaches to the red blood cell, with minimal amounts (3%) detected in the plasma. The half-life in the blood is approximately 21 to 30 days. Excretion is primarily through the kidneys, with small amounts deposited in the hair, nails, and bile. The lead that remains in the body accumulates mostly in the bone (65% to 90%). Lead can enter any cell and toxicity may occur in any tissue or organ. Classically, in severe lead intoxication, gastrointestinal and central nervous system toxicities are the most clinically apparent. Gastrointestinal symptoms include anorexia, nausea, vomiting, abdominal pain, and constipation. The blood lead level is typically 50 mcg/dL or greater when these symptoms are present. Lead poisoning was a lethal disease in the United States decades ago, primarily related to neurotoxic effects. At levels above 100 mcg/dL, children may show evidence of encephalopathy, including a marked change in mentation or activity, ataxia, seizures, and coma. Increased intracranial pressure may be present on examination. These effects are usually permanent with long-term sequelae of retardation, palsies, and growth failure.

Most children who have elevated blood lead levels have subclinical disease. Fewer than 5% of children present with overt symptoms of lead toxicity. An elevated blood lead level, suggesting excessive environmental exposure, is defined as 10 mcg/dL. Many studies have shown associations between blood lead levels and impaired neurocognitive function. These results have provided the primary impetus for current public health efforts. Of note, no lead level is normal and even lead levels below 10 mcg/dL are thought to lead to subtle neurocognitive dysfunction.

Screening for lead toxicity

Prevention and treatment of lead toxicity remains a major public health concern, and efforts for screening have primarily focused on high risk populations. All children

Table 6.2 Recommendations for the treatment of lead toxicity.

Blood lead level (mcg/dL)	Recommendations
<10	Environmental assessment, risk reduction, nutritional guidance, retest in 3 mo if concern for exposure
10–14.9	Environmental assessment, risk reduction, nutritional guidance, report to public health department, confirm result with venous sample
15–19.9	As above, if no improvement on retest, aggressive environmental assessment, abdominal radiographs if ingestion suspected
20–44.9	Aggressive environmental intervention, abdominal radiographs if ingestion is suspected. If blood lead levels persist on retest, chelation with oral succimer (DMSA) should be considered although does not have proven efficacy in reducing blood lead levels at these concentrations and therefore impacting neurocognitive outcomes
45–69.9	Chelation therapy with oral succimer (DMSA) 10 mg/kg TID × 5 d followed by 10 mg/kg BID × 14 d. Abdominal radiograph to assess for enteral lead. If with CNS symptoms, should treat as if lead level >70 mcg/dL. May require hospitalization to monitor for adverse effects, institute environmental abatement, and ensure compliance. Consider alternative regimen of $CaNa_2$ EDTA 25 mg/kg/d for 5 d as IV infusion (continuous or intermittent) with required inpatient administration for hydration and monitoring electrolytes. **Ensure calcium salt is given**
>70	Dimercaprol (BAL) 25 mg/kg/d IM, divided Q4 hours for minimum 72 h; after the second dose of BAL, immediately follow with $CaNa_2$ EDTA 50 mg/kg/d continuous IV for 5 d. Urine should be alkalinized with BAL therapy. In addition, **can cause hemolysis with G6PD deficiency and is dissolved in peanut oil.** Multiple potential side effects. BAL and EDTA cause renal dysfunction, EDTA may also cause hypokalemia. Must give adequate hydration and monitor electrolytes. After the initial treatment, subsequent courses may be BAL and $CaNa_2$ EDTA or $CaNa_2$ EDTA alone based on repeat lead level. **Ensure calcium salt is given**

Abbreviations: CNS, central nervous system; EDTA, ethylenediaminetetraacetic acid; IV, intravenous; IM, intramuscular.

should have a screen of potential environmental exposures by their primary health care provider starting at 1 year of age, and repeated when the child is mobile and attains hand-to-mouth behavior. The Centers for Disease Control (CDC) and the American Academy of Pediatrics (AAP) recommend venous blood lead sampling for children identified to be at high risk (living in housing built prior to 1960, indigent, urban, and minority children) at 1 and 2 years of age. Venous blood samples should be used to assess blood lead levels as capillary samples may give falsely low results. If the screening test confirms an elevated blood lead level, specific management guidelines have been developed by the CDC and AAP and are summarized in Table 6.2. The vast majority of children with elevated lead levels are not candidates for chelation therapy with currently available drugs. Children with low levels (<20 mcg/dL) are asymptomatic and unlikely to have significant increase in lead excretion with chelation. These children benefit primarily from decreased exposure.

Blood lead levels measure the blood concentration at a point in time and may not be able to accurately predict bone stores. Bone lead content may be assessed noninvasively using a radiographic technique called X-ray fluorescence. Measurement of the heme precursor, free erythrocyte protoporphyrin (FEP), may also provide a useful clue about the duration of exposure and the degree of lead accumulation. Excessively high FEP levels classically are seen with severe lead toxicity. Other causes of elevated FEP levels include iron deficiency, inflammatory disorders (due to decreased iron absorption), increased fetal hemoglobin, and rarely, porphyria.

Management of lead toxicity

The primary aims of management are prevention of future lead exposure and resultant absorption as well as enhancement of excretion. The steps to accomplish these goals include:

1. Assessment of the environment to eliminate the sources of exposure or removal of the child from the contaminated environment.
2. Modifying the child's behavior to decrease hand-to-mouth activity.

3. Ensuring adequate nutrition, especially minerals, to limit lead absorption, including evaluation for concomitant iron deficiency.
4. Administering medications (chelators) in children with very high lead levels to increase lead excretion.

After chelation therapy, a period of reequilibration for 10 to 14 days should be allowed, prior to repeat assessment of the blood lead concentration. Subsequent treatments should be based on these levels, using the same criteria specified in Table 6.2. Ongoing efforts should be made to provide the family with education in order to prevent exposure in the child's environment in addition to assuring adequate nutrition. Family members and siblings should be screened as well.

Suggested Reading

Bellinger DC. Very low lead exposures and children's neurodevelopment. Curr Opin Pediatr 20:172–177, 2008.

Brittenham GM. Iron-chelating therapy for transfusional iron overload. N Engl J Med 364:146–156, 2011.

Chandra L, Cataldo R. Lead poisoning: basics and new developments. Pediatr Rev 31:399–406, 2010.

Neufeld EJ. Update on iron chelators in thalassemia. Hematology Am Soc Hematol Educ Program. 451–455, 2010.

7 Approach to the Bleeding Child

Hemostasis is a critical protective response of the body to reverse a loss of vascular integrity and prevent excessive blood loss. It requires a coordinated interaction between platelets, vascular endothelial cells, and plasma clotting factors. The first and primary stage of hemostasis is the formation of a platelet plug that involves a complex interaction between circulating platelets and the exposed vascular subendothelial layer. The steps in the process include platelet adhesion, mediated by an interaction between von Willebrand factor (VWF) and platelet surface glycoprotein (Gp) Ib, and platelet activation, mediated by platelet surface Gp IIb/IIIa and leading to release of platelet contents. Gp IIb/IIIa interacts with VWF and fibrinogen, leading to platelet aggregation and enlargement of the platelet plug. This lays the foundation for the formation of a fibrin clot, the secondary stage of hemostasis caused by activation of the coagulation cascade.

Clinical disorders associated with abnormalities of primary hemostasis include vascular abnormalities, qualitative platelet abnormalities, quantitative platelet abnormalities, and von Willebrand disease. These aberrations in primary hemostasis are characterized by bleeding of the mucous membranes, epistaxis, and superficial ecchymoses. Typical manifestations are prolonged oozing from minor wounds or abrasions, or abnormal intraoperative bleeding. Aberrations in secondary hemostasis are characterized by bleeding from large vessels with subcutaneous, palpable hematomas, hemarthroses, or intramuscular hematomas. The hemophilias are examples of disorders in this category.

Evaluation of the bleeding child

There are three critical questions that must be addressed when faced with a child who is actively bleeding or has experienced a major hemorrhage in the past. The first two questions are, "is the patient continuing to bleed?" and "is the patient hemodynamically stable?" These questions should be answered quickly and simultaneously. Patients who are actively bleeding but are hemodynamically stable should have efforts directed at controlling the bleeding. While therapies that are specific for a particular bleeding disorder should not be provided before a diagnosis is made, more general strategies such as ice, pressure, and elevation can be used. Patients who do not appear to be actively bleeding but are hemodynamically unstable require rapid initiation of

Handbook of Pediatric Hematology and Oncology: Children's Hospital & Research Center Oakland,
Second Edition. Caroline A. Hastings, Joseph C. Torkildson, and Anurag K. Agrawal.
© 2012 John Wiley & Sons, Ltd. Published 2012 by John Wiley & Sons, Ltd.

vascular reexpansion and a search for occult bleeding.

Once the patient is stabilized and bleeding is controlled, the third critical question is whether the child presenting with bleeding warrants an evaluation for a bleeding disorder. Examples of excessive bleeding include epistaxis lasting more than 15 minutes despite the appropriate application of pressure to the side of the nose, significant blood loss following a dental procedure lasting more than 24 hours or requiring blood transfusion, bruising that seems excessive following trauma, or menorrhagia (heavy menstrual bleeding lasting for 7 days or more, or loss of more than 80 mL of blood per cycle). When evaluating a child for "excessive bruising," it is essential to determine whether the bruising could be the result of nonaccidental trauma. Bruising involving the scalp, back, or chest, or having a pattern suggestive of common instruments of abuse such as belts, cords, or wire should be reported. Excessive bruising caused by underlying bleeding disorders occurs on areas more commonly involved in falls or trauma such as shins and bony prominences.

History

Assessment of the child with a suspected or known bleeding diathesis begins with a complete history. The nature of the bleeding should be explored with particular attention to location, duration, frequency, and the measures necessary to stop it. The time of the patient's first episode of bleeding should be documented and a careful history of bruising during the toddler age is important. A previous history of bleeding associated with trauma or surgery, dental extraction, circumcision, or tonsillectomy is also important, as is a history of petechial rash, arthritis with hemarthroses, or blood transfusion. In females, the duration and severity of menstrual bleeding should be documented.

A family history and pedigree are crucial, as many bleeding disorders are hereditary. The history should also address the use of over-the-counter and prescription drugs that can induce bleeding. The most common offenders are aspirin, ibuprofen, and naproxen. It is important to ask the patient specifically about the use of medications for colds, sinus trouble, muscle aches, or headaches, which may contain these medications. Some antibiotics, penicillins in particular, can affect platelet function or be associated with specific inhibitors of clotting. Anticonvulsants can cause thrombocytopenia, and procainamide has been associated with an acquired lupus anticoagulant.

Physical examination

In addition to the routine examination, the skin should be scrutinized carefully for petechiae, purpura, and venous telangiectasias. The joints should be examined for swelling or chronic changes such as contractures or distorted appearance with asymmetry related to repeated bleeding episodes. Mucosal surfaces such as the gingiva and nares should be examined for bleeding.

Initial laboratory evaluation

The purpose of the initial laboratory evaluation is to screen for the presence of a bleeding disorder, hopefully categorize the disorder as primary or secondary, and direct further evaluation. Appropriate screening tests include a complete blood count (CBC), peripheral blood smear, prothrombin time (PT), and partial thromboplastin time (PTT). In certain circumstances, this list will also include a fibrinogen and a thrombin time (TT).

The CBC provides several pieces of useful information. It provides the platelet count, identifying in most cases the presence or absence of thrombocytopenia. However, it is important to review the peripheral blood smear, as a small number of patients with a low measured platelet count will have pseudothrombocytopenia, a condition caused by platelet clumping in the presence of the anticoagulant EDTA. It provides the hemoglobin and mean corpuscular volume (MCV), which can provide clues regarding the duration and severity of the patient's bleeding. The presence of anemia indicates a clinically significant bleeding disorder; the concomitant presence of microcytosis suggests the bleeding has been prolonged and has led to iron deficiency. A normocytic anemia suggests that the bleeding has been more recent and likely more severe, as the blood loss has likely been more significant. Abnormalities in more than one cell line (anemia, thrombocytopenia, and/or neutropenia) suggest the presence of a bone marrow failure state such as aplastic anemia or marrow infiltration as is seen in leukemia. Many analyzers provide a measure of the mean platelet volume which can be useful in evaluating the thrombocytopenic patient. Large platelets are often seen in consumptive thrombocytopenia such as immune thrombocytopenic purpura (ITP), normal-sized platelets in hypoproliferative thrombocytopenia, and small platelets in inherited conditions such as Wiskott–Aldrich syndrome.

The PT evaluates the extrinsic system of coagulation. Factor VII is the only coagulation factor measured by the PT that is not measured by the PTT. Thus, in isolated factor VII deficiency, the PT is prolonged with a normal PTT. Factor VII is vitamin K dependent and has a very short half-life, so the PT is one of the most sensitive measures of oral anticoagulant therapy with vitamin K antagonists such as warfarin. Most laboratories now report an international normalized ratio (INR) along with the PT. The INR is calculated as the patient PT/control PT to the power of the international sensitivity index. This index corrects for the large variation in the sensitivity of thromboplastin reagents to low plasma concentrations of some coagulation proteins. A normal value is 1.00 to 1.10. The INR is used to evaluate the adequacy of oral anticoagulant therapy; the PT should be used to look for the presence of a clotting factor deficiency.

The PTT assesses the integrity of the intrinsic system of coagulation. Depending on the laboratory methods, the PTT will be normal when the activity of all measured coagulation factors is at least 30% of normal. It is prolonged in patients with hemophilia, and in some patients with VWD due to the decreased concentration of factor VIII in the plasma. However, the PTT is much more susceptible than the PT to spurious abnormalities caused by errors in collection or processing of the specimen. These are outlined in Table 7.1.

The most commonly encountered inhibitors of coagulation detected in children are so-called lupus anticoagulants. These are IgG antibodies directed against phospholipids, and while they are commonly identified in adults with autoimmune disease, they occur frequently in children as a post-infectious phenomenon that is short-lived. As phospholipid is an essential cofactor in the PTT assay, antiphospholipid antibodies will commonly cause prolongation of the test. Addition of normal plasma (with additional phospholipid) as is done in mixing studies will often at least partially normalize the test, but it will most often remain abnormal. These antibodies have no effect on clotting *in vivo*, and patients with lupus anticoagulants do not have clinical bleeding; in fact, their most common coagulation problem is thrombophilia rather than bleeding.

The TT is useful in evaluating the terminal steps of coagulation and identifying anticoagulants present in plasma. The TT is abnormal when the plasma concentration of fibrinogen is decreased (hypofibrinogenemia or afibrinogenemia), when the fibrinogen present is dysfunctional (dysfibrinogenemia), or when there are

Table 7.1 Factors affecting the validity of the partial thromboplastin time (PTT) test.

Aspect	Problem	Remarks
Sample collection	Clots	Clots caused by slow blood flow or delay in transferring sample will cause abnormal results
	Plasma volume	Volume of anticoagulant must be corrected for plasma volume. If tube is not completely filled, or patient is extremely anemic or polycythemic, sample will not be appropriately anticoagulated
	Heparin contamination	Very small amounts of heparin will cause the PTT to be abnormal
Interpretation	Age-dependent normal values	Mild prolongation is normal in the newborn period (immaturity of the coagulation system)
	Inhibitor vs. factor deficiency	A number of agents can interfere with the PTT assay and cause a factitious prolongation of the test. If the concentration is high they can lead to a mild prolongation of the PT as well. These are diagnosed by mixing the patient's plasma and normal plasma in a 1:1 ratio and repeating the test. If the PTT is prolonged due to factor deficiency, this maneuver will increase the level of all coagulation factors to at least 50% and normalize the test. If the prolongation is due to an inhibitor, it may improve but will remain prolonged. See the discussion of inhibitors

Abbreviations: PTT, partial thromboplatin time; PT, prothrombin time.

circulating anticoagulants (heparin) or fibrin degradation products. As dysfibrinogenemia is most often asymptomatic, a prolonged TT in the face of a normal fibrinogen level is almost always associated with heparin or an inhibitor.

Abnormalities in one or more of the above screening tests will be noted with most bleeding disorders. An approach to identifying the most likely coagulation disorders given the results of these tests is presented in Table 7.2.

Management

Once the diagnosis is made, specific treatment can be provided based on the recommendations outlined in the following chapters. Two exceptions are management of epistaxis and menorrhagia. These types of bleeding can be caused by a variety of different conditions; yet in most situations, the following management plans will be effective. See also Figure 7.1.

Management of epistaxis

1. Place patient in a sitting position to decrease venous pressure, or if the patient is recumbent in bed, turn head to the side. Keep the head higher than the level of the heart. Do not allow patient to lie flat.

2. Flex neck anteriorly, with the chin touching the chest.

3. With the thumb and index finger, pinch the soft parts of the nose. Hold pressure firmly over the lower half of the nose. Avoid compressing the upper half of the nose.

Table 7.2 Interpretation of screening coagulation tests.

Test results	Differential diagnosis	Follow-up laboratory studies
PT normal PTT normal Platelet count normal	Von Willebrand Disease Platelet function disorder Factor XIII deficiency Fibrinolytic defect	PFA-100 Von Willebrand studies Platelet aggregation studies Urea clot lysis test Euglobulin clot lysis Factor XIII assay Alpha-2-antiplasmin, PAI-1, and TPA

PT normal
PTT prolonged
Platelet count
    normal
	PTT inhibitor
	Von Willebrand disease
	Hemophilia A or
	    Hemophilia B
	Heparin contamination
		PTT mixing study
		Factor assays (VIII, IX, and XI)
		Von Willebrand studies
		TT/reptilase time

PT prolonged PTT normal Platelet count normal	PT inhibitor Vitamin K deficiency Warfarin Factor VII deficiency	PT mixing study Factor assays (II, VII, IX, and X)
PT prolonged PTT prolonged Platelet count normal	Circulating inhibitor Liver dysfunction Vitamin K deficiency Factor deficiency (II, V, X, or fibrinogen) Dysfibrinogenemia	PT/PTT mixing studies TT/reptilase time Fibrinogen Factor assays
PT prolonged PTT prolonged Platelet count low	DIC Liver disease Kasabach-Merritt syndrome	TT Fibrinogen Factor assays D-dimers
PT normal PTT normal Platelet count low	Acute ITP Chronic ITP Collagen vascular disease Early bone marrow failure syndrome	None Antinuclear antibodies Anticardiolipin antibodies Direct antiglobulin test (Coombs) Serum immunoglobulin levels Serum complement levels HIV and hepatitis C antibody testing Bone marrow aspirate Marrow chromosomal analysis

Abbreviations: PT, prothrombin time; PTT, partial thromboplastin time; PFA-100, platelet function analyzer-100; PAI-1, plasminogen activator inibitor-1; TPA, tissue plasminogen activator; TT, thrombin time; DIC, disseminated intravascular coagulation; ITP, immune thrombocytopenic purpura.

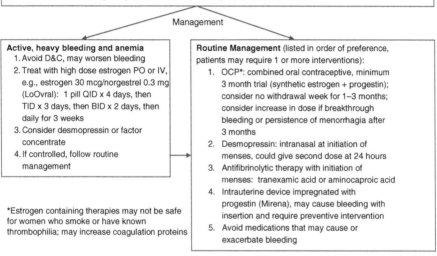

Menorrhagia : >80 mL blood loss/cycle or heavy, regular periods >7 days duration with pad/tampon use >1 per hour or passing >1 inch wide clots

and

Diagnosis or suspicion of von Willebrand disease or other bleeding disorder: type and severity may influence nature of bleeding and intervention

Assessment:
1. **History:** categorize bleeding pattern by duration, regularity, quantification of bleeding
2. **Medication History:** evaluate for drugs associated with bleeding including warfarin, heparin, salicylates, non-steroidal anti-inflammatory drugs, phenytoin, antipsychotics (SSRIs) and tricyclic anti-depressants, prolonged antibiotic use (low vitamin K), herbal supplements
3. **Physical:** evidence of bleeding disorder or gynecologic problem
4. **Laboratory:** assess for degree of anemia and red cell indices with CBC, urine βHCG for pregnancy screen, consider STI (gonorrhea, chlamydia with bleeding and use of OCPs)
5. **Imaging:** assess for anatomic etiology with pelvic ultrasound to look for fibroids, polyps, endometriosis, pregnancy complications, ovarian cysts, endometrial cancer

Management

Active, heavy bleeding and anemia
1. Avoid D&C, may worsen bleeding
2. Treat with high dose estrogen PO or IV, e.g., estrogen 30 mcg/norgestrel 0.3 mg (LoOvral): 1 pill QID x 4 days, then TID x 3 days, then BID x 2 days, then daily for 3 weeks
3. Consider desmopressin or factor concentrate
4. If controlled, follow routine management

*Estrogen containing therapies may not be safe for women who smoke or have known thrombophilia; may increase coagulation proteins

Routine Management (listed in order of preference, patients may require 1 or more interventions):
1. OCP*: combined oral contraceptive, minimum 3 month trial (synthetic estrogen + progestin); consider no withdrawal week for 1–3 months; consider increase in dose if breakthrough bleeding or persistence of menorrhagia after 3 months
2. Desmopressin: intranasal at initiation of menses, could give second dose at 24 hours
3. Antifibrinolytic therapy with initiation of menses: tranexamic acid or aminocaproic acid
4. Intrauterine device impregnated with progestin (Mirena), may cause bleeding with insertion and require preventive intervention
5. Avoid medications that may cause or exacerbate bleeding

Figure 7.1 Menorrhagia in young women with bleeding diathesis: clinical assessment and management strategies. Abbreviations: SSRI, selective serotonin reuptake inhibitors; CBC, complete blood count; STI, sexually transmitted infection; OCP, oral contraceptive pill, D&C, dilatation and curettage.

4. Hold pressure for 20 minutes with the head in a flexed position. If manual pressure is stopped momentarily to examine or change dressings, the 20 minute digital pressure will likely need to start again. Pressure and time allow for clot formation to occur. If bleeding continues, reassess location of digital pressure and reapply. If bleeding stops and recurs, repeat manual pressure for 20 minutes. If bleeding continues and clot(s) can be visualized, remove clot(s) and reapply digital pressure for 20 minutes.

5. Advise patient not to blow nose for at least 12 hours to avoid dislodging the clot.

6. Nasal packing may be indicated if the source of bleeding is not well visualized or bleeding is profuse. Types of packing include compressed sponge, Vaseline gauze packing, gelfoam, or topical thrombin packing. Compressed sponges are compressed when dry and expand when wet. The expansion produces active and passive absorption and places gentle pressure on the mucosa. The nasal sponge should fit snugly through the nare and be placed along the floor of the nasal cavity. Sponges are easy to insert and can be removed with little discomfort. Neosporin can be applied to the sponge for ease of insertion and to act as an antimicrobial agent. Topical thrombin powder (a vasoconstrictor) applied to the inserted end of the sponge can provide additional hemostasis. Anterior packs may be left in place for 1 to 5 days, though should be removed within 24 hours in an immunocompromised patient due to the risk of infection. Humidification and nasal saline spray can help prevent drying and crusting of the oral mucous membranes as a result of mouth bleeding. Broad-spectrum antibiotics, to cover skin flora as well, should be considered in patients who are immunosuppressed with a nasal pack in place. Vaseline gauze packing, when placed correctly and snugly, is a reliable means of packing. Packing may be soaked in 4% topical cocaine or a solution of 4% lidocaine and topical epinephrine (1:1000) to provide local anesthesia and vasoconstriction.

Management of menorrhagia

1. The American College of Obstetricians and Gynecologists and the American Academy of Pediatrics issued a committee consensus report in 2006 in which they defined normal menstruation. This report stated that normal menstruation begins at 11 to 14 years of age, the normal cycle interval is 21 to 45 days, and the normal length of menstrual flow is 7 days or less with product use no more than three to six pads or tampons per day. Based on this, menorrhagia has been defined as heavy menstrual bleeding lasting for more than 7 days or resulting in the loss of more than 80 mL per menstrual cycle. However, attempts to quantify menstrual blood loss in clinical practice can be quite difficult. Variables that have been identified as predicting menstrual blood loss of >80 mL include the passing of clots >1 inch in diameter, a low serum ferritin, or changing a pad or tampon more often than hourly.

2. The most effective management of menorrhagia is prevention. This can often be accomplished with hormonal therapy. The most common approach is the use of combination estrogen–progestin oral contraceptive pills (COCP), both cyclic and extended cycle use. Regular COCPs can been prescribed in an extended cycle pattern, with the patient taking 63 to 84 days of active pills before stopping for 7 days to allow withdrawal bleeding. Young women often prefer this approach despite the occasional breakthrough bleeding that may occur. Table 7.3 lists COCP preparations that have been used successfully in managing menorrhagia in women with bleeding disorders. There are no data that indicate that any of these agents are superior to the others in controlling bleeding.

3. Other hormonal approaches to prevent menorrhagia include the levonorgestrel intrauterine system (Mirena), oral progestogens, and injected progestogens. Mirena has been shown to be as efficacious as endometrial ablation in decreasing the incidence and severity of menorrhagia. It has also been shown in one small study to be well tolerated by nulliparous adolescent females. Oral progestin-only OCPs (Micronor, Nor-QD) contain norethindrone as the active agent. The progestin implant (Implanon) contains etonogestrel. Depo-Provera is an injectable progestin only contraceptive containing medroxyprogesterone as the active agent.

4. Young women presenting with the acute complaint of menorrhagia should have a pregnancy test performed to ensure that they are not having a miscarriage. They should also be carefully evaluated to rule out the presence of severe anemia or hypovolemia. If they are hemodynamically stable, have no prior personal or family history of abnormal bleeding, and are not allergic to

Table 7.3 Preparations of combination oral contraceptive pills used to treat menorrhagia in women with bleeding disorders.

Hormone content	Brand name
150 mcg desogestrel/30 mcg ethinyl estradiol	Apri
	Cyclessa
	Desogen
	Ortho-Cept
	Reclipsen
	Velivet
150 mcg levonorgestrel/30 mcg ethinyl estradiol	Enpresse
	Jolessa
	Levora
	Lutera
	Nordette
	Portia
	Quansense
250 mcg norgestimate/35 mcg ethinyl estradiol	MonoNessa
	Ortho-Cyclen
	Previfem
	Sprintec
3 mg drospirenone/30 mcg ethinyl estradiol	Ocella
	Yasmin

nonsteroidal anti-inflammatory drugs (NSAIDs), ibuprofen 200 mg every 4 to 6 hours can be tried. NSAIDs have been shown to decrease the amount of menstrual flow by 25% to 30% by altering the endometrial prostaglandin balance. However, they are contraindicated in women with known or suspected coagulopathy.

5. "Double-dose" COCPs can be used to treat young women presenting with acute menorrhagia as well. Any of the COCPs in Table 7.3 containing 35 mcg of ethinyl estradiol/tablet can be prescribed twice a day for up to 7 days until the bleeding stops, after which the remainder of the pack is completed on a once daily schedule.

6. If these steps are not effective or the bleeding is more significant, tranexamic acid can be added to any of these treatments at a dose of 1300 mg (two tablets) three times daily for up to 5 days. This antifibrinolytic agent has been successfully used to treat menorrhagia in women both with and without coagulopathies.

7. Women with inherited coagulopathies (Type 1 VWD, hemophilia carriers, platelet function disorders) should ideally be tested for responsiveness to DDAVP prior to menarche. If they are responsive, this should be used as first-line therapy for menorrhagia. It can be given IV at a dose of 0.3 mcg/kg in 50 mL normal saline over 30 minutes. A concentrated nasal preparation is also available (Stimate) containing 150 mcg/spray; it is given at a dose of one spray in each nostril once daily. Either preparation can be repeated daily for up to 3 to 4 days during the heaviest menstrual flow. It should be used in conjunction with tranexamic acid if the bleeding is heavy. Side effects include flushing, headache, nausea, fluid retention, and rarely, hyponatremia.

8. Women with persistent bleeding despite these therapies should be hospitalized for more aggressive therapy, including intravenous estrogen. Consultation with a gynecologist or adolescent medicine physician well versed in the management of this disorder is recommended.

Case study for review

A 4-year-old girl presents to the emergency department with a 3 day history of easy bruising and "rash." She denies any other bleeding including epistaxis, oral bleeding, hematuria, or hematochezia. She has otherwise been well except for an upper respiratory infection 2 weeks ago.

1. What other information would be helpful in evaluating this child?

The girl's parents deny any previous history of easy bruising, hemarthroses, or muscle bleeding in the past. The family history is significant for two older brothers who have never had any bleeding abnormalities. There is no history of epistaxis, gingival bleeding, menorrhagia, or excessive bleeding with surgery or trauma in any other family members. There is no family history of malignancy or autoimmune disorders. The patient has not been taking any medications recently.

2. What will you be looking for on physical examination?

The vital signs are normal, and the patient is at the 50th percentile for height and weight. She appears completely healthy. There are no signs of oral bleeding or purpura. Her heart and lung exam are normal, and she has no tenderness, masses, or hepatosplenomegaly on abdominal exam. You note a diffuse petechial rash over her entire body, with several ecchymoses on her shins and arms, with a few on her back. Her neurological exam is completely normal.

3. What are your first thoughts, and what would you like to do next?

The presence of petechiae and increased superficial bruising suggests a disorder of primary hemostasis. The lack of a previous history and a negative family history suggest this is more likely to be an acute problem rather than a congenital one, although this is not certain. Acquired problems of primary hemostasis include acquired (often immune-mediated) thrombocytopenia or acquired (often drug-induced) platelet function abnormalities. This presentation could also result from a vasculitis, although most patients with such a problem would likely appear more ill. The best next steps would be to obtain a CBC and coagulation studies to see if you can identify where an abnormality might be. The CBC reveals a hemoglobin of 12.3 g/dL, a WBC count of 6.5×10^9/L with a normal differential, and a platelet count of 6×10^9/L. The PT is 12.2 seconds (reference range, 12.6 to 13.5 s) and the PTT is 30 seconds (range, 26 to 33 s).

4. What do you think now, and what is your next step?

The patient has isolated thrombocytopenia with a normal hemoglobin and platelet count, and no evidence of a clotting factor deficiency. The recent history of a viral illness is very consistent with ITP. The absence of any clinically significant bleeding at this point means that no immediate intervention is necessary. The management of ITP is discussed more fully in Chapter 12.

Suggested Reading

Allen GA, Glader B. Approach to the bleeding child. Pediatr Clin N Am 49:1239–1256, 2002.

Hayward CP. Diagnostic approach to platelet function disorders. Trans Apheresis Sci 38:65–76, 2008

Ahuja SP, Hertweck SP. Overview of bleeding disorders in adolescent females with menorrhagia. J Pediatr Adolesc Gynecol 23:S15–S21, 2010.

8 Von Willebrand Disease

Von Willebrand disease (VWD) is the most common inherited bleeding disorder, affecting as much as 1% of the general population, and equally affects both genders as well as all races and ethnicities. The actual prevalence is difficult to determine, as many affected individuals are either asymptomatic or have such mild symptoms that they do not seek medical attention. While most patients with VWD have the inherited form, an acquired form also occurs. The three characteristic clinical features of the inherited form are excessive mucocutaneous bleeding, abnormal von Willebrand factor (VWF) laboratory studies, and a family history of abnormal bleeding.

VWF is a large multimeric glycoprotein that is synthesized in megakaryocytes and endothelial cells. VWD is usually inherited in an autosomal dominant manner, but a rare autosomal recessive form and an X-linked recessive form have also been described. VWD results from either a deficiency or a defect in the VWF protein. This protein plays two critical roles in hemostasis: the large multimers bind to platelet glycoprotein Ib (GPIb) causing platelet activation and adherence to damaged endothelium, and it is the carrier protein for factor VIII (FVIII), stabilizing it and protecting it from degradation and clearance from plasma. This accounts for the prolonged partial thromboplastin time (PTT) seen in some patients.

VWD is classified into three types: Type 1, found in 70% to 80% of cases, is characterized by partial deficiency of normally functioning VWF. Type 2 is characterized by functional defects in VWF. It is divided into four subtypes. Type 2A is characterized by a decreased number of high-molecular-weight multimers and a concomitant decrease in platelet adhesion. The measured amount of VWF:Ag (antigen) is normal or only slightly decreased, but the VWF:RCo (ristocetin cofactor), a measure of VWF activity, is much lower. Type 2B is caused by mutations that pathologically increase platelet–VWF binding, which leads to the proteolytic degradation and depletion of large, functional VWF multimers. Circulating platelets are also coated with mutant VWF, which may prevent the platelets from adhering at sites of injury. The VWF-coated platelets often become sequestered in the microcirculation, leading to thrombocytopenia. Type 2M is characterized by decreased interaction between VWF and platelet GPIb on connective tissue. The ratio of VWF:RCo to VWF:Ag is low as in Type 2A, but the multimer panel appears normal. Type 2N is marked by decreased binding

Handbook of Pediatric Hematology and Oncology: Children's Hospital & Research Center Oakland, Second Edition. Caroline A. Hastings, Joseph C. Torkildson, and Anurag K. Agrawal.
© 2012 John Wiley & Sons, Ltd. Published 2012 by John Wiley & Sons, Ltd.

between VWF and FVIII, resulting in a phenotype of autosomal recessive hemophilia. Type 3, a rare condition, is characterized by the almost complete absence of VWF.

The majority of affected patients experience mucocutaneous bleeding such as epistaxis, easy bruising, and menorrhagia in women. They may also experience posttraumatic or postsurgical bleeding. Patients with severe VWD may experience bleeding into muscles and joints as well. VWD should be suspected in the patient with platelet-type bleeding and a family history of a bleeding diathesis.

Clinical presentation

The clinical features of VWD can be quite variable. In most cases of VWD, the bleeding is mild. Mucosal bleeding, such as epistaxis, gingival bleeding with tooth brushing, ecchymoses, or menorrhagia, are classic. The initial presentation, however, may be postoperative bleeding, such as following a tonsillectomy and adenoidectomy or dental extraction. In retrospect, the child who was thought to have normal childhood complaints (bruising and epistaxis) is realized to actually have a bleeding disorder. Recurrent or severe epistaxis, particularly in the older child or adult, is unusual and warrants investigation. It is important to obtain a thorough medical history of bleeding from the family as this may provide clues. Since other affected family members are often unaware that they have the condition, simply inquiring about a history of bleeding problems often yields negative results. Specific questions such as "Have any women in the family had hysterectomies during their child-bearing years because of intractable uterine bleeding?" or "Do any men in the family insist on shaving with an electric razor?" (because of the prolonged oozing they experience if they nick themselves with a safety razor) can be more informative. Often, the child is diagnosed with VWD and then a parent or sibling is found to have the disorder after screening.

In patients with mild VWD, the stress associated with serious operations or childbirth may prevent symptoms. VWF is an acute phase reactant and the level will frequently increase into the normal range following surgery, in pregnancy, or in patients with active liver disease or collagen vascular disease. It can be reduced in hypothyroidism. Even the stress of phlebotomy can increase the level of VWF, which can make it difficult to confirm the diagnosis even with repeat testing. Neonates have elevated VWF levels following vaginal delivery, making it difficult to diagnose in the neonatal period. VWF levels can be up to 25% lower in individuals who are blood type O, increasing the difficulty in distinguishing between VWD and normal individuals with a low VWF level.

Diagnosis

Screening tests are of little value in making the diagnosis of VWD. The complete blood count (CBC) may demonstrate iron deficiency anemia if the patient's blood loss has been significant, but it is nonspecific. The rare patient with Type 2B VWD may have mild thrombocytopenia. If the level of VWF is sufficiently low, the PTT may be prolonged due to decreased concentration of FVIII, but this is neither sensitive nor specific. The PFA-100 platelet function analyzer is a more useful screening test for VWD. It measures the time required for blood, drawn through a fine capillary, to block a membrane coated with collagen and epinephrine or collagen and ADP. Its sensitivity in identifying patients with VWD is fairly high, but its specificity is low. Four specific tests are used to diagnose VWD:

1. Factor VIII coagulant (FVIIIc): functional measurement of FVIII coagulant activity, which is carried in the circulation by VWF.

2. Von Willebrand factor antigen (VWF: Ag): VWF protein as measured by protein assays; does not imply functional ability. Immunologic quantitation of VWF by either the quantitative immunoelectrophoretic assay (Laurell assay) or the enzyme-linked immunosorbent assay.

3. Von Willebrand factor activity (VWF: RCo): ristocetin induces the binding of VWF to the GPIb receptor on formalin-fixed platelets. The slope of the platelet agglutination curve correlates with the level of plasma VWF.

4. Multimeric analysis: an agarose gel electrophoretic study used to identify quantitative or qualitative multimer abnormalities. The most common type of VWD (Type 1) has a normal multimeric analysis.

The classification of patients with VWD based on the results of these tests is presented in Table 8.1.

Even with these test results, it can be difficult to determine whether a child has VWD or not, especially in mild cases. Unlike hemophilia, there are not clearly defined levels of VWF antigen or activity that separate normal patients from those with VWD. The National Heart, Lung, and Blood Institute (NHLBI) of the National Institutes of Health published an algorithm, presented in Figure 8.1, to assist in identifying affected individuals while at the same time avoiding overdiagnosis. Except for patients with clearly abnormal VWF levels (<30%), the diagnosis should be made after consultation with a hematologist.

Treatment

The goal of treatment in VWD is to control or prevent serious or life-threatening bleeding. There are no effective therapies to limit the chronic bruising that many active children experience, and parents need to be given assistance to accept that reality. Many children and adults with Type 1 VWD, especially males, never require therapy. Individuals with Type 2 or Type 3 VWD are much more likely to need treatment at various times throughout life.

Three strategies are used to treat patients with VWD: increase the plasma concentration of VWF by releasing endogenous VWF stores through stimulation of endothelial cells with desmopressin, replace VWF by using human plasma-derived, viral-inactivated concentrates, and use agents that promote hemostasis and wound healing but do

Table 8.1 Classification of von Willebrand disease.

VWD subtype	VWF:Ag	VWF:RCo	FVIII:C	RCo:Ag ratio (%)	Multimer pattern
1	↓	↓	↓ or N	>60	Normal
2A	↓	↓↓	↓ or N	<60	Abnormal
2B	↓	↓↓	↓ or N	<60	Abnormal
2M	↓	↓↓	↓ or N	<60	Normal
2N	↓ or N	↓ or N	10–40%	>60	Normal
3	↓↓↓	↓↓↓	<10%	–	–

Abbreviations: VWD, von Willebrand disease; VWF:Ag, von Willebrand factor antigen; VWF: RCo, von Willebrand factor ristocetin cofactor activity; FVIII:C, Factor VIII coagulant; N, normal.

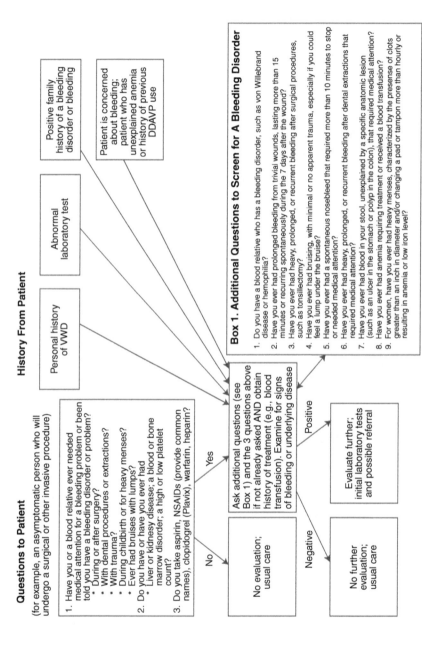

Figure 8.1 Algorithm for diagnosis of von Willebrand disease. Abbreviations: VWD, von Willebrand disease; DDAVP, desmopressin.

not substantially alter the plasma concentration of VWF. These strategies are not mutually exclusive; different bleeding episodes may require a combination of two or even all three of these strategies to be effective.

Desmopressin (DDAVP) is the treatment of choice in mild Type 1 disease (65% to 80% of all cases) and may be of benefit with some of the other variants. It stimulates endogenous release of VWF from endothelial cells, with most patients experiencing a two- to fourfold increase in their plasma VWF and FVIII levels within 15 to 30 minutes of the infusion. The approximate half-life of these released factors is 8 to 10 hours. Occasionally, patients do not respond to this therapy (especially children younger than 18 months of age). The peak effect is observed in 30 to 60 minutes. A therapeutic trial of DDAVP should be given to determine individual responsiveness to this therapy with measurement of FVIII and VWF levels before and after administration. After baseline levels are obtained, a standard dose of 0.3 mcg/kg is administered intravenously in 30 to 50 mL of normal saline over 15 to 30 minutes, and levels are measured again 60 minutes after completion of the infusion. A positive trial is defined as at least a twofold increase in the VWF:Ag and VWF:RCo activity. Ninety percent of patients with Type 1 VWD demonstrate a positive response to intravenous (IV) DDAVP.

A unique **intranasal form of DDAVP** (Stimate, 1500 mcg/mL) is also available to treat bleeding in VWD. A more dilute form of DDAVP (100 mcg/mL) is approved for use in patients with diabetes insipidus but should not be prescribed for VWD, as it is impossible to deliver an adequate dose with this preparation. Stimate is most useful for individuals with more frequent episodes of bleeding requiring therapy, such as women with menorrhagia not controlled using other measures. Given its high cost and relatively short shelf life (6 months after the bottle is opened), it is less suitable for individuals with very infrequent bleeding episodes. Although effective, there is some variability in response due to inconsistent absorption. Therefore, patients should be tested for responsiveness prior to prescribing. The dose for children weighing less than 50 kg is one spray (150 mcg) once daily. The effective dose in adolescents and adults is one spray in each nostril (total dose of 300 mcg) once daily. The peak effect is observed 60 to 90 minutes after administration.

Patients undergoing surgical procedures such as tonsillectomy or dental extractions may need extended therapy to maintain increased levels of VWF and FVIII until healing has occurred. Studies have demonstrated that DDAVP can be repeated daily for up to 4 days with little loss of efficacy as measured by VWF levels or PFA-100. Pre- and postinfusion measurements of VWF:Ag or VWF:RCo can be done to establish continued clinical responsiveness. However, it may be difficult to obtain the results of these tests quickly.

Patients with Type 1 VWD who have severe bleeding manifestations unresponsive to DDAVP or those patients with desmopressin-unresponsive Type 2 or 3 disease require treatment with exogenous VWF. Unlike FVIII replacement products, there are no recombinant VWF products yet in clinical use, although one product is being evaluated in animal models. The FDA has approved three plasma-derived FVIII/VWF products, Humate-P, Wilate, and Alphanate for the treatment of VWD. A fourth plasma-derived product, Koate DVI, is licensed in the United States for the treatment of hemophilia and is used off-label to treat VWD. These agents are not identical, and have differing ratios of FVIII to VWF, so should not be considered interchangeable.

Humate-P contains 50 to 100 IU/mL VWF: RCo activity and 20 to 40 IU/mL FVIII activity. It has the highest ratio of VWF: RCo to FVIII activity and the highest concentration of high-molecular-weight multimers. Alphanate contains 40 to 180 IU/mL FVIII activity and at least 16 IU/mL VWF: RCo activity. The FDA approved Wilate, the most recently licensed product, in 2010. It was approved specifically for use in VWD, and has essentially equal amounts of VWF: RCo and FVIII activity. It has demonstrated both safety and efficacy in patients with VWD. There are no head-to-head studies comparing the efficacy of any of these products. Wilate's packaging promotes more frequent dosing with lower doses of product, which the company states is more physiological and more cost-effective.

The goal of factor replacement therapy is to reach a therapeutic level of VWF:RCo of 100 IU/mL and nadir of >50 IU/mL. Recommended starting doses are 40 to 60 IU/kg of VWF:RCo activity, followed by 20 to 40 IU/kg every 8 to 24 hours as needed to maintain desired levels. Major surgical procedures should only be performed at centers that have the capability of measuring VWF activity levels in-house on a daily basis. To decrease the risk of thrombotic events, VWF:RCo levels should be <200 IU/mL, and FVIII levels should be <250 to 300 IU/mL.

Other adjuvant therapies are available that are often helpful in managing bleeding in patients with VWD. Direct pressure is very effective in managing epistaxis and bleeding from tooth sockets or lacerations. Family members must be taught to maintain continuous pressure "without peeking" for at least 20 minutes for best results. If the bleeding remains uncontrolled, a single dose of desmopressin is usually effective to stop bleeding in patients who have shown responsiveness. Low-estrogen oral contraceptives have been very helpful in controlling menorrhagia as they minimize the

amount of endometrial development that takes place. Minor surgical procedures such as laceration repairs or dental extractions can frequently be managed with a single treatment of desmopressin or factor concentrate followed by antifibrinolytic therapy for 7 to 10 days. Two antifibrinolytic agents are available, epsilon aminocaproic acid (Amicar) and tranexamic acid; Amicar is the more widely used agent. The oral dose of aminocaproic acid is 100 to 200 mg/kg (maximum dose, 10 g) as the initial dose, followed by 100 mg/kg (maximum dose, 5 g) every 6 hours. To maintain effectiveness, families must be instructed to adhere to the every 6 hour schedule. The dose of tranexamic acid is 25 mg/kg/dose every 6 to 8 hours. Both drugs are available in oral and intravenous forms. These drugs are particularly effective in minimizing bleeding from mucosal surfaces due to the increased level of fibrinolytic activity present in these areas.

Patients with Type 3 VWD have plasma VWF and FVIII levels that are extremely low (typically less than 5 IU/dL). Desmopressin is usually ineffective in these cases, but a therapeutic trial of desmopressin may be given, as occasionally patients will respond appropriately. These patients often have significant bleeding including profound epistaxis or hemarthroses similar to that seen in patients with hemophilia due to their low levels of both FVIII and VWF. With bleeding, such patients should be managed similarly to patients with hemophilia, using the previously mentioned FVIII concentrates that contain adequate levels of VWF and FVIII.

Patients with Type 2A VWD have abnormally small VWF multimers, and desmopressin, though frequently effective, often has only a transient effect. Serious bleeding should be treated with plasma-derived FVIII/VWF concentrates. These patients may do well with desmopressin for the treatment of minor bleeds or dental extractions.

Type 2B VWD is often associated with mild thrombocytopenia due to excessive platelet binding to an abnormal VWF molecule and rapid clearance. Stress can exacerbate the thrombocytopenia. Desmopressin is usually contraindicated due to the potential for worsening thrombocytopenia and failure to demonstrate a therapeutic response. However, in mild bleeding, desmopressin may be effective. For internal bleeding or surgery, patients should receive FVIII/VWF concentrate. If profound thrombocytopenia exists, concomitant administration of platelets may be necessary.

Patients with 2M VWD will demonstrate an increase in VWF:Ag but not in VWF:RCo in response to DDAVP, due to the defective binding of their VWF to GPIb. These patients routinely require replacement with FVIII/VWF concentrates for bleeding episodes or for surgery. Patients with Type 2N VWD similarly require factor replacement; although they produce normal amounts of FVIII, it is destroyed prematurely due to the inability of their VWF to bind to the FVIII molecule and protect it. Replacement with functional VWF will typically normalize their FVIII levels even if the relative concentration of FVIII in the product is low since they are able to produce normal amounts.

Acquired von Willebrand syndrome

Acquired von Willebrand syndrome (AVWS) refers to defects in VWF concentration, structure, or function that are not inherited directly but are consequences of other medical disorders. It is usually caused by one of three mechanisms: autoimmune clearance or inhibition of VWF, increased shear-induced proteolysis of VWF, or increased binding of VWF to platelets or other cell surfaces. Autoimmune causes of AVWS in children include postviral antibody production similar to immune

thrombocytopenic purpura (ITP), lymphoproliferative diseases, systemic lupus erythematosus, other autoimmune disorders, and some cancers, most commonly Wilms tumor. Pathologic increases in fluid shear stress can occur with cardiovascular lesions such as ventricular septal defect and aortic stenosis, or with primary pulmonary hypertension. This leads to increased destruction of VWF, particularly the larger multimers; the multimer panel often resembles that seen in Type 2A VWD. Its occurrence in Wilms tumor and other malignancies is believed to be due to expression of platelet GPIb on the tumor cell surface, leading to binding of VWF to the tumor with subsequent degradation. Hyaluronic acid secretion by nephroblastoma cells is another potential mechanism in Wilms tumor patients leading to decreased efficacy of VWF. Patients may present with classic signs and symptoms of VWD and their levels of VWF, VWF:Ag, and FVIII are typically quite low.

Desmopressin may induce a transient rise in VWF in AVWS. One small study demonstrated that intravenous immunoglobulin (IVIG) at a dose of 1 g/kg/d for 2 days was beneficial in improving VWF levels and decreasing clinical bleeding, but this is only beneficial in immune-mediated AVWS. Plasmapheresis, corticosteroids, and immunosuppressive agents have also been successful in these patients. For serious bleeding, treatment with factor concentrate (high VWF content) should be given. The antibodies typically disappear with control or resolution of the underlying disease.

Other considerations

As a general precaution, all children with bleeding disorders should be immunized with the hepatitis B vaccine, with boosters given at appropriate time intervals, since these children have a lifelong potential for receiving blood products. Patients and families should be counseled to avoid aspirin, NSAIDs, and other platelet-inhibiting drugs. Also, it is generally recommended that children wear MedicAlert bracelets and have information readily available (at school, home, and doctor's office) specifying the diagnosis and treatment for bleeding.

Suggested Reading

Nichols WL, Hultin MB, James AH, et al. Von Willebrand disease: evidence based diagnosis and management guidelines, the National Heart, Lung, and Blood Institute Expert Panel report. Haemophilia 14:171–232, 2008.

9 Hemophilia

Hemophilia is defined as an inherited bleeding disorder caused by low levels, or absence, of a blood protein that is essential for clotting. The congenital hemophilias are uncommon disorders, with a total incidence of 10 to 20 per 100,000 births. The most common form is factor VIII (FVIII) deficiency (hemophilia A or classic hemophilia), with an estimated incidence of 1 in 5000 males. The second most common form is factor IX (FIX) deficiency (hemophilia B), with an incidence of approximately 1 in 25,000 males. Both the FVIII and FIX genes are carried on the X chromosome; thus, both hemophilia A and B are X-linked recessive disorders. Approximately 80% of hemophilia patients have hemophilia A and 20% have hemophilia B. Both disorders are found throughout the world and do not appear to have any ethnic or racial predisposition.

Hemophilia A and B are clinically indistinguishable since both FVIII and FIX are essential factors in the intrinsic clotting pathway for activating factor X (FX). Factor levels are measured in comparison to a reference standard that is assumed to have a factor level of 100% (1.0 IU/mL). In the normal individual, FVIII and FIX levels range from 50% to 200% (0.50 to 2.0 IU/mL). Disease severity is defined as severe (<1%), moderate (1% to 5%), and mild (6% to 50%). The frequency of bleeding symptoms generally correlates well with the measured residual factor activity. Boys with severe hemophilia bleed with minimal trauma and bleeding symptoms are usually apparent by the time the infant begins to crawl or walk, whereas those with mild hemophilia usually bleed only with significant trauma or surgery and may have a delayed diagnosis.

Several other congenital factor deficiencies have been described as well, but are all very uncommon. They are described in Table 9.1.

Afibrinogenemia is associated with frequent and serious bleeding. Spontaneous bleeding is rare if the fibrinogen level is >50 mg/dL. The thrombin time (TT) is the most sensitive test to diagnose this disorder. **Hypoprothrombinemia** is an autosomal recessive disorder associated with mild bleeding. All patients have some prothrombin activity. Prothrombin deficiency also occurs in patients with vitamin K deficiency, liver disease, and warfarin use. **Factor V (FV) deficiency** is often characterized by bleeding from mucous membranes including epistaxis, menorrhagia, and bleeding after dental procedures. Congenital deficiency of both FV and FVIII can occur as a result of a mutation in the ERGIC-53 gene, which acts as a chaperone for intracellular transport of these factors through the endoplasmic reticulum.

Handbook of Pediatric Hematology and Oncology: Children's Hospital & Research Center Oakland, Second Edition. Caroline A. Hastings, Joseph C. Torkildson, and Anurag K. Agrawal.
© 2012 John Wiley & Sons, Ltd. Published 2012 by John Wiley & Sons, Ltd.

Table 9.1 Rare coagulation factor deficiencies.

Deficiency	Estimated prevalence	Source of replacement	Biological half-life	Gene on chromosome
Fibrinogen	1/1,000,000	Cryoprecipitate	90 h	4
Prothrombin	1/2,000,000	Activated PCCs	60 h	11
Factor V	1/1,000,000	FFP	12 h	1
Factor VII	1/500,000	rFVIIa	2–6 h	13
Factor X	1/1,000,000	Activated PCCs	24 h	13
Factor XI	1/1,000,000	FFP	40 h	4
Factor XIII	1/2,000,000	FFP	3–5 days	1 and 6

Abbreviations: PCC, prothrombin complex concentrate; FFP, fresh frozen plasma; rFVIIa, recombinant factor VII.

Patients with **factor VII deficiency** who have levels less than 1% have bleeding symptoms similar to that of classic hemophilia with hemarthrosis, intramuscular hemorrhage, and intracranial hemorrhage (ICH). Heterozygotes are typically asymptomatic. Two-thirds of patients with **factor X (FX) deficiency** have hemarthroses and hematomas. The proportion of patients with FX deficiency who require treatment is higher than that of the other rare coagulation deficiencies. **Factor XI (FXI) deficiency** is characterized by mucocutaneous and genitourinary tract bleeding; the likelihood of bleeding does not correlate well with measured FXI levels. Only individuals with **factor XIII (FXIII) deficiency** whose levels are <1% are symptomatic. Bleeding manifestations include soft-tissue hemorrhages, hemarthroses, and hematomas, and patients undergoing surgery or trauma may experience poor wound healing.

Alpha2-antiplasmin deficiency, factor XII deficiency, prekallikrein (Fletcher's factor) deficiency, and high-molecular-weight kininogen (Fitzgerald's factor) deficiency have also been identified using appropriate clotting measurements. Alpha2-antiplasmin is the primary inhibitor of plasmin, a key component of the fibrinolytic pathway. Patients with α2-**antiplasmin deficiency** are unable to effectively inhibit plasmin, and therefore lyse clots abnormally quickly leading to abnormal bleeding. As clots are formed normally, all the usual screening coagulation tests are normal except for the euglobulin and urea clot lysis tests. **Factor XII (FXII) deficiency, prekallikrein deficiency, and high-molecular-weight kininogen deficiency** all cause prolongation of the PTT but are not associated with clinical hemorrhage.

Clinical presentation

Boys with hemophilia may develop symptoms very early in life, experiencing a hemorrhage after circumcision or with separation of the umbilical cord. However, up to 50% of affected male infants have no difficulty during the neonatal period, and a negative history of bleeding after circumcision does not rule out the diagnosis of hemophilia. Mild hemophilia may go unsuspected for years until the patient experiences trauma or has a surgical procedure. Conversely, patients with severe hemophilia often experience spontaneous hemorrhages, both externally and internally, into the head, joints, muscles, and retroperitoneum. Bleeding from the mouth or frenulum often occurs during infancy, and minimal lacerations may cause very prolonged bleeding. Intramuscular injections (as with immunizations) often result in large hematomas. Joint hematomas (hemarthroses) can result in secondary joint degeneration. Life-threatening blood loss can occur with intramuscular bleeds. ICH occurs in 2% to 14% of hemophilia patients and is associated with an 18% mortality. Although ICH is much more common in severe hemophilia, it has been reported in patients with mild hemophilia as well.

ICH is the most serious complication in hemophilia. A history of trauma is elicited in only 20% to 25% of patients with central nervous system (CNS) hemorrhages, and there may be a delay of days or weeks before symptoms develop. Bleeding can be intracerebral, subdural, subarachnoid, or epidural. Patients who survive these episodes frequently experience complications such as mental retardation, seizure disorders, or motor impairment. Any history of head trauma should be considered emergent. A nonfocal neurologic examination does not exclude a diagnosis of an intracranial bleed. Any suspicion of a significant intracranial injury should prompt a head CT and close neurological observation. Immediate treatment to achieve a factor level of 80% to 100% should be provided and maintained until an intracranial bleed can be fully excluded. An intraspinal hemorrhage should be excluded with any back trauma or symptoms of a peripheral neuropathy. A lumbar puncture should never be performed in a hemophilia patient without factor therapy to avoid this complication.

Hemarthroses appear in young children as they become mobile. The elbows are often first affected as the infant begins crawling, followed by shoulders, wrists, hips, knees, and ankles. The hands and spine are rarely involved. The initial signs of a hemarthrosis are vague and difficult to detect, especially in the nonverbal infant. Early, aggressive

treatment of an acute hemarthrosis is recommended to relieve symptoms and hopefully prevent recurrent bleeding into the same joint, setting up the situation of a "target" joint.

Bleeding into muscle is characterized by pain and limitation of mobility. They can be difficult to evaluate, particularly if they occur in deep muscles such as the iliopsoas muscle (see below). They can result in long-term complications such as permanent muscle contractures. It is important to exclude any potential neurovascular compromise that can result from compression of adjacent nerves.

An **iliopsoas hemorrhage** can be quite devastating due both to the long-term consequences and to the large volume of blood loss that can occur acutely into this large muscle bed and into the retroperitoneal space. The presenting signs of groin or lower abdominal/upper thigh pain can be difficult to differentiate from a hip bleed. With an iliopsoas bleed, examination reveals inability to extend the hip, with normal internal and external hip rotation. Radiologic confirmation by CT scan is recommended.

Soft tissue hemorrhages occur very commonly and do not require therapy unless their location is near vital structures. For instance, a retropharyngeal bleed with potential airway compromise should be aggressively treated. Vigorous examination of the oropharynx with a tongue blade or other manipulations should be avoided to prevent injury with subsequent hemorrhage. A "straddle" injury resulting in a hematoma of the perineal/perirectal area should be closely evaluated for neurologic compromise as evidenced by either bladder or bowel dysfunction.

About 70% of hemophilia patients will have at least one episode of **hematuria**. Usually, these episodes are painless, thus if there is severe pain associated with hematuria, a thrombosis in the renal pelvis should be excluded. Increased fluid intake and bed rest is recommended. Factor replacement may be warranted with persistent symptoms. Treatment with antifibrinolytic drugs is contraindicated given the risk of upper urinary tract obstruction caused by clot.

Epistaxis occurs in hemophilia patients, most commonly in those with severe disease. Gastrointestinal bleeding can also occur but is atypical; an underlying gastrointestinal lesion should be excluded. Intramural bleeding into the bowel wall can occur, with signs of severe pain and possible intestinal obstruction. Appropriate therapy may avoid an unnecessary laparotomy.

Prolonged gingival oozing is common after shedding of deciduous teeth, eruption of new teeth, or instrumentation. Treatment with an antifibrinolytic medication is recommended for prolonged symptoms. Routine dental care is particularly important in the patient with a bleeding disorder to prevent the need for restorative care in the future where extensive factor replacement therapy is often indicated. Regional block anesthesia is discouraged, even with factor coverage, given the risk of hemorrhage that can lead to nerve damage and extension into the neck causing airway compromise.

Diagnosis

The diagnosis of FVIII deficiency should be suspected in males presenting with a characteristic bleeding history, especially if there is a family history of males with abnormal bleeding. However, 30% of patients with hemophilia A and B have spontaneous mutations and no family history of abnormal bleeding. A prolonged PTT in conjunction with a normal PT and platelet count is suggestive of the diagnosis; this can be confirmed by specifically measuring levels of FVIII and FIX.

Newborn males with a possible or confirmed diagnosis of hemophilia should be carefully evaluated for an intracranial hemorrhage, especially if delivered via assisted vaginal delivery (vacuum extraction or forceps). However, infants delivered via cesarean section are also at risk for severe bleeding. The initial PTT can be performed on cord blood, but it must be remembered that the upper limit of normal for newborns is longer than for adults. The normal range for FVIII levels in the newborn is the same as for adults, but FIX levels are lower until the concentrations of factors produced by the liver mature to adult levels (approximately 6 months of age). Therefore, the diagnosis of hemophilia B may be more difficult initially. Confirmatory studies should be performed on a sample obtained by venipuncture if a cord blood sample was initially obtained. Arterial as well as femoral or jugular venous sites to obtain plasma samples should be avoided if possible. Prenatal testing for both conditions is available to pregnant women who are known carriers.

Treatment

After the newborn period, affected infants rarely require treatment until they become more mobile with increasing age. Treatment recommendations for the hemophilia patient depend on several factors: the type and severity of disease (mild, moderate, or severe; FVIII or FIX deficiency); the site of the bleed (proximity to vital structures) with consideration of long-term debilitating consequences; and therapy response (factor recovery/survival and inhibitor status).

Treatment of patients with hemophilia and bleeding is by replacement of factor in a concentrated form. Many high-purity plasma-derived preparations are currently available, as are recombinant FVIII and FIX products. Most experts feel that hemophilia patients who have not been previously treated with plasma-derived products should be treated with only recombinant products.

There are two treatment strategies currently used for patients with hemophilia. Episodic or on-demand treatment involves providing treatment at the time a bleeding episode occurs. Prophylactic therapy is the periodic infusion of factor replacement to prevent such bleeding episodes. A number of single institutional case series have demonstrated the superiority of prophylaxis regimens in the prevention of joint disease, but widespread adoption of this strategy for all patients has been limited by the high cost of factor replacement therapy and the challenge of adequate vascular access, particularly in young patients.

When providing on-demand therapy, the duration, frequency, and doses of factor provided depend on the severity of the hemophilia and bleeding episode. Factor vials vary in the number of units of factor activity they contain. The required factor dose should be calculated, and vials should then be selected that come closest to the calculated target dose. Doses are calculated using the following formula:

$$\text{Dose (units of FVIII)} = \text{Weight (kg)} \times \text{desired \% rise of FVIII level} \times 0.5$$

For FIX, multiply result by 2, for recombinant FIX, multiply by 2.4.

Round up to the whole vial since factor is expensive and not uniformly dispersed in suspension. Table 9.2 outlines the dose and duration of therapy for commonly encountered bleeding episodes in hemophilia patients. More serious bleeding episodes should be treated using doses at the higher end of the range.

Other important interventions for a hemarthrosis include initial immobilization and application of ice to the area or use of a cryocuff. For particularly critical joints such as the shoulder or hip, where long-term consequences of pressure-induced avascular necrosis can be debilitating, a longer treatment course is recommended. Iliopsoas bleeds should be treated as retroperitoneal rather than as muscle bleeds.

Table 9.2 Guidelines for factor replacement in hemophilia A and B.

Site of hemorrhage	Optimal factor level (%)	Dose (units/kg body weight)		Minimum duration of treatment (days)
		Factor VIII	Factor IX*	
Muscle	30–50	20–30	30–40	1–2
Joint	50–80	25–40	50–80	1–2
Gastrointestinal tract	40–60	30–40	40–60	10–14
Oral mucosa	30–50	20–30	30–40	2–3
Epistaxis	30–50	20–30	30–50	2–3
Hematuria	30–100	25–50	70–100	1–2
Retroperitoneal	80–100	50	100	7–10
Central nervous system	80–100	50	100	14
Trauma or surgery	80–100	50	100	14

*Recombinant FIX should be dosed 1.2 times higher.

Inhibitors

The development of an inhibitor, an antibody that inactivates the coagulant function of replacement factor, is one of the most serious complications of hemophilia treatment. FVIII inhibitors develop in 20% to 30% of boys with severe hemophilia A, whereas FIX inhibitors develop in 3% to 5% with severe hemophilia B. These usually develop within the first 50 exposures to factor replacement. Risk factors for inhibitor development include the nature of the underlying mutation, with those leading to substantial loss of coding information representing greater risk, high-intensity product exposure, CNS bleeding, and African-American race. Inhibitors are quantitated by Bethesda titers: one Bethesda unit (BU) is the amount of inhibitor that inactivates 50% of FVIII function in a one-stage clotting assay. Low-titer inhibitors (<5 BU) can be managed by using larger doses of factor replacement; higher titer inhibitors require the use of alternative hemostatic agents. Alternative agents include prothrombin complex concentrates (PCCs), activated PCCs (aPCCs), and recombinant factor VIIa (rFVIIa). Immune tolerance induction with high, frequent doses of FVIII or FIX has also been successful. Management of patients with inhibitors is difficult and complex and should be performed only by experienced hematologists.

Other considerations

In addition to aggressive factor replacement when bleeding has occurred and the use of physical therapy programs to prevent or minimize chronic joint disease, comprehensive medical care must be provided to all patients with hemophilia. All immunizations including hepatitis B vaccine should be given on schedule. Regular dental care is essential to prevent excessive decay and gingival disease that may predispose to complications. Psychological support is essential to assist patients and families cope with the emotional and social burden imposed by the disease. A comprehensive program of patient and family education will prevent complications caused by failure to recognize or understand warning signs of hemorrhage as well as empower family members and eventually the patient to take an active role in the management of the disease. Education in home treatment is vital, and should be used whenever possible, as speed in the treatment of bleeding, especially hemarthroses, is directly related to minimizing long-term complications of the disease.

Suggested Reading

Kessler CM. New perspectives in hemophilia treatment. Hematology Am Soc Hematol Educ Prog 429–435, 2005.

Manco-Johnson MJ. Advances in the care and treatment of children with hemophilia. Adv Pediatr 57:287–294, 2010.

10 The Child with Thrombosis

Virchow's triad describes risk factors for thrombus (blood clot) formation: (1) venous stasis, (2) endothelial injury, and (3) hypercoagulability. Hypercoagulability, also called thrombophilia or a prothrombotic state, is defined as a propensity to develop thrombosis secondary to aberrations in the coagulation system. Thrombophilia is becoming increasingly recognized in pediatric patients and can refer to multiple potential conditions: (1) spontaneous thrombus formation, (2) recurrent thrombosis, (3) thrombosis out of proportion to the underlying risk factor, and (4) thrombosis at a young age.

Optimal prevention and treatment in pediatric patients with thrombosis differs from adult patients for several reasons. These include physiologic age-dependent differences in the hemostatic system that influence the risk for venous thromboembolism, differing underlying etiologies and location of clots, and differing responses to antithrombotic agents. Little evidence exists as how best to manage pediatric patients with thrombosis, both from a diagnostic and from a treatment standpoint. Much of the currently utilized data is based on adult studies, and here we summarize the generally accepted recommendations in lieu of evidence-based pediatric guidelines (see Figure 10.1).

Evaluation of thrombosis

Pediatric patients may have both congenital and acquired risk factors underlying thrombus formation. The single most common acquired risk factor for venous thromboembolism is the presence of a central venous catheter (e.g., endothelial injury). Other acquired risk factors include trauma, surgery, infection, nephrotic syndrome, inflammatory syndromes, diabetes, complex congenital heart disease, liver disease, and malignancy (e.g., acute lymphoblastic leukemia in association with the use of asparaginase or solid tumors with tumor thrombus). Asymptomatic patients may be found to have an incidental clot on imaging, or the patient may be symptomatic, most often with swelling, pain, or erythema in an extremity. Venous ultrasonography with Doppler flow remains the cornerstone of evaluation for thrombosis, as in adults. Lack of venous compression or Doppler flow is diagnostic for thrombus. This imaging modality is limited to the extremities, neck, distal subclavian veins, and potentially, distal iliac veins. Echocardiography can be utilized to evaluate for atrial clots and the proximal superior and inferior vena cava. Imaging of the abdomen and pelvis as well as the upper venous system requires CT or magnetic

Handbook of Pediatric Hematology and Oncology: Children's Hospital & Research Center Oakland, Second Edition. Caroline A. Hastings, Joseph C. Torkildson, and Anurag K. Agrawal.
© 2012 John Wiley & Sons, Ltd. Published 2012 by John Wiley & Sons, Ltd.

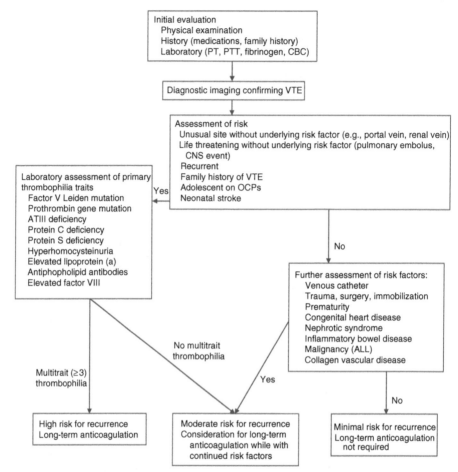

Figure 10.1 Evaluation of the child with venous thromboembolism (VTE). (Abbreviations: PT, prothrombin time; PTT, partial thromboplastin time; CBC, complete blood count; CNS, central nervous system; OCP, oral contraceptive pill; ATIII, antithrombin III; ALL, acute lymphoblastic leukemia).

resonance venography (MRV). Similarly, sinus venous thrombosis must be evaluated by magnetic resonance imaging/ arteriography (MRI/MRA). Pulmonary emboli or thrombosis can be identified with a helical CT scan.

Testing for thrombophilia

Although often undertaken, clear guidelines are lacking as to the utility of testing for an underlying hypercoagulable state. In the patient with a known acquired risk factor and secondary thrombosis, it is unclear that testing for thrombophilia will aid in the management of the patient (e.g., asymptomatic catheter-related thrombosis). Patients might have a single-trait thrombophilia on testing, but this alone may not contribute significantly to thrombus development. Patients with a consumptive process (e.g., disseminated intravascular coagulation and sepsis) and secondary thrombosis such as with deficiencies in protein C and S and antithrombin III could benefit from testing and factor replacement if found to be deficient. For patients with spontaneous thrombosis, often found in adolescents (e.g., adolescent female starting oral contraceptives) and in neonates (secondary to stroke or sinus venous thrombosis), testing should be considered. For patients with a symptomatic catheter-related thrombosis or for an asymptomatic patient with a positive family history, the decision to test for thrombophilia must be made on an individual basis after appropriate family counseling. The family must be advised that a positive screen for a single thrombophilia trait will not result in a change in management and may lead to unnecessary anxiety. Similarly, negative testing may give false reassurance and does not completely abrogate the potential for thrombosis. The primary thrombophilia traits are listed in Table 10.1.

Table 10.1 Primary thrombophilia traits.

Thrombophilia trait	Description
Factor V Leiden	G1691A polymorphism, present in ~5% of Caucasian population, leads to inherited activated protein C resistance
Prothrombin gene mutation	PT G20210A polymorphism, present in ~2% of Caucasian population, leads to elevated prothrombin levels
Antithrombin III deficiency	Can be seen in consumptive process (sepsis, DIC, active clot), liver disease, heparin therapy, complex congenital heart disease, asparaginase use in acute lymphoblastic leukemia
Protein C deficiency	Can be seen in consumptive process (sepsis, DIC, active clot), liver disease, warfarin therapy, nephrotic syndrome, complex congenital heart disease
Protein S deficiency	Can be seen in consumptive process (sepsis, DIC, active clot), liver disease, warfarin therapy, nephrotic syndrome, complex congenital heart disease
Hyperhomocysteinemia	Check fasting homocysteine, can be secondary to underlying MTHFR mutation
Elevated lipoprotein (a)	Poorly understood, competes with plasminogen, thus decreasing fibrinolysis, also activates PAI-1 decreasing fibrinolysis and potentially leading to increased thrombogenesis
Antiphospholipid antibodies	Antibodies against cell membrane phospholipid, called lupus anticoagulant, paradoxically leads to elevated PTT without correction on 1:1 mix. Secondary confirmatory testing includes anticardiolipin antibodies and $\beta2$ glycoprotein, must be confirmed on two separate occasions 12 weeks apart as can be seen transiently with infection
Elevated factor VIII	An acute phase reactant, can be constitutively elevated

Abbreviations: DIC, disseminated intravascular coagulation; MTHFR, methylenetetrahydrofolate reductase; PAI-1, plasminogen activator inhibitor-1; PT, prothrombin time; PTT, partial thromboplastin time.

Management of thrombosis

Management of pediatric thrombosis is again based on adult studies and expert guidelines. Removal of the precipitating agent should be done as possible in cases with an acquired risk factor. Treatment of thrombosis is undertaken to prevent clot propagation, pulmonary embolus, and the postthrombotic syndrome (PTS). Although reported frequently in adults, PTS is poorly understood in children but can potentially lead to chronic pain, swelling, skin changes, and collateral venous formation. The decision to initially utilize a thrombolytic (tissue plasminogen activator, TPA) versus an anticoagulant (unfractionated heparin, UH or low-molecular-weight heparin, LMWH) must be made in consultation with a pediatric hematologist. In some cases, thrombectomy or thrombolysis by intervention radiology should be considered.

Thrombolysis

In general, a thrombolytic should be considered in patients with an occlusive thrombus without significant risk factors for bleeding (recent surgery, central nervous system hemorrhage). Patients with a long-standing occlusive thrombus (i.e., >14 days) or without evidence of improvement on imaging studies after 24 to 48 hours of TPA therapy may benefit from thrombectomy or thrombolysis by interventional radiology. Although not evidence based, we typically treat with low-dose systemic TPA as suggested by Manco-Johnson (see suggested further reading) at a dose of 0.03 to 0.06 mg/kg/h with a maximum of 2 mg/h for 24 to 48 hours to decrease the risk of significant hemorrhage that is seen with bolus TPA, unless there is a life-threatening clot (e.g., massive pulmonary embolism). Arterial clots may benefit from a higher systemic dose for a shorter time period. Also if possible, TPA should be instilled distal to the clot in order to decrease first-pass liver metabolism, although this is mitigated with the use of systemic TPA as it is expected that much of the TPA will bypass the obstruction through collateral circulation. Patients receiving systemic low-dose TPA therapy should have close monitoring of coagulation studies (prothrombin time [PT], partial thromboplastin time [PTT], and fibrinogen), platelets, and plasminogen to ensure hemostatic and fibrinolytic potential and the need for potential repletion with fresh frozen plasma (FFP).

Anticoagulation

If TPA is thought to pose significant risk, or if the patient has a nonocclusive thrombus or transient risk factors, UH or LMWH may be started. UH is a natural anticoagulant and works by complexing to the physiologic inhibitor antithrombin III (ATIII), accelerating the inhibition of thrombin and other coagulant proteins. It is therefore important to ensure adequate levels of ATIII when administering heparin. Many potential issues are present with UH usage in children: (1) rapid clearance, (2) low ATIII levels in the first few months of life, (3) greater variability in dosing compared to adults, and (4) lack of evidence assessing the optimal target PTT range for the prevention and treatment of venous thromboembolism. The patient must also be monitored for the development of heparin antibodies that can most notably lead to heparin-induced thrombocytopenia (HIT). Long-term usage can also lead to osteoporosis. LMWH is more widely utilized now due to a more narrow dosing range and wide therapeutic window secondary to direct targeting of Factor Xa as well as reduced incidence of HIT and osteoporosis.

In general, we utilize LMWH unless there is potential need for immediate reversal of anticoagulation. Although protamine can be utilized with LMWH, the reversal effect is not complete (thought to be about two-thirds effective) and therefore a risk of bleeding can still be present if, for instance, surgical intervention is required emergently. In these cases, UH should be utilized due to its short half-life and ability to be fully reversed. UH is generally given at a loading dose of 75 U/kg followed by a maintenance dose of 20 U/kg/h with a goal PTT of 2 to 3× the upper limit of the reference range or, preferably, anti-Xa levels of 0.3 to 0.7 U/mL, if available in a timely manner. Currently, the only LMWH approved by the FDA for pediatric patients is enoxaparin, with a half-life of 4 hours and subcutaneous dosing. For treatment of thrombosis, enoxaparin must be given every 12 hours, usually starting at 1.0 to 1.25 mg/kg (see Formulary and Manco-Johnson for more specific dosing guidelines). Treatment effectiveness is followed by anti-Xa levels, with goal levels of 0.5 to 1.0 U/mL (checked 4 hours after the second or subsequent dose). For prophylaxis, 0.5 mg/kg is typically given twice daily. Anti-Xa levels do not need to be checked with prophylactic dosing. In practice, some hematologists utilize 1 mg/kg once daily for prophylaxis, although available data suggest this may undertreat a group of patients, especially those <5 years of age.

Concomitant use of TPA and UH or LMWH may also be beneficial in clot lysis without significantly increasing hemorrhagic risk, although again this recommendation is not evidence-based in pediatric patients and must be determined on a per patient basis in consultation with a pediatric hematologist, weighing the potential risks of hemorrhage and potential benefits of clot lysis. Therapeutic efficacy can simply be followed with repeat imaging, although this can be difficult with central venous clots that may require multiple CT or MRI with resultant increased radiation exposure and cost, respectively. Other potential markers to follow for clot lysis include d-dimers or fibrin-split products which should increase with lysis, although

marker elevation may be confounded by continuing inflammation.

Duration of therapy

Duration of therapy depends on multiple factors including the time to removal of inciting agents such as central venous catheters, presence of thrombophilia traits, and time to clot resolution. Patients initially treated with TPA or UH therapy should be transitioned to LMWH or warfarin therapy for long-term maintenance. Because of the time required to reach an appropriate therapeutic level, warfarin therapy should begin at least 48 hours prior to discontinuation of heparin therapy. Maintenance with LMWH is frequently used due to the difficulty in maintaining a therapeutic international normalized ratio (INR) with warfarin therapy.

For patients with clot resolution, anticoagulation should be continued at prophylactic dosing for 6 weeks to 3 months after removal of the inciting agent (e.g., central venous catheter) due to the likelihood of continued endothelial injury. For patients without clot resolution (potentially after ineffective interventional thrombectomy and/or thrombolysis), anticoagulation should be continued for 6 to 12 months to potentially decrease or resolve the clot and prevent the development of PTS. Patients that had a spontaneous or recurrent thrombus and were found to have multitrait thrombophilia (≥ 3 traits) or antiphospholipid syndrome should continue life-long anticoagulation.

New agents

Multiple new agents will be available in the near future for pediatric patients and are summarized in Table 10.2.

Case study for review

You are seeing a 17-year-old female in clinic who is deciding on whether to start oral

Table 10.2 Novel anticoagulants.

Name	Comments
Factor Xa inhibitors	
Fondaparinux	Selective factor Xa inhibitor, mediates its effects through ATIII, decreased HIT, half-life 17 hours, once daily SC dosing
Idraparinux	Hypermethylated analogue of fondaparinux, 80-hour half-life (once weekly SC dosing)
Rivaroxaban	Oral factor Xa inhibitor, once daily dosing in adults for thromboprophylaxis, has shown noninferiority to warfarin
Direct thrombin inhibitors	
Argatroban	Approved in adult patients with HIT, narrow therapeutic window and short-acting IV formulation
Dabigatran	Oral formulation, approved in adult patients, has shown noninferiority to warfarin, currently approved in the United States for stroke prevention in patients with atrial fibrillation, in the United Kingdom as an alternative to warfarin for thromboprophylaxis

Abbreviations: ATIII, antithrombin III; HIT, heparin-induced thrombocytopenia; SC, subcutaneous; IV, intravenous.

contraceptive pills (OCPs). She has an aunt that had a "blood clot" when she was in her fifties. Your patient does not know any further details about the incident but does know about the potential increased risk of blood clots with oral contraceptive pills.

1. What advice would you give the patient?
2. She asks about testing for clotting risk factors, what do you advise her?

All patients who are starting OCPs should be made aware of the increased risk of blood clots with estrogen-containing contraceptives (about a three times increased risk). This risk is thought to be about 2 to 3 per 10,000 per year on OCPs, or about 0.02% to 0.03% incidence per year (baseline risk being approximately 0.008% per year). Single-trait thrombophilias, most commonly Factor V Leiden mutation, increase this risk significantly. Specifically for Factor V Leiden, the risk for a heterozygous carrier increases the risk approximately 30 times to a yearly incidence of 0.6% to 0.9%. This

incidence is also highest in the first year of OCP usage.

Thrombophilia testing can be considered on an individual basis for the patient wishing to start OCPs who has a family member with a known thrombophilia. Additionally, the patient should be offered alternative lower risk forms of contraception. In this case, the practitioner should try to get more information regarding the episode of thromboembolism in the aunt. Were there acquired risk factors such as trauma, surgery, or immobility? Was the clot thought to be spontaneous? If so, was the aunt tested for thrombophilia?

Current recommendations would not advise testing your patient without further information. If the aunt had a spontaneous thrombus, one could advise that she should be tested for thrombophilia, and if found to be positive your patient could be tested as well. If it was determined that there was an underlying risk factor in the aunt's thromboembolism, testing her and/ or your patient would not be advised. In the situation where thrombophilia testing of your patient is not advisable (the most likely scenario in general), you should counsel your patient closely on the risks and benefits of OCPs and the potential lower risk alternative therapies such as progesterone-only preparations (e.g., Depo-Provera).

Suggested Reading

Bounameaux H, Perrier A. Duration of anticoagulation therapy for venous thromboembolism. Am Soc Hematol Educ Prog 252–258, 2008.

Goldenberg NA. Thrombophilia states and markers of coagulation activation in the prediction of pediatric venous thromboembolic outcomes: a comparative analysis with respect to adult evidence. Am Soc Hematol Educ Prog 236–244, 2008.

Manco-Johnson MJ. How I treat venous thromboembolism in children. Blood 107:21–29, 2006.

Raffini L. Thrombophilia in children: who to test, how, when, and why? Am Soc Hematol Educ Prog 228–235, 2008.

Rosendaal FR. Venous thrombosis: the role of genes, environment, and behavior. Am Soc Hematol Educ Prog 1–12, 2005.

11　The Neutropenic Child

Neutrophils are a key component in the defense against infection. They contain toxic cytoplasmic granules that, following ingestion of infecting bacteria and fungi, are released into the phagocytic vacuole and destroy them. Once released from the bone marrow, they circulate in the blood for a brief time (4 to 6 hours) before leaving the circulation and entering the tissue where, in response to the presence of infection, they act to control the infection while sending chemotactic signals to recruit additional neutrophils to the area and stimulate the accelerated production of neutrophils in the bone marrow. While the presence of adequate neutrophil numbers in the tissue is the best predictor of the patient's ability to fight infection, there is no easy clinical method to determine the number of tissue neutrophils, so the number present in the blood is used as a surrogate marker.

Neutropenia has traditionally been defined as a decrease in the absolute neutrophil count (ANC) to $<1.5 \times 10^9$/L. The ANC is calculated by multiplying the white blood cell count by the total percentage of segmented (mature) neutrophils plus bands. Mild neutropenia is defined as an ANC of 1.0 to 1.5×10^9/L, moderate neutropenia is an ANC of 0.5 to 1.0×10^9/L, and severe neutropenia is an ANC below 0.5×10^9/L. This division is useful for determining the individual's risk for infection and the urgency of medical intervention. However, this definition fails to take into account important variations in normal neutrophil number related to age and ethnicity. Up to 25% of young African-American children will have an ANC between 1.0 and 1.5×10^9/L, and this level should be considered normal in this group. Also, the normal range for ANC extends down to 1.0×10^9/L in infants between 2 weeks and 6 months of age, and should not be considered abnormal if less than this.

Risk assessment

The first question when evaluating a child with neutropenia is: "What is the risk that this patient has or will develop a life-threatening infection?" This is particularly pertinent if the patient presents with fever. The susceptibility to bacterial infection in neutropenic patients is quite variable and depends on a number of factors. The first is the severity of neutropenia, as described above. Patients with mild neutropenia have minimal to no increased risk of infection, those with moderate neutropenia have a mildly increased risk of frequent or severe infections, and those with severe neutropenia are highly susceptible to bacterial infection.

Handbook of Pediatric Hematology and Oncology: Children's Hospital & Research Center Oakland, Second Edition. Caroline A. Hastings, Joseph C. Torkildson, and Anurag K. Agrawal.
© 2012 John Wiley & Sons, Ltd. Published 2012 by John Wiley & Sons, Ltd.

However, patients who are neutropenic as a result of cytotoxic therapy (e.g., chemotherapy and radiation) may be at an increased risk of infection because of the rate of decline of the neutrophil count or other immunosuppressive effects of chemotherapy, even before the ANC falls below 0.5×10^9/L. Another factor is the cause of the neutropenia, if known. Patients with neutropenia caused by intrinsic bone marrow failure or hypoplasia have a greater risk of infection than those whose neutropenia is due to factors extrinsic to the bone marrow such as excessive neutrophil destruction or sequestration (immune neutropenia and splenomegaly, respectively). While patients with extrinsic neutropenia may have a low circulating neutrophil count, their tissue counts are near normal and they are more protected from infection. A third factor is the presence or absence of other phagocytic cells.

Many patients with chronic neutropenia have an elevated circulating monocyte count, which provides some additional protection against pyogenic organisms. Conversely, patients being treated with steroids or other immunosuppressive therapy will have treatment-related abnormalities in cell-mediated, humoral, and macrophage–monocyte immunity and may be at increased risk of invasive infection even with a normal neutrophil count. Patients with a history of splenectomy have an increased risk of overwhelming infection caused by encapsulated bacteria regardless of their neutrophil count.

The age at presentation with neutropenia is an important factor in risk assessment. The younger the child is at the time of diagnosis, the greater the concern that the patient could have a severe form of chronic neutropenia, whereas children who are found to be neutropenic later in life and who do not have a history of frequent bacterial infections or chronic illness are more likely to have a more benign form of neutropenia.

Etiology of neutropenia

A large variety of conditions can lead to neutropenia in childhood. They can be classified as being either acquired causes or inherited causes. Of these, acquired causes are much more frequent. These are presented in Table 11.1.

Viral infection is the most common cause of mild-to-moderate neutropenia. Transient marrow suppression is seen in children with Epstein-Barr virus (EBV), respiratory syncytial virus, influenza A and B, hepatitis, human herpesvirus-6 (HHV6), varicella, rubella, and rubeola. This typically lasts for 3 to 8 days. Neutropenia can also be seen in the setting of overwhelming **bacterial infection** as well as with typhoid fever, Rocky Mountain spotted fever, and tuberculosis. Phagocytosis of microbes leads to release of toxic metabolites, which then activate the complement system, inducing neutrophil aggregation and adherence of leukocytes to the pulmonary capillary bed. Tumor necrosis factor and interleukin-1, released by macrophages, likely accelerate this process. Activated granulocytes sequestered in the lungs may cause acute cardiopulmonary complications. **Neonates** have a limited granulocyte pool in their bone marrow, which can be exhausted rapidly during overwhelming bacterial sepsis.

Replacement of the bone marrow (as occurs with hematologic malignancies, glycogen storage diseases, granulomas associated with infection, and fibrosis related to chemical or radiation injury or osteoporosis) results in neutropenia. Frequently, the erythroid and megakaryocytic lines are also affected.

Medications are a common cause of neutropenia. Neutropenia is a common and expected side effect of anticancer therapy. Many chemotherapeutic agents have a direct toxic effect on the early marrow stem cells. The severity and duration of the neutropenia depend on the particular medication and

Table 11.1 Acquired causes of neutropenia.

Condition	Pathogenesis	Occurrence	Associated findings
Infection	Viral marrow suppression, viral-induced immune neutropenia	Common	EBV, parvovirus, HHV6, other viruses
	Bacterial sepsis-endotoxin suppression	Less common	Severe infection
Bone marrow replacement	Infiltration of marrow with malignant cells, fibrosis, granulomas	Uncommon	Vary depending on underlying cause
Drug-induced	Direct marrow suppression	Common	Underlying condition
	Immune destruction	Less common	
Autoimmune	Primary (molecular mimicry)	Common	Monocytosis common
	Secondary (SLE, Evans syndrome)		
Newborn immune	Alloimmune-maternal sensitization	Rare	Antigen difference in newborn and mother
	Due to maternal autoimmune neutropenia		Maternal neutropenia
Chronic idiopathic	Ineffective or decreased production	Common	Consider also familial benign neutropenia Often asymptomatic
Sequestration	Hypersplenism	Common if spleen is enlarged	Mild neutropenia Enlarged spleen— many causes
Nutritional	Vitamin B_{12} or folate deficiency	Rare in children	Hypersegmented neutrophils
	Copper deficiency		Zinc excess
	Impaired DNA processing		

Abbreviations: EBV, Epstein-Barr virus; HHV6, human herpesvirus-6; SLE, systemic lupus erythematosus.

dosage as well as the patient's underlying disease, state of nutrition, and general health. Many other medications can induce neutropenia, including antibiotics (chloramphenicol, cephalosporins, penicillins, and sulfonamides), anticonvulsants (phenytoin and valproic acid), anti-inflammatory agents, cardiovascular agents, tranquilizers, and hypoglycemic agents. The severity and duration of drug-induced neutropenia are variable. The underlying mechanism is not known, although studies with certain drugs have led to various hypotheses including immune-mediated destruction, toxic effect of the drug or metabolites on the marrow stem cells, and toxic effects on the marrow microenvironment. After withdrawal of the drug, the marrow can repopulate with early myeloid forms within 3 to 4 days and appear morphologically normal by 1 to 2 weeks. The duration of neutropenia is likely related to the underlying mechanism; some chronic idiosyncratic drug reactions can last from months to years.

Autoimmune neutropenia is another common cause of neutropenia following a viral infection, and may be difficult to distinguish from virus-associated marrow suppression due to the difficulty in identifying antineutrophil antibodies. Unlike viral suppression, autoimmune neutropenia can persist for 7 to 24 months, and affected children occasionally suffer from infections of the ear, lung, skin, or other sites.

Neonatal alloimmune neutropenia is analogous to Rh-related hemolytic disease of the newborn; mothers generate IgG antibodies against paternal neutrophil antigens expressed on fetal neutrophils. These antibodies cross the placenta and cause neutropenia in the fetus and newborn.

"Chronic idiopathic" neutropenia, also known as chronic benign neutropenia of childhood, is likely caused by a variety of disorders without a unifying etiology. It is likely that many of these children in fact have autoimmune neutropenia or familial benign neutropenia. They often have mild-to-moderate neutropenia; the susceptibility to infection is roughly proportionate to the degree of neutropenia. The blood neutrophil count remains stable over years, and becomes elevated in response to an infection in a subset of children. Spontaneous remissions at 2 to 4 years of age have been reported. Affected individuals have normal life expectancies. Evaluation of the bone marrow shows decreased myelopoiesis (often with monocytosis), and there is considerable variability in the stage at which maturation is arrested. These patients are at low risk for the development of serious infections, and no treatment is required except during infectious episodes.

Splenomegaly from any cause including chronic hemolytic anemia, portal hypertension, liver disease, and storage disorders can cause mild neutropenia, as well as anemia and thrombocytopenia. If severe, splenectomy may be necessary.

Deficiencies of folate and B$_{12}$ are rare in children; the presence of hypersegmented neutrophils caused by impaired neutrophil nuclear maturation is a clue to this condition. Similarly, copper deficiency is a rare cause of neutropenia often secondary to an underlying malabsorptive process or due to zinc excess. These patients usually present with concomitant anemia and thrombocytopenia.

A number of **inherited conditions** have neutropenia as one of their characteristic features. The more common of these conditions are presented in Table 11.2.

Children with **severe congenital neutropenia (SCN)** often present in early infancy with umbilical infection, skin infections, oral ulcers, pneumonia, or perineal infections. There are two forms: an autosomal recessive form (Kostmann syndrome) involving mutations in the *HAX1* gene that is involved in signal transduction and an autosomal dominant form involving mutations in the neutrophil elastase gene (*ELA2*) or, more rarely, in the *GFI1* gene that targets *ELA2*. Bone marrow aspiration reveals a maturational arrest at the promyelocyte stage. In addition to the risk of death due to overwhelming infection, patients with either of these conditions have an increased risk of developing myelodysplastic syndrome (MDS) or acute myelogenous leukemia (AML).

Cyclic neutropenia is characterized by approximately 21-day cycles of changing neutrophil counts, with frank neutropenia developing at regular intervals and lasting 3 to 6 days. Fever and oral ulcerations usually are seen during the nadir, as well as gingivitis, pharyngitis, and skin infections. Diagnosis is often delayed because the neutrophil count may have improved by the time the patient seeks medical attention. These patients also demonstrate mutations in the *ELA2* gene, but at different locations than in those with SCN. They do not have the same risk of developing MDS or AML. Diagnosis is made by obtaining serial complete blood counts (CBCs) 2 to 3 times/week over 4 to 6 weeks to demonstrate the periodicity of

Table 11.2 Inherited causes of neutropenia.

Condition	Inheritance	Pathogenesis	Occurrence	Associated findings
Severe congenital (Kostmann)	AR	HAX1 mutations causing disturbed regulation of myeloid homeostasis with marrow arrest at the promyelocyte stage	Rare ($1/1–2 \times 10^5$)	ANC $< 0.5 \times 10^9$/L Leukemia risk 15–20%
Severe congenital	AD and sporadic	ELA2 mutations on the face of the molecule opposite the active site causing accelerated apoptosis	Rare ($1/1–2 \times 10^5$)	ANC $< 0.5 \times 10^9$/L Leukemia risk 5–10% ↓T and B cells Marrow: immature myeloid cells
		GFI1 mutations target ELA2	Two families	
Cyclic	AD	ELA2 mutations clustering near the active site of the molecule	$0.5–1/10^6$	21-day cycle with fever and mouth ulcers
Shwachman–Diamond syndrome	AR	SDS gene conversion from the pseudogene, resulting in the failure of neutrophil production	1/50,000	Pancreatic exocrine insufficiency, short stature, metaphyseal dysplasia, marrow failure
		Defect in RNA processing Decreased CD34 cells		Leukemia risk (15%)
Familial benign	AD	Decreased marrow release	Common	Africans and Yemenite Jews Periodontal disease
Marrow failure syndromes: Fanconi anemia	AR	Gene (FANC) defects in DNA repair	$1/10^6$	Dysplastic thumbs, pancytopenia, other anomalies 10% risk of MDS, AML

Dyskeratosis congenita	Usually XR (also AR and AD)	DKC1 mutations (TERC or TERT in AD) Telomerase defect, ribosomal dysfunction		Abnormal skin pigmentation, leukoplakia, dystrophic nails
Diamond–Blackfan anemia	Sporadic 75% AR and AD	RPS19 mutations that affect a ribosomal protein in 25% of families Many patients respond to glucocorticoids		Erythroid failure syndrome Neutropenia in 25–40% Thumb and craniofacial anomalies Increased RBC adenosine deaminase Leukemia risk of 2–3%
Glycogen storage disease 1b	AR	G6PT1 mutations (glucose-6 phosphate translocase)	$1/10^5$	Hypoglycemia, dyslipidemia, hyperuricemia, lactic acidemia, and neutropenia in most patients
Selective IgA deficiency	Unknown or multifactorial	Antineutrophil antibodies?	Common (1/600)	Infections of the upper and lower respiratory tracts in one-third of patients
Wiskott–Aldrich syndrome	XR	Unique "gain of function" missense mutations in the GTPase-binding domain of WASp	$1–10/10^6$	Impaired lymphoid development and maturation of monocytes Associated with eczema, thrombocytopenia, and immune deficiency

Abbreviations: AR, autosomal recessive; AD, autosomal dominant; XR, X-linked recessive; ANC, absolute neutrophil count; AML, acute myelogenous leukemia; MDS, myelodysplastic syndrome.

the cycle. Granulocyte colony-stimulating factor (G-CSF) has been used in patients who develop recurrent infections during their nadir.

Shwachman–Diamond syndrome includes exocrine pancreatic insufficiency, short stature, metaphyseal dysplasia, and bone marrow failure with typically mild-to-moderate neutropenia. Affected patients also have an increased risk of MDS and AML. Intestinal malabsorption with failure to thrive commonly occurs, especially in infancy and early childhood.

Benign familial neutropenia is characterized by moderate neutropenia with minimal risk of invasive bacterial infections. It has been postulated that the underlying cause is a defect in neutrophil mobilization from the bone marrow, but the etiology is as yet unknown. It occurs more commonly in individuals of African, Arabic, and Yemenite Jewish descent. Periodontal disease is the most frequent complication.

Fanconi anemia is characterized by a defect in DNA repair leading to extensive chromosomal breakage. Affected patients have mutations within the *FANC* family of genes, including *FANC A, C,* and *G*. It presents most commonly during the early school age years; patients with the characteristic physical findings may be diagnosed sooner. Thrombocytopenia is often the presenting hematologic abnormality, with anemia and neutropenia developing later. Up to 10% of patients ultimately develop MDS or AML. Bone marrow transplantation is curative, but challenging to complete successfully given the underlying chromosomal fragility.

Dyskeratosis congenita (DKC) is characterized clinically by the triad of abnormal nails, reticular skin pigmentation, and oral leukoplakia. Bone marrow failure occurs during early adulthood and is associated with a high risk of developing aplastic anemia, MDS, leukemia, and solid tumors. Patients have very short germ line telomeres, and approximately half have mutations in one of six genes encoding proteins that maintain telomere function. Affected patients rarely present with hematologic abnormalities during childhood.

Diamond–Blackfan anemia is a congenital anemia that presents in infancy. There is typically a failure of erythropoiesis with preservation of myeloid and platelet production. Only 20% to 25% of cases are inherited; the rest are sporadic. Approximately 50% of affected persons have developmental abnormalities including growth retardation and craniofacial, upper limb/hand, cardiac, and genitourinary malformations. Neutropenia is seen in 25% to 40% of affected children. Patients also have an increased risk of MDS, AML, and osteogenic sarcoma. Genetic studies have identified heterozygous mutations in at least one of eight ribosomal protein genes in up to 50% of cases. Mutations in ribosomal protein L5 (RPL5) are associated with multiple physical abnormalities including cleft lip/palate, thumb, and heart anomalies. The diagnosis is often difficult due to incomplete phenotypes and a wide variability of clinical expression. Up to 80% of patients respond to a course of steroids with improvement in their cytopenias.

The etiology of neutropenia in **glycogen storage disease 1b** is not definitively known, but appears to be related to increased neutrophil apoptosis caused by an excess of reactive oxygen species due to a defect in neutrophil energy metabolism.

Almost one-third of patients with **selective IgA deficiency** have evidence of autoimmune disease; neutropenia in this condition is felt most likely related to the presence of antineutrophil antibodies.

Patients with a mild form of **Wiskott–Aldrich syndrome (WAS)** known as **X-linked neutropenia** have a unique "gain of function" mutation in the GTPase-binding domain of the WAS protein (WASp) that leads to increased actin polymerization in neutrophils, causing defective mitosis and cell movement and ultimately severe neutropenia.

Initial evaluation of the child with neutropenia

Evaluation of the child with neutropenia begins with a thorough history and physical examination. It is critical to know whether the child has had recent or recurrent bacterial infections, and whether there is a family history of neutropenia or recurrent bacterial infections. On examination, attention should be paid to any phenotypic abnormalities, adenopathy, splenomegaly, evidence of a chronic or underlying disease, and meticulous evaluation of the skin and mucous membranes (particularly in the oral and perirectal areas). A CBC must be done to determine if the patient has isolated neutropenia or neutropenia associated with anemia and/or thrombocytopenia. The approach to a child with bi- or trilineage abnormalities is different than that in a child with isolated neutropenia; multiple abnormal lineages increase the likelihood of a more generalized marrow failure state such as aplastic anemia or a marrow infiltrative process such as leukemia. It is valuable to repeat the CBC at least once, especially if the child appears well, to avoid proceeding with a major evaluation due to a laboratory error.

Well-appearing children with mild-to-moderate neutropenia can typically be observed over the next 2 to 3 weeks with serial CBCs. Children with persistent or worsening neutropenia require further evaluation. Patients with recurrent neutropenia should have blood counts checked 2 to 3 times per week for 6 weeks to evaluate for cyclic neutropenia. Additional studies include antineutrophil antibodies, assessment of cellular and serum immune status, and careful review of the peripheral smear for morphologic abnormalities of the white cells. If severe congenital neutropenia or Kostmann syndrome is suspected, assessment for *ELA2* and *HAX1* mutations should be made. A bone marrow aspirate and biopsy may be necessary to identify granulocyte precursors and to search for defects in myeloid maturation. In addition, the bone marrow aspirate and biopsy can be used to exclude hematologic malignancies, marrow infiltration, or fibrosis.

Management of the child with neutropenia and fever

Children identified with neutropenia but who are free of fever or other signs of infection should be evaluated as outlined above, but require no other therapy at that time. Managing the child with neutropenia and fever is more complex and depends on many factors including the nature of the neutropenia (acute or chronic), its severity, and the association with immune defects, underlying illnesses, or malignancies. Patients with acquired neutropenia arising from malignancy or chemotherapeutic drugs have a diminished inflammatory capability and have a greater susceptibility to sepsis. Fever may be the earliest and only warning sign. Sepsis related to chemotherapy-induced neutropenia remains a leading cause of mortality in these patients. Aggressive management of the febrile, neutropenic cancer patient in the hospital has markedly reduced morbidity and mortality due to infection. For management of oncology patients with fever and neutropenia, see Chapter 27.

The management of the febrile child who is discovered to be neutropenic depends on several factors. Patients with fever and mild or moderate neutropenia and signs and symptoms suggestive of a viral illness that otherwise look well may be managed supportively without antibiotics, although in most cases they will receive a long-acting cephalosporin such as ceftriaxone prior to discharge from the clinic or emergency department. Their parents should be instructed to bring them back in 24 hours for further evaluation, or sooner if they develop additional symptoms or begin to appear unwell. If they become afebrile, their neutropenia should be evaluated as outlined above. Patients with fever and mild or moderate neutropenia who have evidence of localized bacterial disease (otitis media, sinusitis, or local skin infections) may be treated with appropriate oral antibiotics in the outpatient setting. Patients with mild neutropenia and evidence of bacterial pneumonia, GU tract infections, lymphadenitis, or systemic symptoms should have cultures of the infection site and of the blood. They may be treated with appropriate oral antibiotics if their appearance is not concerning, but should be seen back for reevaluation within 24 hours. Similar patients with moderate neutropenia can also be treated in the outpatient setting if they appear totally well.

Febrile patients with moderate or severe neutropenia who appear in any way unwell require emergent medical assessment and initiation of therapy, as do children who are known to have severe forms of neutropenia such as severe congenital neutropenia or Kostmann syndrome. These children require:

- Hospital admission.
- Coverage with broad-spectrum antibiotics due to their increased risk of mortality due to sepsis. These should provide coverage for Gram-negative and Gram-positive organisms. A combination of an aminoglycoside and a β-lactam antibiotic provides initial broad coverage and is synergistic for *Pseudomonas* species, but several different antibiotic choices are appropriate and depend on local practice.
- Careful physical evaluation, paying meticulous attention to potential sites of occult infection (e.g., the oral cavity and perineum).
- Laboratory studies: CBC with differential, blood cultures, urinalysis and urine culture, and cultures from sites of suspected infection such as the skin, throat, and stool.
- Chest radiograph if any pulmonary symptoms are present.
- Daily blood cultures and a CBC with differential every 24 hours in the persistently febrile patient to help determine further management.
- CT scan of the chest $(+/-)$ sinuses, abdomen, and pelvis) looking for evidence of occult infection in any patient remaining febrile for >96 hours without a specific cause being identified. They should be started on empiric antifungal coverage due to the increased risk of invasive fungal infection in this patient population.

Prophylactic antibiotics have been used in the past in an attempt to decrease the frequency of serious infections in patients with severe neutropenia. However, this has generally fallen out of favor. Exceptions include the use of prophylactic penicillin or amoxicillin in patients following splenectomy and the use of trimethoprim-sulfamethoxazole prophylaxis to prevent *Pneumocystis jiroveci* (previously known as *Pneumocystis carinii*) pneumonia in patients with T-cell dysfunction in addition to neutropenia.

The use of cytokines, particularly G-CSF, has become increasingly popular in the management of symptomatic neutropenia. It is particularly useful in patients with symptomatic cyclic neutropenia or in the neutropenia-accompanying disorders such as glycogen storage disease 1b, as these patients typically respond well to low dose therapy (1 to 2 mcg/kg/dose) on a daily or alternate day schedule with a goal of maintaining an ANC between 1.0 and 1.5 $\times$ 10^9/L. It is also used frequently in patients with severe chronic neutropenia. However, the doses required to raise the ANC into the desired range vary significantly between patients. A typical starting dose is 3 to 5 mcg/kg/day, and the dose is increased slowly until the desired ANC is achieved. Patients with severe neutropenia who fail to respond to doses as high as 50 to 100 mcg/kg/day are considered poor responders. These patients are candidates for bone marrow transplantation given their high likelihood of mortality due to infection as well as an up to 30% chance of developing myeloid malignancy.

Case study for review

A 7-week-old girl presents to your clinic for evaluation of a fever to 38.6 °C. She had been seen 4 weeks earlier for a well child visit and was noted to have a small ulcer on her vulva. This was treated with oral antibiotics and resolved. Her parents report that the vulvar lesion had recurred 24 hours before she developed the fever. She had no blood work performed at the previous visit. Her physical examination reveals her to be alert and nontoxic appearing. A 6-mm shallow ulceration is present on her vulva with minimal surrounding erythema, drainage, or induration. It is mildly tender, however. Her physical examination is otherwise normal.

1. What additional information would you like?

The patient was born at term via spontaneous vaginal delivery after an uncomplicated pregnancy. Her weight, height, and head circumference were appropriate for gestational age. Her nursery course was unremarkable, and she was discharged from the nursery at 24 hours of life. She is an only child. There is no family history of recurrent fevers, or severe or unusual infections. Her parents are unaware of any "blood problems" in other family members.

2. What additional studies would you like to obtain?

Given her age and degree of fever, a sepsis workup is indicated. A CBC reveals a WBC count of 12.4 $\times$ 10^9/L, a hemoglobin of 11.7 g/dL, and a platelet count of 423 $\times$ 10^9/L. The differential reveals 0% neutrophils, 73% lymphocytes, and 27% monocytes. A urinalysis is normal. Because of her severe neutropenia she is admitted to the hospital and started on broad-spectrum antibiotics. A blood culture is performed and is negative. The vulvar lesion is cultured and grows *Pseudomonas aeruginosa*. The lesion resolves with intravenous antibiotics. A bone marrow aspiration is performed and reveals an adequately cellular specimen with normal megakaryocytes and erythroid precursors. The myeloid lineage shows a maturational arrest at the myelocyte stage, however.

3. What are you thinking now? What would you do next?

The isolated neutropenia in the face of a normal hemoglobin and platelet count makes congenital aplastic anemia unlikely. The young age at presentation, the significant degree of neutropenia, and the unusual organism identified raise concern that this child may have a severe form of congenital neutropenia. Once her active infection has resolved and she is afebrile she can be discharged from the hospital, but should have regular follow-up to determine what her neutrophil count does over time. More importantly, her parents need to understand the importance of bringing her immediately to you or to the emergency room if she develops another fever.

Twice weekly CBCs are performed over the next 6 weeks and reveal a consistent pattern of severe neutropenia, with ANCs ranging from 0 to 170. Serum immunoglobulins are measured and are normal, as are T-cell subset studies. Over that time period, she has several episodes of oral mucosal ulcers.

4. What would be your next step?

The persistent, noncyclic nature of her neutropenia provides further evidence that this infant is suffering from a form of severe congenital neutropenia. Given the lack of a family history, the autosomal recessive form (Kostmann syndrome) would be more likely, although she may have a new *ELA2* mutation. Genetic testing for *HAX1* and *ELA2* mutations can be sent for confirmation. A trial of G-CSF can also be initiated to see if it will result in an increase in the ANC.

Suggested Reading

Berliner N, Horwitz M, Loughran TP. Congenital and acquired neutropenia. Hematol Am Soc Hematol Educ Prog 63–79, 2004.

James RM, Kinsey SE. The investigation and management of chronic neutropenia in children. Arch Dis Child 91:852–858, 2006.

Klein C. Congenital neutropenia. Hematol Am Soc Hematol Educ Prog 344–350, 2009.

12 Thrombocytopenia

Thrombocytopenia, or low platelets, can occur as an isolated finding or in conjunction with a multitude of underlying clinical conditions. Normal platelet counts range from 150 to 400 × 10⁹/L and thrombocytopenia is generally defined as a platelet count of less than 100 × 10⁹/L. Thrombocytopenia may further be defined as mild (50 to 100 × 10⁹/L), moderate (20 to 50 × 10⁹/L), and severe (<20 × 10⁹/L). Other sources define thrombocytopenia as a platelet count of <150 × 10⁹/L or in patients with a drop of >50% from their baseline platelet counts (if known). Thrombocytopenia is typically subdivided into immune and nonimmune causes. Immune causes generally cause increased platelet destruction. Nonimmune causes may cause increased destruction or decreased bone marrow production. In patients with splenomegaly, platelet sequestration may also lead to thrombocytopenia.

Acute immune thrombocytopenic purpura

Immune thrombocytopenic purpura (ITP; also referred to as immune thrombocytopenia or idiopathic thrombocytopenic purpura) is an acquired, isolated disorder in which the patient typically presents with a low platelet count and symptoms of mucocutaneous bleeding. Most cases are considered idiopathic whereas others are secondary to coexisting conditions. The diagnosis of ITP is one of exclusion (see Table 12.1, Figures 12.1, 12.2, and 12.3).

The most common cause of destructive thrombocytopenia is autoimmunity. Shortened platelet survival is due to platelet autoantibody production (usually IgG), often stimulated by infection or drug exposure. IgM antibodies and complement activation are less frequently found but can also be seen in childhood ITP. It is an acute, self-limited disease of isolated thrombocytopenia that usually occurs in children aged 2 to 5 years (though may occur at any age from infancy to adolescence), typically resolving in more than 80% of children within 6 weeks to 6 months. When ITP occurs in the child over 10 years of age, especially females, the course may be chronic and associated with an autoimmune disorder. The otherwise healthy child presents with sudden onset of severe thrombocytopenia (usually < 20 × 10⁹/L), manifested by petechiae and purpura and less frequently mucosal bleeding such as epistaxis, menorrhagia, hematuria, and hematochezia. There is a history of an antecedent viral illness within the past 1 to 3 weeks in up to 60% to 70% of children. It may also follow vaccination with

Handbook of Pediatric Hematology and Oncology: Children's Hospital & Research Center Oakland, Second Edition. Caroline A. Hastings, Joseph C. Torkildson, and Anurag K. Agrawal.
© 2012 John Wiley & Sons, Ltd. Published 2012 by John Wiley & Sons, Ltd.

Table 12.1 Differential diagnosis of thrombocytopenia.

Destructive thrombocytopenias	
Immunologic	ITP
	Drug-induced (valproic acid, amphotericin B, digoxin)
	Infection-induced (HIV, CMV, EBV, parvovirus B19)
	Postvaccination (MMR, Varivax)
	Posttransfusion purpura
	Autoimmune disease (SLE, JIA)
	Evans syndrome (AIHA/ITP)
	Posttransplant
	Hyperthyroidism
	Lymphoproliferative disorders (ALPS)
Nonimmunologic	Microangiopathic disease
	Cyclic thrombocytopenia
	Hemolytic uremic syndrome
	Thrombotic thrombocytopenic purpura
Platelet consumption/ destruction	Sepsis/DIC
	Giant hemangioma (Kasabach–Merritt syndrome)
	Cardiac (prosthetic heart valves, repair of intracardiac defects)
	Malignant hypertension
Neonatal problems	Neonatal alloimmune (NAIT)
	Neonatal autoimmune (maternal ITP)
	Pulmonary hypertension
	Polycythemia
	RDS
	Infection (viral, bacterial, protozoal, spirochetal)
	Sepsis/DIC
	Prematurity
	Meconium aspiration
	Erythroblastosis fetalis (Rh incompatibility)
	Maternal hypothyroidism
Impaired production	
Congenital and hereditary disorders	TAR syndrome
	Fanconi anemia
	Bernard–Soulier syndrome
	Wiskott–Aldrich syndrome
	Glanzmann thrombasthenia
	MYH9 disorders (May-Hegglin anomaly)
	CAMT
	Rubella syndrome
	Von Willebrand disease, type II
	ATRUS
	Dyskeratosis congenita
	Agenesis of the corpus callosum
Associated with chromosomal defect	Trisomy 13 or 18

Table 12.1 (*Continued*)

Metabolic disorders	Marrow infiltration
	Malignancies (leukemia, neuroblastoma, metastatic solid tumors)
	Storage disease
	Myelofibrosis
Acquired processes	Aplastic anemia
	Liver disease/failure
	Drug-induced
	Radiation-induced
	Severe iron deficiency
Sequestration	Hypersplenism (portal hypertension, neoplastic, infectious, glycogen storage disease, cyanotic heart disease)
	Hypothermia

Abbreviations: ITP, immune thrombocytopenic purpura; SLE, systemic lupus erythematosis; JIA, juvenile idiopathic arthritis; AIHA, autoimmune hemolytic anemia; ALPS, autoimmune lymphoproliferative syndrome; DIC, disseminated intravascular coagulation; NAIT, neonatal alloimmune thrombocytopenia; CAMT, congenital amegakaryocytic thrombocytopenia; TAR, thrombocytopenia absent radii; ATRUS, amegakaryocytic thrombocytopenia radio-ulnar synostosis; RDS, respiratory distress syndrome.

MMR or Varivax (live virus vaccines). Severe bleeding such as protracted epistaxis, hemoptysis, or gastrointestinal bleeding leading to severe anemia and need for transfusion is rare. Intracranial hemorrhage (ICH) is the most feared complication with an estimated incidence of 0.1% to 0.5%; more than 50% of patients with ICH present with this finding at diagnosis or within 1 week of diagnosis. More than 75% of patients with ITP and ICH survive. It has yet to be defined what risk factors predispose children with ITP to sustain this rare but extremely serious complication.

Evaluation

The initial evaluation of the child with suspected ITP begins with a complete history and physical examination. Other than a possible antecedent illness and the acute onset of minor bleeding and bruising, the child should be otherwise clinically well appearing. More significant bleeding may be associated with trauma. Bleeding into joints (hemarthroses) should lead one to consider an alternative bleeding disorder (e.g., congenital or acquired factor deficiency such as hemophilia). There should be no history of unexplained fevers, bone pain, or weight loss which would be concerning for an underlying malignancy or chronic infection. A medication history is critical as many drugs have been implicated in inducing drug-mediated immune thrombocytopenia. Implicated drugs include heparin, aspirin, aspirin-containing cold medications, nonsteroidal anti-inflammatory drugs (NSAIDs), and seizure medications such as valproic acid. Chronic infections with HIV, CMV, and hepatitis C may cause a low platelet count and appropriate screening should be done. *Helicobacter pylori* has been implicated in adults with ITP and there are some reports of this association in children as well. Family history should include an assessment for autoimmune diseases,

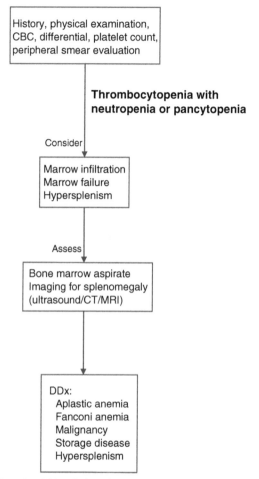

Figure 12.1 Approach to the child with thrombocytopenia and additional cytopenias. Abbreviations: CBC, complete blood count; DDx, differential diagnosis.

immune deficiency, or congenital syndromes associated with thrombocytopenia (see Table 12.1). The physical exam should assess for lymphadenopathy, hepatosplenomegaly, short stature, dysmorphic features, or the presence of congenital anomalies (e.g., radius, thumb, and fingers).

The laboratory features of ITP include a low platelet count in the face of an otherwise normal complete blood count (CBC). However, the hemoglobin, white blood cell count, and/or absolute neutrophil count may be altered due to a recent infection, and the hemoglobin may be low due to bleeding. Coagulation screening tests including PT, PTT, and fibrinogen and the complete metabolic panel should be normal. Therefore, no studies other than a CBC truly need to be done if the diagnosis of ITP is strongly suspected. The platelet count should be confirmed to be low on a second evaluation if the physical findings do not correlate with the laboratory value.

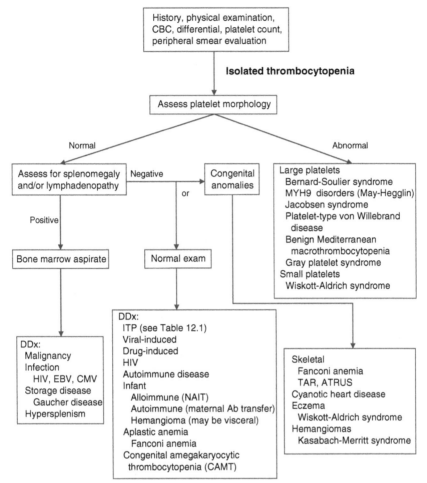

Figure 12.2 Approach to the child with isolated thrombocytopenia. Abbreviations: CBC, complete blood count; DDx, differential diagnosis; ITP, immune thrombocytopenia purpura; HIV, human immunodeficiency virus; EBV, Epstein-Barr virus; CMV, cytomegalovirus; NAIT, neonatal alloimmune thrombocytopenia; Ab, antibody; TAR, thrombocytopenia absent radius; ATRUS, amegakaryocytic thrombocytopenia radio-ulnar synostosis.

If two cytopenias are present with any findings on the history or physical suggestive of another diagnosis, consideration should be given to performing a bone marrow aspiration (BMA). However, a bone marrow evaluation is rarely necessary to confirm the diagnosis. BMA in ITP typically demonstrates the presence of immature megakaryocytes in normal or increased numbers with normal erythroid and myeloid lineages. By convention, a BMA is done on individuals with suspected ITP only if steroids are to be part of the treatment plan due to the small chance the thrombocytopenia may be an early manifestation of leukemia. However, even this practice is controversial.

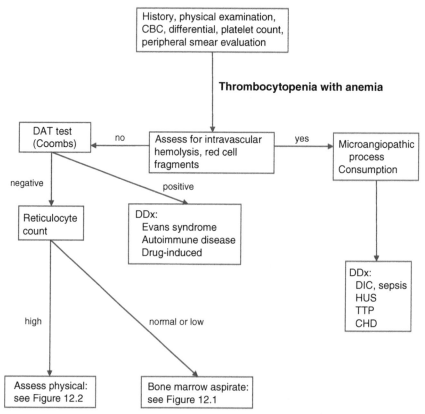

Figure 12.3 Approach to the child with thrombocytopenia and anemia. Abbreviations: CBC, complete blood count; DAT, direct antiglobin test (Coombs); DDx, differential diagnosis; DIC, disseminated intravascular coagulation; HUS, hemolytic uremic syndrome; TTP, thrombotic thrombocytopenic purpura; CHD, congenital heart disease.

Additional laboratory evaluations may be required for specific clinical indications (e.g., screening for autoimmune or thyroid disease, viral testing for HIV, hepatitis C, CMV, or parvovirus B19; direct antiglobulin testing [DAT; Coombs] and reticulocyte count if concern for autoimmune hemolytic anemia; and immunoglobulin levels and T/B cell numbers if concern for underlying immunodeficiency syndrome). Antiplatelet antibody tests are not sensitive or specific and not required for diagnosis or for routine clinical management.

Review of the peripheral blood smear confirms a low platelet count, and the few remaining platelets typically are large. If platelet size is determined by an automated cell counter (Coulter), it is usually elevated, consistent with young platelet age (due to early marrow release associated with rapid peripheral platelet destruction). Oftentimes the platelet count is underestimated as very large immature platelets (megakaryocytic fragments) are not counted by the Coulter. This may in part explain the relative lack of bleeding symptoms in children with very low platelet counts. The erythrocyte and leukocyte counts and morphology should be normal and there should be no evidence of hemolysis or microangiopathic disease (e.g., schistocytes and/or burr cells).

False values for platelet counts can result from aggregation of platelets in the syringe or collection tube, counting of small non-platelet particles (fragmented red or white cells) by automated cell counters, and pseudothrombocytopenia due to *in vitro* platelet agglutination by anticoagulant-dependent ethylenediaminetetraacetic acid (EDTA) antibodies. Review of the blood film should assess for clumps of agglutinated platelets at the periphery of the slide.

Treatment

The **natural history of acute ITP** is complete resolution in the majority of children. Despite the relatively benign course experienced by most children with ITP, the sudden onset, concern for a possible serious condition such as leukemia or aplastic anemia, and concern for life-threatening bleeding often guide the initial treatment decision making. Parents often bring their child to see the primary care or emergency physician, many of whom are not accustomed to encountering such severe thrombocytopenia. Risk factors for the rare life-threatening hemorrhage have yet to be elucidated and dogma has been to treat the patient according to platelet count rather than being guided by the degree of clinical symptoms. This clinical scenario has led to significant controversy as to whether intervention is warranted, when it is warranted, and with what treatment. Contemporary therapies have not been shown to alter the course or outcome of children with acute ITP. As such, the concept of nontreatment in ITP is increasingly becoming the standard of care in most pediatric hematology/oncology centers.

All patients and families should be counseled regarding rough play, contact sports, and general anticipatory guidance such as the use of protective gear (helmets) and seat belts. Intramuscular injections should be withheld until platelet counts increase. Specific medications that interfere with platelet function (such as NSAIDs, SSRIs [selective serotonin reuptake inhibitors], anticonvulsants, and aspirin) should not be given.

The use of a bleeding score as the framework for a consistent treatment strategy is gaining in popularity and several scoring systems have been published to date. Patients are categorized by the presence of clinical signs and symptoms of bleeding; more than 80% present with **mild** clinical bleeding (manifested by bruising, petechiae, mild epistaxis, and no anemia). **Moderate** clinical bleeding is characterized by more significant mucosal bleeding such as more severe epistaxis or menorrhagia and **severe** bleeding (usually < 5% of patients) is marked by unusual or severe bleeding requiring hospitalization for control and/ or blood transfusion support with symptoms seriously interfering with quality of life. All patients may present with very low platelet counts (e.g., 1 to 20×10^9/L) though those with severe symptoms tend to have initial platelet counts < 10×10^9/L.

Utilizing the bleeding score, many patients with clinically mild or moderate bleeding can be effectively managed with **observation**. The anxiety of patients, families, and other caregivers can often be alleviated with education on the pathophysiology and natural history of ITP in addition to general preventive measures and periodic clinical and laboratory assessments. Platelet counts do not need to be checked more often than every 1 to 2 weeks (or even less often in the clinically stable child). Disruption of school or work is not necessary, though participation in contact sports or other situations that could lead to head or abdominal injury should be avoided until the platelet count is known to have returned to a safe levels (typically $>50 \times 10^9$/L). With observation, the majority of patients with ITP will have resolution of symptoms and the underlying thrombocytopenia while avoiding unnecessary costs and side effects of medications and hospitalization.

Pharmacological treatments to raise the platelet count in children with moderate-to-severe bleeding include two first-line therapies: **intravenous immune globulin (IVIG)** and **RhoGAM** (anti-Rh [anti-D] immune globulin, also Rhophylac). IVIG is thought to function by saturating the Fc receptors on the reticuloendothelial cells in the spleen and liver, thereby decreasing the clearance of opsonized platelets. These treatments typically provide a quick yet transient increase in the platelet count, often sustained 2 to 4 weeks. More than 80% of patients respond with an increase in the platelet count, which is sufficient to decrease or eliminate bleeding symptoms. Patients and families should be counseled as to the transitory effect of IVIG treatment due to the misconception that a subsequent decrease in platelet count is indicative of increased disease severity. The dose of IVIG is 0.8 to 1 g/kg over 4 to 6 hours. If necessary, IVIG may be repeated two to three times for a total dose of 2 to 3 g/kg; doses should be given at least 24 hours apart to allow sufficient time to determine response. A rise in the platelet count is usually seen within 24 to 72 hours and peaks at approximately 9 days. A good initial response is an increase in platelet count by 20 to 50×10^9/L. Side effects of IVIG are usually immediate, relate to the rate of infusion, and include nausea, lightheadedness, and headache. At times, onset of a severe headache can prompt an emergent head CT to assess for potential intracranial hemorrhage. These symptoms can be alleviated by slowing the rate of infusion and premedicating with diphenhydramine if further doses are needed. Fever may also occur, and

premedication with acetaminophen is advisable. Rare side effects include anaphylaxis in an IgA-deficient patient, aseptic meningitis, acute renal failure, pulmonary insufficiency, and thrombosis. Although IVIG is a pooled blood product, it is thought to be safe with regard to viral transmission and does not require consent as with blood product administration. Subsequent dosing with IVIG may be indicated depending on clinical symptomatology and continued thrombocytopenia.

RhoGAM is a less-expensive alternative therapy to IVIG. The dose is 75 mg/kg IV over 20 to 30 minutes. Response rate and time to onset are similar to IVIG. Anti-D works by binding the RhD antigen expressed on the surface of red blood cells, leading to their recognition by Fc receptors on cells of the reticuloendothelial system. The coated red cells are thought to compete with the antiplatelet–antibody coated platelets for the activated Fc receptor sites, thereby slowing platelet clearance. Side effects include fever and chills, intravascular hemolysis, headache, emesis, and rarely anaphylaxis. Premedication with acetaminophen and diphenhydramine may prevent these adverse effects with subsequent infusions. A response is typically seen within 24 to 48 hours. Patients must be Rh positive, have a functional spleen (at least not known to be splenectomized or asplenic), and not be anemic (i.e., > 2 to 4 g/dL below expected hemoglobin for age). RhoGAM does cause transient hemolysis and a decrease in hemoglobin of 1 to 2 g/dL over the ensuing 3 to 4 days should be expected. The hemoglobin should subsequently recover within 10 days. Though rare, the U.S. Food and Drug Administration currently mandates that patients be monitored for 8 hours with serial urinalysis after administration of anti-D due to cases of severe, life-threatening hemolysis.

Amicar (ε-aminocaproic acid) may be utilized in patients with prolonged thrombocytopenia and persistent mucosal bleeding without anemia (mild bleeding). Reports of efficacy with minimal side effects make low-dose therapy a good option (10 mg/kg/dose every 6 to 8 hours). Another option is low-dose prednisone which may benefit the patient with a long course of ITP who secondarily develops alteration in vascular integrity. Low-dose steroids would not be expected to raise the platelet count; however, they would have minimal side effects.

Corticosteroids may be used in the initial medical management of ITP, though typically are considered a second-line therapy in pediatrics. Response is slower than with IVIG or RhoGAM and is usually within 3 to 4 days. The first steroid prescribed is prednisone, 1 to 2 mg/kg/day for 2 to 4 weeks, tapering the dose post-platelet response (i.e., $>100 \times 10^9$/L) over several weeks. The initial response rate is 70% to 90%. An immune rebound may occur with a taper that is too rapid and patients will often require prolonged steroid therapy to maintain the desired platelet count. There are several mechanisms by which steroids affect the platelet count: inhibition of phagocytosis of the antibody-coated platelets leading to prolonged platelet survival; inhibition of antibody production by B-lymphocytes; improvement of capillary integrity reducing clinical bleeding; and an increase in platelet production. Many patients respond to this treatment, although side effects may occur with repeated treatment or chronic use such as gastritis, fluid retention, weight gain, mood lability, acne, striae, high blood pressure, and elevated serum glucose. An alternative to oral steroids is high-dose pulse infusion of intravenous methylprednisolone. Some patients become thrombocytopenic again after therapy and require retreatment. A relapse may be managed safely by observation and restriction of activity and medications, or with intermittent IVIG and/or pulse steroids.

Dexamethasone has also been used with efficacy in refractory patients.

Emergency therapy

Patients with known or suspected life-threatening hemorrhage such as central nervous system hemorrhage from ITP (usually with concomitant platelet count $< 10 \times 10^9$/L) should be treated emergently with combination therapy including IVIG 1 g/kg daily for 2 to 3 days and intravenous high-dose methylprednisolone 30 mg/kg/day (up to 1 g/day) for 1 to 3 days. Active life-threatening hemorrhage with refractory thrombocytopenia is one of the only current indications for emergency splenectomy. Continuous infusion of platelets should be considered in an emergent situation and during surgery or childbirth in a severely thrombocytopenic patient, in conjunction with other therapies. Off-label recombinant factor VIIa (rFVIIa) may also be considered.

Chronic immune thrombocytopenic purpura

Acute and chronic ITP are defined based on disease duration, with chronic ITP defined as persisting for > 6 months. Approximately 10% to 20% of children with acute ITP that persists will go on to have chronic ITP. The child with chronic ITP is still likely to have complete resolution within 6 months to 2 years or may have an associated autoimmune disease or underlying immunodeficiency state. Some practitioners define chronic ITP as that lasting beyond a 1 year period. Most patients with chronic ITP do not need treatment as the platelet count is often above 20×10^9/L and bleeding is minimal. Platelet count alone does not correlate with the risk of hemorrhage as platelets are large due to a healthy marrow response to peripheral thrombocytopenia and, as a consequence, have greater than normal procoagulant activity. In the rare patient with chronic, refractory ITP who has clinical hemorrhage or cannot tolerate the living restrictions imposed by the thrombocytopenia, intervention with medical or surgical therapies should be considered.

ITP may be the initial manifestation of aplastic anemia including Fanconi anemia before progression to pancytopenia, Evans syndrome (association of ITP with autoimmune hemolytic anemia), systemic lupus erythematosis (SLE), or autoimmune lymphoproliferative syndrome. HIV infection should be considered in all patients with isolated thrombocytopenia as this is frequently the first manifestation of disease in children. ITP may also be present in children years before the diagnosis of immunodeficiency (i.e., common variable immunodeficiency) is evident.

Therapies utilized in the treatment of acute ITP may be utilized for chronic ITP, though continued administration, cost, and side effects frequently limit their use. Other considerations include additional medical and surgical approaches.

Rituximab is a chimeric human–mouse monoclonal antibody directed against the transmembrane CD20 antigen present on B cells, leading to apoptosis and antibody-dependent cellular cytotoxicity. Children with chronic ITP may have a 30% to 50% response rate with rituximab. The standard dosage is 375 mg/m^2 IV weekly infusion (over 4 to 6 hours) for 4 weeks. Most patients start to show a response by the second week, though delayed responses several weeks later may occur. Responses may be short-lived or last for years. Acute toxicity is minimal though patients may experience fever and chills (often abates with subsequent infusions), serum sickness, headache, nausea, emesis, and mucocutaneous reactions (continuum from hives and dermatitis to rarely reported Stevens-Johnson syndrome and toxic epidermal necrolysis). B-cell depletion lasts for approximately 6 months with a significant decrement in humoral response, although decreased total IgG immunoglobulin levels and increased infections have not been frequently reported. For the treatment of ITP without an underlying immunodeficiency, it remains unclear if increased infection is a risk in pediatric patients after rituximab. Although considered a T-cell-dependent infection, B-cell depletion may lead to an increased risk of PCP (*Pneumocystis jiroveci* pneumonia) and cotrixomazole prophylaxis should be considered. Hepatitis B reactivation and progressive multifocal leukoencephalopathy secondary to JC virus are rare considerations in this population.

Splenectomy may be considered for patients with chronic ITP with bleeding and/or limitation in activities negatively impacting quality of life. Splenectomy is successful in 60% to 85% of patients; however, relapse of ITP may occur due to immune-mediated platelet destruction in other organs, especially the liver. Patients should ideally receive appropriate immunization several weeks prior to surgery due to the risk of infection with encapsulated organisms (pneumococcus, *haemophilus influenza*, or meningococcus). Lifelong penicillin prophylaxis is recommended postsplenectomy.

Vinca alkaloids (vincristine and vinblastine), danazol (a virilizing androgen), and immunosuppressive agents such as azathioprine and cyclophosphamide have also been used with some success. Ascorbic acid, cyclosporine, and interferon α-2b are other agents that have also been investigated for use in chronic ITP. Long-term management of chronic ITP includes periodic assessments for development of other manifestations of immunodeficiency or autoimmune disease, counseling regarding activities and medications, and periodic assessments of the platelet count to assess for continuation or resolution of the underlying process.

The thrombopoietin (TPO) mimetics are currently under investigation for the treatment of childhood chronic ITP, following successful clinical trials in adults. As ITP is likely the result of impaired production in addition to peripheral immune-mediated destruction, these drugs may have some role in treatment to stimulate increased production, even in patients with normal thrombopoietin levels. Drugs currently under investigation are romiplostim (Nplate®) and eltrombopag (Promacta®). Concerning toxicities include marrow reticulin fibrosis and thromboembolism. It is likely that these drugs or subsequent generations will provide potential new therapeutic options in the future.

Neonatal alloimmune thrombocytopenia

Neonatal alloimmune thrombocytopenia (NAIT) is caused by the transplacental passage of maternal alloantibodies directed against fetal platelets, similar in pathophysiology to hemolytic disease of the newborn. Unlike hemolytic disease of the newborn, NAIT often affects the first-born offspring. Although rare, NAIT is the most common cause of severe thrombocytopenia in the first few days of life. Alloantibodies are secondary to human leukocyte antigen incompatibility as fetal platelet antigens are inherited from the father. Immunization in the mother against fetal platelet antigens can occur during the current or a previous pregnancy or secondary to a previous platelet transfusion and may lead to severe thrombocytopenia in the fetal-newborn period, with a high risk of fatal hemorrhage. Thrombocytopenia leading to fetal loss and hemorrhage has been reported as early as 16 to 24 weeks of gestation. Although several platelet antigens have been implicated, the large majority of cases can be related to human platelet antigen 1a (HPA-1a) incompatibility (HPA-1a-negative mother with an HPA-1a-positive fetus). HPA-1a resides on the GP IIb/IIIa complex that is responsible for fibrinogen receptor activity and thus important in aggregation and platelet-plug formation. Therefore, development of anti-HPA-1a antibodies may interfere with normal platelet aggregation in addition to decreasing platelet number, resulting in a qualitative platelet defect as well as in addition to a quantitative one. This may in part explain the high incidence of serious bleeding in these infants as compared with those born to mothers with ITP with alloantibodies directed against alternate antigens. HPA-1a is common in the Caucasian population in addition to HPA-5b. HPA-4 incompatibility is more common in Asian populations.

The infant with NAIT typically presents with moderate-to-severe thrombocytopenia (<20 to 50×10^9/L) and may rapidly develop petechiae, purpura, and bleeding. ICH is common, occurring in 10% to 20% of neonates and may occur prenatally or antenatally. Therefore, head ultrasound should always be part of the initial diagnostic workup. Complications of early central nervous system hemorrhage include hydrocephalus, porencephaly, seizures, and fetal loss. Early jaundice occurs in 20% of cases owing to resolution of intracranial or intraorgan hemorrhage. The infant should otherwise be generally healthy without other perinatal complications and the mother should have an unremarkable hematologic history. For a mother with a previous low platelet count, the differential diagnosis should include maternal idiopathic, autoimmune, and drug-dependent thrombocytopenias, infection, and preeclampsia. Infants may also be thrombocytopenic secondary to birth asphyxia, infection, congenital bone marrow hypoplasia, or from prematurity. The presence of hepatosplenomegaly, intrauterine growth retardation, and/or intracranial calcifications with thrombocytopenia should suggest a congenital viral infection. However, if a secondary diagnosis is not clearly delineated, it is important to exclude alloimmune thrombocytopenia by appropriate immunologic testing as future-affected pregnancies tend to be more severe and require close antenatal monitoring.

Early **platelet alloantigen evaluation** of the newborn and parents is important, both in offering the affected infant appropriate treatment and in order to minimize the risk of devastating complications with future pregnancies. Evaluation includes platelet typing on the mother and father, specifically looking for antigens responsible for alloimmunization such as HPA-1a. Serum from the mother and infant is screened for antiplatelet antibodies against either the infant's or the father's platelets. We send blood for the NAIT workup to the Blood Center of Wisconsin™.

Several **treatment** options are available for the infant with neonatal alloimmunization. Transfusion with antigen-negative platelets has been the mainstay of treatment, when available. Since HPA-1a-negative platelets are present in only 2% of the Caucasian population, the most available source of platelets is from the mother. Random platelet transfusions (10 to 20 mL/kg) may provide a transient increase, lasting 1 to 2 days, and should be used in cases of serious hemorrhage, while antigen-negative platelets are being obtained and prepared. If random donor platelets are ineffective, then cross-matched donor platelets or washed maternal platelets may be used if available. An excellent alternative treatment is IVIG. The recommended dose is 1 g/kg/24 hours for 1 to 2 doses (until the platelet count is $\geq 50 \times 10^9$/L). Platelet transfusion may still be necessary with IVIG if immediate correction of the thrombocytopenia is needed. Corticosteroids can be effective in reducing platelet destruction and increasing vascular integrity. Methylprednisolone, 1 mg/kg IV

every 6 to 8 hours, with IVIG is frequently effective. Regular head ultrasounds should be done while the infant remains severely thrombocytopenic ($<50 \times 10^9$/L). If intracranial bleeding is present, platelets should be kept at $\geq 100 \times 10^9$/L. Head MRI is necessary to further define the hemorrhage. Ultrasound should be repeated at 1 month in children with ICH to identify early hydrocephalus. Resolution of thrombocytopenia typically occurs within 2 to 6 weeks.

Mothers with an affected infant should be counseled on the need for aggressive monitoring with future pregnancies due to the risk of increasingly severe NAIT. Fetal platelet counts should be obtained starting around 20 weeks of gestation, with ultrasound monitoring for hemorrhage. Maternal antiplatelet titers cannot be used to accurately predict affected fetuses. IVIG 1 g/kg/week given to the mother from mid-gestation until near term has been shown to effectively increase fetal platelet counts in the majority of cases. Delivery should be planned near term with an elective cesarean section or planned induced vaginal delivery after documented increase in fetal platelet count following administration of maternal IVIG. Antigen-negative platelets, which can be obtained from the mother by apheresis, should be obtained and prepared prior to delivery in the event of extreme thrombocytopenia or hemorrhage. The infant's platelet count should be checked at birth and every 6 to 12 hours for 1 to 2 days and be kept $\geq 50 \times 10^9$/L. Frequency of monitoring can be decreased depending on the stability of the platelet count and the clinical status of the infant.

Neonatal autoimmune thrombocytopenia

Neonatal autoimmune thrombocytopenia occurs due to the passive transfer of autoantibodies from mothers with ITP and may be idiopathic, caused by other disorders including autoimmune diseases such as systemic lupus erythematosis, hypothyroidism, and lymphoproliferative states, or secondary to medications. Unlike NAIT, these antibodies recognize both maternal and fetal platelet antigens. Maternal ITP should be distinguished from gestational thrombocytopenia that tends to occur late in pregnancy and leads to mild thrombocytopenia in the mother (e.g., 70 to 100×10^9/L) without the development of antibodies. Therefore, the infant is not at risk for thrombocytopenia. Maternal platelet counts return to normal shortly after birth. The degree of thrombocytopenia seen in neonates born to mothers with ITP is less severe than with NAIT, with only 10% to 15% having platelet counts $<50 \times 10^9$/L. Bleeding is minimal and ICH is rare (<1% to 2%). The platelet count may be normal at birth but falls within 1 to 3 days of delivery. Platelet counts should be monitored closely and a head ultrasound obtained to exclude ICH. Treatment should be initiated if the platelet count falls below 30 to 50×10^9/L with the same treatment regimen as for NAIT: IVIG, IV methylprednisolone, and random donor platelet transfusion if necessary for hemorrhage. The duration of thrombocytopenia is usually 3 to 6 weeks.

Drug-induced thrombocytopenia

In addition to immune-mediated mechanisms induced by drugs, many bone marrow suppressive agents such as chemotherapy cause thrombocytopenia, though usually in the face of pancytopenia. Management is usually with platelet transfusion, to prevent or treat bleeding. The bone marrow effects of these agents often define their dose-limiting toxicity, and thrombocytopenia is a common effect. Patients usually respond well to platelet transfusion but can become refractory because of the underlying illness, organomegaly and sequestration, development of alloimmunization, sepsis, and other medications. Other potential offending drugs include anticonvulsants such as valproic acid, chlorothiazides, estrogenic hormones, ethanol, ristocetin, and protamine sulfate.

Heparin-induced thrombocytopenia (**HIT**) is caused by antibody formation to complexes of heparin and platelet factor 4 leading to platelet activation, often resulting in severely low counts as well as risk for thrombosis. It is much less common in children than adults. HIT should be suspected in the child receiving heparin (usually secondary to unfractionated but can also occur with low molecular weight) who develops unexplained thrombocytopenia of any degree within 5 to 10 days of exposure, often defined as a decrease of ≥ 50% from baseline (even if still in the normal range). Testing for heparin-induced antibodies is not very specific as many patients without HIT will have circulating antibody. If suspected, based on clinical scoring that defines likelihood, functional studies of platelet activation under the presence of heparin can be done by specialized laboratories. These tests include the serotonin release assay and heparin-induced platelet aggregation assay. Heparin should be discontinued and replaced by an anticoagulant that does not lead to antibody formation such as argatroban. Warfarin should not be utilized immediately due to associated protein C deficiency with risk of microthrombosis leading to skin necrosis and gangrene.

Nonimmune thrombocytopenia

Many nonimmune-mediated processes lead to **increased platelet consumption**. Generalized platelet activation with trapping of microaggregates in the small vasculature contributes to **microangiopathic hemolytic anemia** (**MAHA**) occurring in congenital heart disease, **hemolytic uremic syndrome (HUS)**, and **thrombotic thrombocytopenic purpura (TTP)**. HUS is primarily associated with a prothombotic state induced by exposure to shiga-toxin producing *Escherichia coli* (usually O157:H7), particularly affecting the renal vasculature and leading to the triad of MAHA, platelet consumption, and renal failure. HUS is the most common cause of acute renal failure in children. Patients may present with abdominal pain and bloody diarrhea and are treated with supportive care (i.e., red cell transfusions, dialysis as necessary). Platelet transfusion may worsen the clinical status and should be used with caution.

Idiopathic TTP is a rare disease in children, characterized by the pentad of thrombocytopenia, hemolytic anemia, renal impairment, neurologic symptoms, and fever, although few patients present with the full gamut of symptoms. Idiopathic TTP is often clinically indistinguishable from diarrhea-negative HUS. There is also a rare congenital form in which affected neonates present with jaundice and thrombocytopenia, although patients may not have an episode of overt TTP for years until triggered by infection, pregnancy, or stress. Patients with congenital TTP have low levels of ADAMTS13, a protein that cleaves unusually large multimers of von Willebrand factor into a biologically less-active form. Absence of ADAMTS13 inhibits cleavage of these large multimers allowing spontaneous platelet adhesion and aggregation.

Patients with acquired TTP, which is often idiopathic, commonly demonstrate antibodies to the protein, unlike the congenital form in which there is a constitutive deficiency. Affected individuals are more commonly female, of African descent, and diagnosis can be associated with pregnancy, autoimmune disease, infection, or transplantation. The hallmark of disease is the presence of segmental hyalin microthrombi in the microvasculature that can also be seen in the lymph nodes and spleen. Classic signs and symptoms include fever, malaise, nausea and vomiting, abdominal and chest pain, arthralgia and myalgia, pallor, jaundice, purpura, progressive renal failure, and fluctuating neurologic signs and symptoms. Laboratory features include thrombocytopenia and MAHA. The peripheral blood smear will show polychromasia, basophilic stippling, schistocytes, microspherocytes, and nucleated red cells. The DAT (Coombs) should be negative as TTP is not an autoimmune hemolytic anemia. The LDH and unconjugated bilirubin will be elevated and haptoglobin reduced due to the MAHA, with associated hemoglobinuria. Without treatment, mortality is >90%. Plasmapheresis is the mainstay of therapy in the acquired form. Fresh frozen plasma is usually sufficient to treat the congenital form. Patients may also benefit from rituximab and other immunosuppressive drugs including steroids, cyclosporine, cyclophosphamide, vincristine, and azathioprine.

Increased utilization of platelets may occur in active bleeding, infection, or sepsis. In **disseminated intravascular coagulation (DIC)**, there is an imbalance between intravascular thrombosis and fibrinolysis, with increased platelet consumption, depletion of plasma clotting factors, and formation of fibrin. DIC can be initiated by many events, including sepsis due to bacteria, viruses, or fungi; malignancy, particularly acute promyelocytic leukemia and neuroblastoma; hemolytic transfusion reactions; and trauma. Therapy is aimed at treating the underlying etiologic process. Supportive care consists of platelet transfusion to maintain platelet counts $>50 \times 10^9$/L and plasma protein replenishment to correct coagulopathies and maintain fibrinogen >100 mg/dL.

Thrombocytopenia can occur in the **sick newborn** for many reasons, most commonly with infection, prematurity, asphyxia, respiratory distress syndrome, pulmonary hypertension, or meconium aspiration. These infants appear to have normal to increased platelet production, but a decreased platelet life span for reasons that are unclear. Thrombocytopenia is a frequent occurrence in congenital cyanotic heart disease associated with compensatory polycythemia. Therapeutic phlebotomy may lessen the thrombocytopenia.

The association of thrombocytopenia and **giant hemangiomas** occurs in the infant with **Kasabach–Merritt syndrome** and represents a form of localized intravascular coagulation. The hemangiomas may be multiple and may involve only viscera. Therefore, in an infant with unexplained thrombocytopenia, imaging studies should be done to look for a vascular anomaly. Hemangiomas are proliferative lesions that grow rapidly for several months and then regress spontaneously. Platelet thrombi may develop in these lesions and platelet life span may be decreased. These infants may also have a consumptive coagulopathy with low fibrinogen levels and elevated concentrations of fibrin degradation products. The lesions are also prone to necrosis and infection. A particular hemangioma's size or location cannot predict whether it will lead to platelet trapping and thrombocytopenia. These infants should be managed by close observation and hematologic monitoring while waiting for regression to occur. However, the lesions may become large enough to compromise the infant by impinging on the airway or vital organs, leading to compartment syndrome, and resulting in serious illness or death. External compression of hemangiomas by firm bandaging, when possible due to location, may reduce blood flow and platelet trapping. Corticosteroid treatment at a dose of 1 to 2 mg/kg/day may bring about regression of the lesion and normalization of the platelet count.

Interferon α-2a has been shown to be beneficial in correcting the platelet count and shrinking the lesion. Recent fortuitous discovery of propanolol as a treatment for hemangiomas has now made it first-line therapy; although not clearly delineated, the mechanism of action is likely related to the inhibition of angiogenesis. Supportive transfusion therapy is indicated with active bleeding due to thrombocytopenia. Platelet transfusion as well as infusion of coagulation factors (fresh frozen plasma, cryoprecipitate, and antifibrinolytic drugs) may be helpful but usually are of only transitory benefit. Antiplatelet medications (aspirin and dipyridamole) have been used in the past to interfere with platelet trapping within the hemangioma but carry the risk of causing platelet dysfunction in addition to the existing thrombocytopenia.

A variety of conditions that result in **splenomegaly** are associated with thrombocytopenia. The large spleen sequesters and destroys circulating platelets. Anemia, leukopenia, and neutropenia may also be present. Megakaryocytic production in the marrow is normal, and may be accelerated in response to a decrease in the circulation. Storage diseases, early portal hypertension, hemolytic conditions (red cell membrane defects), infections such as with HIV, EBV, and CMV, and malignancies are frequently associated with splenomegaly and may result in **hypersplenism** (increased splenic activity and resultant red cell destruction).

Decreased platelet production

Thrombocytopenia due to decreased production may be a result of an acquired or inherited disease process. Decreased production may be a direct effect of marrow crowding due to malignancy (leukemia or metastatic solid tumors such as lymphoma, neuroblastoma, medulloblastoma, and rhabdomyosarcoma) or storage diseases (Gaucher, Neimann-Pick, etc.). Drugs may be implicated in decreased production. The liver is the site of TPO production and liver disease is associated with chronic severe thrombocytopenia. Severe iron deficiency can result in decreased production, though early iron deficiency states are associated with an elevated platelet count likely due to marrow stress. Diseases affecting the marrow matrix (aplastic anemia and myelofibrosis) cannot support stem cell growth and maturation with resultant thrombocytopenia.

Thrombocytopenia related to an inherited condition is frequently distinguished by characteristic clinical features, early presentation and chronic course, family history, platelet morphology, and lack of response to classic treatments for ITP. A number of these conditions are associated with macrothrombocytes and mild-to-moderate thrombocytopenia including Bernard-Soulier syndrome, MYH9-related disorders (May-Hegglin anomaly with bluish cytoplasmic inclusions including Sebastian, Fechtner, Epstein, and Alport-like syndromes), platelet-type von Willebrand disease, gray platelet syndrome (storage pool disease), benign Mediterranean macrothrombocytopenia, Paris-Trousseau type thrombocytopenia, and more poorly defined syndromes such as Montreal platelet syndrome. Microthrombocytes are seen in Wiskott-Aldrich syndrome, an X-linked disorder resulting from a mutation on the WAS gene. Wiskott–Aldrich syndrome is characterized by thrombocytopenia, recurrent bacterial and viral infections secondary to T-cell dysfunction, chronic eczema, and a propensity to develop autoimmune disorders. Patients with defects in the WAS gene may also have a milder syndrome called X-linked thrombocytopenia with small platelets and immune dysregulation which may develop over time. Of note, it is difficult to appreciate small platelets in the newborn and the mean platelet volume reported on the CBC is unreliable in the face of thrombocytopenia.

Patients with inherited thrombocytopenia may have normally sized platelets in certain conditions including congenital amegakaryocytic thrombocytopenia (CAMT), thrombocytopenia with absent radii (TAR), familial platelet disorder and predisposition to AML (acute myelogenous leukemia), amegakaryocytic thrombocytopenia with radio-ulnar synostosis (ATRUS), and autosomal dominant thrombocytopenia. CAMT, a rare cause of neonatal thrombocytopenia, is a bone marrow failure syndrome inherited in an autosomal recessive manner due to deficiency in the TPO receptor c-mpl. Bleeding symptoms lead to diagnosis in infancy although CAMT is often initially confused with other more common neonatal causes of thrombocytopenia such as alloimmune- and autoimmune-mediated processes. However, unlike these other conditions, the thrombocytopenia does not resolve with time. There are no classic physical features. Diagnosis is based on markedly reduced megakaryocytic precursors in the bone marrow with normal erythroid and myeloid lineages with elevated TPO levels. Current treatment is supportive care, platelet transfusion as needed, and consideration for curative hematopoietic stem cell transplantation. Gene therapy is being developed.

Children with ATRUS present similarly to CAMT with severe thrombocytopenia at birth, but with the addition of associated skeletal anomalies and sensorineural hearing loss. Skeletal abnormalities are fusion of the radius and ulna at the elbow, often associated with minor clinodactyly. The disease may progress to aplastic anemia or leukemia. TAR syndrome is also thought to be secondary to a defective response to TPO with variable thrombocytopenia and normal erythroid and myeloid lineages.

Most cases are diagnosed at birth or in utero due to bilateral absence of the radii manifested as a shortening of the forearms and flexion at the elbows. The thumbs are present, which distinguish TAR from the skeletal anomaly associated with Fanconi anemia. Patients may have additional platelet dysfunction and are at risk for significant bleeding episodes. Typically, the thrombocytopenia improves through childhood. Associated clinical features include additional skeletal limb defects, renal and cardiac anomalies, facial capillary hemangiomas, and cow's milk intolerance. Fanconi anemia is an inherited disorder characterized by chromosomal instability with skeletal anomalies and hypoproductive thrombocytopenia, although other cell lines are eventually affected. These patients have an increased susceptibility to develop leukemia and may benefit from early hematopoietic stem cell transplantation if a suitable donor is available.

Case study for review

A 9-year-old previously well Hispanic boy presents to the emergency department with a 2-hour history of profuse epistaxis. On presentation he is noted to be well-developed and well-nourished, frightened, fatigued, and pale, with numerous ecchymoses and blood pouring from both nares. He is emergently triaged and has bilateral nasal packing placed. He continues to have massive bleeding and has repeated emesis of digested and bright red blood. His vitals are T 37.2°C, HR 156, RR 30, and BP 62/38.

1. What are your immediate thoughts regarding possible diagnosis? How do you confirm this and what steps do you take in treatment and stabilization of your patient?
2. What pertinent history should you obtain?

3. What findings do you look for on examination to either confirm or dispute your suspected diagnosis?

Obviously, the first concern is to try to stop the bleeding and treat him for acute, symptomatic hemorrhage. You suspect a bleeding disorder and see this is an otherwise healthy child with no known inherited bleeding diathesis. Although ITP presents with acute massive bleeding in fewer than 5% of cases, you are appropriately concerned that he has mucosal type bleeding associated with either an acquired or inherited platelet problem, which may be qualitative or quantitative. You order a STAT CBC to determine both platelet and hemoglobin levels and initiate fluid resuscitation awaiting the results.

Additional historical points to elicit include recent illness, medication exposure, underlying disease, and prior symptoms. You are contemplating other diagnoses such as von Willebrand disease and acute leukemia and ask questions related to these possibilities. In this case, the mother states that he has been healthy, with no prior medications, illnesses, hospitalizations, or other comorbidities. There is no family history of a diagnosed bleeding disorder (though you make a mental note to pursue these questions later as family members may not have been evaluated for symptoms suggestive of von Willebrand disease). The mother states that he on awakening this morning had unexplained bruises over his torso and extremities and blood blisters in his mouth. He complained of feeling sick to his stomach and began to have simultaneous emesis and nose bleeding, which led to her calling an ambulance as she could not stop it.

On examination, you note he is alert and oriented, though frightened to see so much blood and expresses to you he thinks he is going to die. You provide reassurance and quickly note his oral and skin findings of diffuse petechiae and purpura. Purpuric lesions on the torso are very unusual and frequently not associated with trauma, reflecting more spontaneous bleeding. He has no adenopathy, organomegaly, other skin rashes, and no pain on palpation of the extremities and abdomen with full range of motion of all joints, and in general appears well developed and appropriate for age. All these findings are supportive of a diagnosis of ITP.

Your patient's CBC comes back with a platelet count of 2×10^9/L, hemoglobin 6.2 g/dL, and white blood cell count of 7.4×10^9/L with a normal differential. You explain the anemia as secondary to massive epistaxis.

Your patient now has evidence of gross hematuria and melena, with a further drop in blood pressure despite having received a unit of packed red blood cells and volume support. The complete metabolic panel and coagulation studies are normal.

4. What is your next thought for treatment?
5. How do you counsel the family?

As you are now certain that this is acute ITP and your patient is experiencing life-threatening hemorrhage, you initiate therapy with IVIG 1 g/kg IV over 4 hours, methylprednisolone 1 mg/kg IV every 8 hours, continuous infusion of packed red blood cells, and fluid support with Lactated Ringer's or normal saline. Consideration should also be given to continuous infusion of platelets. Consultation with an ENT surgeon should be obtained for nasal packing and control of the bleeding in the posterior pharynx.

The prognosis of ITP, even in the face of such a dramatic presentation, is excellent. However, this situation is tenuous due to lack of therapies that could cause an immediate rise in the platelet count. At this time, his prognosis is guarded.

Your patient is hospitalized in the PICU and continues to received red cell transfusions, continuous platelet transfusion

(1 pheresed unit every 2 to 3 hours), FFP infusion, further doses of methylprednisolone, and a second dose of IVIG. On day 3, the hemoglobin drops to 4.6 g/dL and the decision is made to perform an emergent splenectomy. The family is counseled that he may not survive this procedure. Fortunately, however, he does very well and is supported with transfusions without a worsened clinical course. Unfortunately, there is no immediate response to splenectomy. Typically, in patients that do respond there is an immediate increase in postoperative platelet count, often to above normal levels due to an exaggerated marrow response that persists after the source of peripheral destruction or sequestration has been removed. Splenectomy is not successful in $\geq$30% of cases and it cannot be predicted who will respond. Our patient continues to receive massive blood product support for one week, then starts to stabilize with an increase in hemoglobin to 8 g/dL and platelet count of 54×10^9/L. He continues on a course of steroids, eventually transitioning to oral prednisone, and tapering off by 6 weeks. By this time his platelet count normalizes, and several years later he continues to have a normal platelet count.

Of interest, the patient re-presents with moderate epistaxis, no anemia, and a normal platelet count 1 year later. Further diagnostic workup reveals a diagnosis of type 1 von Willebrand disease.

6. How would the knowledge of this comorbidity have influenced your management of the patient with the initial presentation of ITP and massive epistaxis?

Knowledge of this disease may have led to the use of additional therapies such as DDAVP to stimulate release of von Willebrand factor, and Humate-P, a Factor VIII concentrate that also contains von Willebrand factor and is used for von Willebrand factor replacement. It is unknown whether such additional therapies may have impacted the clinical course.

Suggested Reading

Buchanan GR. Bleeding signs in children with idiopathic thrombocytopenic purpura. J Pediatr Hematol Oncol 25:S42–S46, 2003.

Bussel JB, Sola-Visner M. Current approaches to the evaluation and management of the fetus and neonate with immune thrombocytopenia. Semin Perinatol 301:35–42, 2009.

Cines DB, Bussel JB, Liebman HA, Luning Prak ET. The ITP syndrome: pathogenic and clinical diversity. Blood 113:6511–6521, 2009.

Israels SJ. Diagnostic evaluation of platelet function disorders in neonates and children: an update. Semin Thromb Hemost 35:181–188, 2009.

Neunert CE, Buchanan GR, Imbach P, et al. Severe hemorrhage in children with newly diagnosed immune thrombocytopenic purpura. Blood 112:4003–4008, 2008.

Neunert C, Lim W, Crowther M, et al. The American Society of Hematology 2011 evidence-based practice guidelines for immune thrombocytopenia. Blood 117:4190–4207, 2011.

Segel GB, Feig SA. Controversies in the diagnosis and management of childhood acute immune thrombocytopenic purpura. Pediatr Blood Cancer 53:318–324, 2009.

13 Evaluation of the Child with a Suspected Malignancy

Each year approximately 15,000 children and adolescents under 20 years of age are diagnosed with cancer in the United States. The likelihood of a young adult having a history of childhood cancer is approximately 1 in 300. Although cancer remains the leading cause of death in children except for accidents, survival continues to steadily increase. In adolescents, cancer deaths are less common than those caused by accidents, homicide, and suicide. More than 80% of children diagnosed with cancer are now expected to be cured of their disease. That being said, cancer remains a devastating diagnosis. The initial approach to the child and family must be with a heightened sensitivity to the emotional impact. Once a diagnosis of cancer is suspected, an immediate and thorough evaluation should proceed.

Initial symptoms of cancer may be somewhat elusive, given the subtle and overlapping symptoms and signs that may be present in both malignant and nonmalignant disease. Many pediatricians and clinicians may only see a new case of childhood cancer every 5 to 7 years, and each case may be so unique as to not allow for the increased awareness of this possibility.

The history is the first step in the diagnostic process, with the chief complaint providing the most important clue. Most of the symptoms of childhood cancer are either due to a mass and its effect on the surrounding tissues, invasion of the marrow, or secretion of a substance by the tumor that disturbs normal function. A careful family history should be elicited and include familial cancers. Certain conditions can predispose to malignancy such as genetic diseases (e.g., Down syndrome, Beckwith–Wiedemann syndrome, neurofibromatosis), prior history of a malignancy, or radiation therapy. Environmental and genetic factors have been associated with the development of malignancy; genetic factors are known to play a significant role in the development of pediatric cancer, whereas environmental factors are postulated to play a role in the increasing incidence of certain cancers.

Timely diagnosis is critical though can be difficult due to the nonspecific symptoms and rarity of the diseases. Though highly curable in many circumstances, earlier diagnosis may play a factor in improved prognosis. Consideration should be given to the nature of the complaint by the child and

Handbook of Pediatric Hematology and Oncology: Children's Hospital & Research Center Oakland, Second Edition. Caroline A. Hastings, Joseph C. Torkildson, and Anurag K. Agrawal.
© 2012 John Wiley & Sons, Ltd. Published 2012 by John Wiley & Sons, Ltd.

Table 13.1 Presenting signs and symptoms of some common pediatric cancers and their differential diagnoses.

Presenting signs or symptoms	Common diagnoses (nonmalignant conditions)	Potential malignancy
Headache, morning vomiting	Migraine, sinusitis	Brain tumor
Lymphadenopathy	Infection	Lymphoma, leukemia
Bone pain/limping	Infection, trauma, growing pains	Bone tumor, leukemia, neuroblastoma
Abdominal mass	Constipation, kidney cyst, full bladder	Wilms tumor, neuroblastoma
Extremity mass	Cyst, infection, trauma	Bone tumor, soft tissue sarcoma
Mediastinal mass	Infection, cyst	Lymphoma, leukemia
Pancytopenia	Infection	Leukemia
Bleeding	Coagulation disorders, platelet disorders, ITP	Leukemia (APL), neuroblastoma
Back pain	Trauma	Leukemia, lymphoma, CNS tumor, extension of abdominal tumor into spinal cord
Chronic ear drainage	Otitis media/externa	Langerhans cell histiocytosis
Feminizing/masculinizing symptoms	Precocious puberty	Adrenocortical carcinoma, brain tumor, germ cell tumor

Abbreviations: APL, acute promyelocytic leukemia (AML M3); ITP, immune thrombocytopenic purpura; CNS, central nervous system.

family, potential explanations for the complaint (or lack thereof), persistence of symptoms, and lack of response to common interventions (see Table 13.1).

Headache is one of the most common complaints in the pediatric population, the majority of which are attributable to nonmalignant conditions. Although few headaches are caused by intracranial masses, primary brain tumors or metastases must be ruled out when dealing with a patient with repeated or persistent headaches. Headaches are often the first symptom of a brain tumor and, dependent on location, are frequently accompanied by more subtle findings on neurologic examination. History should include questions to characterize the headache including worrisome signs such as recurrent morning headache, headache that awakens the child, intense incapacitating headache, associated vomiting, or changes in the quality, frequency, and pattern of the headaches. Associated neurologic symptoms or signs should warrant an emergent evaluation for a tumor in the central nervous system. These include, but are not limited to, localizing symptoms such as focal weakness, cranial nerve palsies, ataxia, failure to thrive, and developmental delays or regression. A thorough neurologic examination, including evaluation for papilledema, should precede radiographic imaging. Other important historical points include an assessment of changes in visual acuity, behavior, and academic performance. MRI is recommended to evaluate for the presence of an **intracranial mass** in children with symptoms suggestive of a brain tumor. CT may be appropriate as an initial test in certain settings depending on the availability of MRI. CT is a good, rapid tool for the assessment of acute

Table 13.2 Conditions suggesting need for brain imaging in children with headache.

Presence or onset of neurologic abnormality
Ocular findings such as papilledema, decreased visual acuity, or loss of vision
Vomiting that is persistent, increasing in frequency, or preceded by recurrent headaches
Change in character of headache such as increased severity and frequency
Recurrent morning headaches or headaches that repeatedly awaken child from sleep
Short stature or deceleration of linear growth
Precocious puberty
Diabetes insipidus
Age 3 years or less
Neurofibromatosis
History of acute lymphoblastic leukemia with irradiation of central nervous system

hemorrhage or increased intracranial pressure (see Table 13.2).

Lymphadenopathy is a common finding on examination in children. Enlarged lymph nodes are a frequent presenting sign in association with malignancies or infection, and differentiation requires a meticulous and systematic approach. Lymph nodes become large in response to infection or infiltration. Generally, a lymph node is considered enlarged if it measures greater than 10 mm, although inguinal nodes may be 15 mm or greater before being considered worrisome and epitrochlear nodes are concerning once greater than 5 mm. In addition to size, other factors to consider in establishing a differential between infection and malignancy include persistence or rate of growth, quality of the node, location and distribution (e.g., adenopathy that is symmetric, localized, regional, or disseminated), and presence of other signs or symptoms of infection. Adenopathy in the supraclavicular, axillary, or epitrochlear areas is considered an abnormal finding. Adenopathy that persists longer than 6 weeks is concerning for malignancy as is a unilateral location. Nodes that are hard, nonmobile, and nontender are worrisome for malignancy. Nodes associated with fluctuance, tenderness, warmth, or overlying erythema are more consistent with infection. However, these are only generalizations as rapidly growing malignant nodes may be tender and infectious nodes may be quite firm and nonmobile.

Important **historical points** to elicit include:
• Duration of lymphadenopathy or localized mass
• Presence of a recent infectious illness
• Skin lesions, cuts, or abrasions (and relationship to nodal drainage patterns)
• Recent immunizations
• Medications
• Animal contact (e.g., cat scratch, rodent bite, tick bite)
• Recent transfusion
• Travel
• Possible sexually transmitted infection
• Presence of symptoms such as arthralgias, weight loss, and night sweats

The differential diagnosis of lymphadenopathy includes infectious etiologies (viral, bacterial, spirochetal, and protozoan), connective tissue disease, hypersensitivity states, lymphoproliferative disorders, immunodeficiency states, storage diseases, and malignancy. In infants, the differential diagnosis of head and neck lumps includes lymphadenopathy and congenital malformations such as cystic hygroma, thyroglossal duct cyst, branchial cleft cyst, epidermoid cyst, and neonatal torticollis. Localized adenopathy may be infectious in origin including bacterial causes such as *Staphylococcus aureus*, beta-hemolytic strep, cat-scratch disease (*Bartonella henselae*), and tuberculous and nontuberculous mycobacteria, in addition to nonbacterial causes such as HIV, EBV, cytomegalovirus (CMV), and toxoplasmosis.

The **physical examination** of the child with lymphadenopathy includes an assessment of the size, location, and quality of the node(s). A full examination should include assessment of the skin and mucocutaneous tissues draining to the particular node in question, and evidence of other signs related to an underlying disease process such as hepatomegaly and splenomegaly. Nodes should be measured in largest diameter, the quality should be assessed as to mobility, firmness, tenderness, and overlying skin changes, and these findings should be documented. Children with mildly enlarged nodes should be monitored with frequent examinations, and when not associated with malignancy, most of these nodes will revert to normal size.

If infection is considered the cause of the adenopathy, as in localized cervical adenitis, it is reasonable to **treat** the patient with a 2 week course of antibiotics. Dependent on the history, physical, and clinical suspicion, a particular antibiotic regimen can be chosen in addition to sending serology or further testing for likely organisms. A baseline complete blood count (CBC) with differential and peripheral blood smear should be done if there is any concern for a diagnosis other than infection. The patient should be seen again following completion of the antibiotics and if the node has not changed or has increased in size, consideration should then be given to biopsy. Many cases of infection-related adenopathy resolve spontaneously in 2 to 6 weeks or as a result of antibiotic treatment (see Figure 13.1).

For the large node (i.e., >2.5 cm in size) or in the patient without response to antibiotics, further evaluation is required. Additional studies should include a PPD (or quantiferon gold), chest radiograph, CBC with differential (if not already done), chemistries including lactate dehydrogenase (LDH) and uric acid, and serologies as indicated by history and examination. A biopsy should be done on enlarging or persistently large nodes or if adenopathy is also seen on chest radiography. It is recommended that excisional biopsies (i.e., removal of intact node) be performed when malignancy is suspected to evaluate the architecture of the node in addition to the cellular infiltrate. The largest node should be biopsied when possible, with avoidance of the upper cervical and inguinal areas. Studies to be performed on the tissue include Gram stain and culture (bacterial, mycobacterial, viral, and/or fungal); histology and immunohistochemistry for suspected malignancy; and if malignancy is confirmed, flow cytometry and specific cytogenetic testing for further classification.

Splenomegaly is the finding of a palpable spleen edge on examination. A 1 to 2 cm splenic tip is found in 30% of full-term neonates and in as many as 10% of healthy children. Approximately 3% of healthy college students have palpable spleens. Therefore, this finding on a routine physical examination of an otherwise healthy child should not create great concern. Children with other signs of systemic disease, however, should have their splenomegaly evaluated.

Splenomegaly is associated with many disease states, both congenital and acquired:
- *Hemolytic anemia*: hereditary spherocytosis, thalassemia, splenic sequestration in sickle cell disease, and autoimmunity
- *Immunological disease*: common variable immune deficiency, connective tissue disorders, and autoimmune lymphoproliferative disease
- *Infection*: viral (EBV, CMV, HIV, hepatitis), bacterial (tularemia, abscesses, tuberculosis, infective endocarditis), spirochetal, protozoan, and fungal
- *Storage disease*: Gaucher, Neimann-Pick, and mucopolysaccharidoses

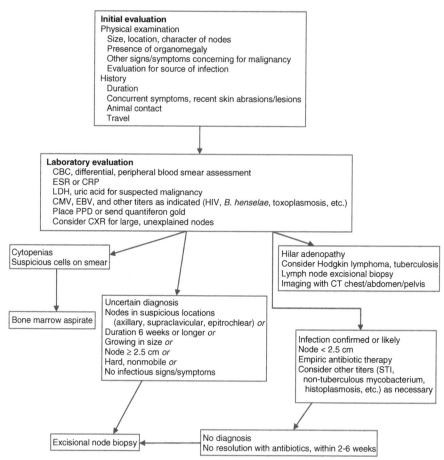

Figure 13.1 Evaluation of the child with adenopathy. (Abbreviations: CBC, complete blood count; ESR, erythrocyte sedimentation rate; CRP, C-reactive protein; LDH, lactate dehydrogenase; CMV, cytomegalovirus; EBV, Epstein-Barr virus; CXR, chest X-ray; CT, computed tomography; STI, sexually transmitted infection).

- *Malignancy*: leukemias as well as Hodgkin and non-Hodgkin lymphoma

A detailed **history** should be obtained to gain clues as to the etiology of the enlarged spleen. The patient should be questioned regarding current or recent infectious symptoms, fevers or rigors (e.g., in subacute bacterial endocarditis, infectious mononucleosis, and malaria), jaundice (with hemolytic anemia or liver disease), abnormal bleeding or bruising (malignancy), travel to endemic areas (malaria), trauma (splenic hematoma), and family history (hemoglobinopathies, thalassemia, and hereditary spherocytosis with prior splenectomy or cholescystectomy). The **physical examination** should include a measurement of the spleen size (centimeters below the midcostal margin), consistency, and presence of tenderness (which suggests rapid increase in size) in addition to the presence of adenopathy or hepatomegaly. The vitals should be reviewed for evidence of fever or hypotension and the skin assessed for cutaneous bleeding. Other considerations include evaluation for stigmata of specific disease states including jaundice, cardiac murmurs, arthritis, as well as specific findings of endocarditis including Roth spots (retinal hemorrhages), Janeway lesions (nontender hemorrhagic lesions on the palms/soles), and Osler nodes (tender microemboli on the fingers and toes).

The **laboratory and imaging** assessment is determined based on suspicion of the underlying etiology of splenomegaly. Consideration should also be given to a secondary effect of hypersplenism in which the child may have cytopenias due to a large spleen. Persistent splenomegaly should be fully investigated as follows:

• *CBC*: evaluate red cell indices, reticulocyte count, platelet count, white blood cell count, and review peripheral blood smear (all to help rule out hematologic disorders such as hemolytic anemia; membrane disorders with spherocytes or elliptocytes; increased red cell indices and anemia in thalassemia; atypical lymphocytes as in EBV; leukemic blasts; and cytopenias secondary to leukemia or hypersplenism)

• *Infection*: blood culture, viral studies, PPD (or quantiferon gold), thick and thin smear, and serologies to rule out EBV, CMV, HIV, histoplasmosis, tuberculosis, and malaria

• *Hemolytic evaluation*: CBC, reticulocyte count, direct antiglobulin test (Coombs), haptoglobin, serum bilirubin, LDH, red cell enzyme assays (G6PD, pyruvate kinase deficiency), osmotic fragility testing or ektacytometry, and urinalysis

• *Liver disease*: complete metabolic panel, coagulation studies, hepatitis panel, α-1 antitrypsin, ceruloplasmin (Wilson disease), and 24-hour urine copper

• *Connective tissue disease*: ESR, complement (C3, C4, CH50), antinuclear antibody, and rheumatoid factor

• *Infiltrative diseases*: bone marrow aspirate and biopsy (looking for blasts, storage cells) and enzyme study for Gaucher (glucocerebrosidase)

• *Lymph node biopsy*: can be done if performed with coexistent lymphadenopathy

• *Imaging*: volumetric and heterogeneity assessment with ultrasound, CT, or MRI; liver–spleen scan with ^{99m}Tc-sulfur colloid for functional analysis; can also send pit count for pitted red blood cells.

Bone pain is unusual in children and adolescents except when associated with trauma. Growing pains are a common complaint and consist of bilateral (80% of cases) lower extremity pain occurring in the afternoon, evening, or night, affect children between 3 and 14 years of age, occur most commonly on a weekly or monthly basis and much less frequently daily, and are relieved with massage in the majority of cases. Children presenting with this complaint have an excellent prognosis. Pain is otherwise usually due to bone, bone marrow, or nerve infiltration. Back pain in young people is pathologic and may be due to a tumor in the spinal cord or one causing external compression such as neuroblastoma, rhabdomyosarcoma, or a leukemic chloroma. This finding should prompt an MRI of the spine, as these conditions typically result in no abnormalities on plain film.

Patients with primary bone tumors often present with localized pain, frequently in association with a growing mass. Pain may be attributed to recent mild trauma or growing pains. In some cases, patients sustain a pathological fracture after seemingly mild trauma due to infiltration of the periosteum and weakening of the bone. Bone pain is typically a presenting symptom in patients with osteogenic sarcoma and Ewing sarcoma. Langerhans cell histiocytosis very often involves bone and may present with localized bone pain anywhere in the body, often with overlying soft tissue swelling.

Diffuse or multifocal bone pain is a common presenting symptom in acute leukemia. It is reported in more than 25% of patients diagnosed with acute lymphoblastic leukemia (ALL), but is seen less commonly in acute myelogenous leukemia (AML). It is due to marrow crowding with leukemic cells. Patients will often complain of back or leg pain that is persistent and increasing in intensity and very young children may become irritable and refuse to walk or participate in normal activities. Musculoskeletal pain in children is often diagnosed as arthritis or bone or joint infection. Pain may be asymmetric and often children present with a limp with pain seemingly disproportionate to the findings on examination. In contrast to children with arthritis, children with leukemia will have worsened pain at night, severe pain that may shift to other locations, no morning stiffness or swelling, and may have associated constitutional symptoms such as weight loss and night sweats. Associated laboratory findings that may suggest malignancy include an elevated erythrocyte sedimentation rate, elevated serum LDH, anemia, thrombocytopenia, neutropenia, and/or leukopenia. Any of these findings should prompt an examination of the bone marrow.

Bone pain may also be a direct result of bony metastatic disease or marrow infiltration secondary to other tumors including neuroblastoma, rhabdomyosarcoma, Ewing sarcoma, and non-Hodgkin lymphoma. Localized bone pain warrants radiographic evaluation (two-view plain radiographs) for the assessment of a lesion or leukemic changes.

Cytopenias and/or abnormalities on the peripheral blood smear are suspicious for a marrow infiltrative process, primarily leukemia. Isolated anemia, leukopenia, or thrombocytopenia can occur in leukemia but much more commonly the patient will present with bi- or pancytopenia. Pancytopenia may also indicate the lack of blood cell production as in aplastic anemia, or is caused by the proliferation of malignant cells in the marrow with resultant crowding. The anemia is frequently characterized as one of chronic diseases (i.e., normochromic and low reticulocyte count). Leukocyte counts are variable at presentation in acute leukemia and may be normal, decreased, or elevated. The cell differential, however, is likely to show neutropenia and the peripheral blood smear will likely, though not always, demonstrate blasts or immature cells. Unless metastasis to the marrow has occurred, leukopenia and thrombocytopenia are rarely associated with extramedullary malignancies (see Table 13.3).

Patients with bi- and pancytopenia require bone marrow aspiration and possibly biopsy for suspected diagnosis of a marrow infiltrative process, most likely acute leukemia. The situation can be more complex in the case of a single depressed lineage. Children with persistent or worsening normocytic, normochromic anemia without manifestations of hemolysis, clinical suspicion of transient erythroblastopenia of childhood, or renal disease with low erythropoietin production should have diagnostic bone marrow studies performed. Those with isolated severe thrombocytopenia suspected of having immune thrombocytopenic purpura (ITP) with no clinical signs or symptoms of malignancy should be followed closely and, if with the development of additional cytopenias or the need to start corticosteroids as part of their treatment for ITP, should also have a bone marrow examination. The necessity of bone marrow examination prior to the initiation of steroids for the treatment of ITP is controversial.

Table 13.3 Evaluation of the child with suspected leukemia.

History and physical examination

Assess life-threatening conditions including severe anemia, thrombocytopenia, DIC, infection, compression of vital organs, hyperleukocytosis, and metabolic derangements

Laboratory studies

CBC with manual differential, reticulocyte count, examination of peripheral blood smear

Metabolic panel with electrolytes, BUN, creatinine, uric acid, LDH, AST, ALT, alkaline phosphatase, total bilirubin, magnesium, calcium, and phosphorus

Serologies: varicella, CMV, HSV, hepatitis A, B, and C (obtain prior to transfusion if possible)

Coagulation studies (PT, PTT, fibrinogen, FDP, or D-dimers) in suspected AML (especially APL)

Type and screen for red cell transfusion, if necessary

If febrile or ill-appearing: blood and urine cultures

Radiographic studies

Chest radiograph (assess for mediastinal mass)

Plain bone films of sites of bone pain (assess for pathological fractures)

Diagnostic studies

Bone marrow aspiration

Specimens for morphology, immunophenotyping, and karyotype

    Extra "pulls" as per protocol for biological studies (Children's Oncology Group or local institutional studies)

    For "dry" tap, obtain bone marrow biopsy for diagnostic studies

Lumbar puncture (platelet count ≥ 50–100×10^9/L per institutional protocol)

    Cytology, chamber count (WBC, RBC, protein, and glucose), and CSF culture if patient is febrile

    Initial procedure should be done by an experienced clinician, after careful evaluation for elevated ICP

Abbreviations: DIC, disseminated intravascular coagulation; CBC, complete blood count; BUN, blood urea nitrogen; LDH, lactate dehydrogenase; PT, prothrombin time; PTT, partial thromboplastin time; AML, acute myelogenous leukemia; APL, acute promyelocytic leukemia (AML M3); WBC, white blood cell; RBC, red blood cell; CSF, cerebrospinal fluid; ICP, intracranial pressure; FDP, fibrin degradation products; CMV, cytomegalovirus; HSV, herpes simpex virus.

Bone marrow examination with aspirate and/or biopsy is indicated in the following situations:

• Significant depression of one or more peripheral blood lineages (white cells, red cells, and platelets) without an obvious explanation

• Presence of circulating blasts on the peripheral blood smear

• Any cytopenias associated with unexplained lymphadenopathy, splenomegaly, hepatomegaly, anterior mediastinal mass, or bone pain.

Bleeding as a presenting sign in cancer is usually related to severe thrombocytopenia and occurs commonly in children with acute leukemia. Manifestations typically involve mucocutaneous tissues with clinical signs including petechiae, purpura, epistaxis, and menorrhagia. Patients with acute promyelocytic leukemia (APL; AML M3) are at risk for severe bleeding at presentation due to underlying coagulation abnormalities and disseminated intravascular coagulation (DIC), whereas Wilms tumor patients may have acquired von Willebrand disease at presentation increasing bleeding risk. Patients with extensive marrow involvement such as advanced stage neuroblastoma may also present with significant purpura.

Mediastinal masses may lead to compression of respiratory, vascular, or other structures and can range from an asymptomatic incidental finding to significant compromise and an emergent situation. Most mediastinal masses in children are malignant. Imaging with chest radiography and chest CT yields information with respect to location in the mediastinum and potential for compromise.

Anterior mediastinal masses are more typically seen in older children and adolescents and frequently are associated with lymphomas, T-cell leukemia, thymic tumors, thyroid tumors, and some benign tumors (teratomas, lipomas, and angiomas). Malignant tumors, especially lymphomas and leukemia, may have rapid growth rates and quickly lead to compromise with presentation of superior vena cava syndrome, airway obstruction, dysphagia, and symptoms of increased intracranial pressure due to decreased cerebral venous return. The mass may cause a pericardial effusion or directly obstruct cardiac outflow leading to cardiac compromise. See Chapter 14 for assessment and management.

Middle mediastinal masses are also more likely malignant. Infections should be in the differential diagnosis and one should consider tuberculosis or histoplasmosis in addition to pericardial cysts, bronchogenic cysts, esophageal lesions, or direct extension of an abdominal mass. Malignant tumors common in this location include Hodgkin lymphoma and nodal masses of neuroblastoma, rhabdomyosarcoma, and germ cell tumors.

Posterior mediastinal masses are generally neurogenic in origin and include benign and malignant tumors. These include ganglioneuroma, neurofibroma, and neuroblastoma. Most of these lesions are asymptomatic, but may present with symptoms of spinal cord compression such as pain or focal neurological signs.

A palpable **abdominal mass** is one of the most common presenting findings of a malignant solid tumor in children. Nonmalignant etiologies include impacted stool, intussusception, abdominal aorta, a distended bladder, hydronephrotic kidneys, and pregnancy.

The **age** of the child can provide a clue to diagnosis. In the newborn, an abdominal mass is most likely to be a congenital abnormality of renal origin. The most common malignant tumors in young children are neuroblastoma and Wilms tumor. Children with Wilms tumor most often present well appearing and the mass is an incidental finding by a family member or during a well-child check. Unlike Wilms tumor, neuroblastoma will often present with evidence of spread and systemic symptoms including weight loss, fever, and bone pain. In older patients, the mass may be related to leukemia or lymphoma with enlargement of the spleen and liver. The most common lymphoma in children is Burkitt lymphoma that may present as a rapidly enlarging abdominal mass leading to pain and obstructive symptoms (gastrointestinal and urinary tracts) in association with metabolic derangements from tumor lysis. Burkitt and other lymphomas, as well as primary gastrointestinal tumors, may also occur in the ileocecal area and serve as a lead point for intussusception.

The **history** is important to determine if the symptoms are related to the mass. A careful genitourinary history should be obtained to determine if the mass may be of renal origin. Historical points may provide suspicion of catecholamine production such as flushing, palpitations, diarrhea, and sweating (very rare). Constitutional symptoms such as failure to thrive, fever, night sweats, and sudden weight loss should lead one to suspect a disseminated process such as neuroblastoma in young children or lymphoma in older children and adolescents.

A meticulous and careful **physical examination** of the child should be done by first attempting to have the child relax. When examining the abdomen, keep in mind the normal structures that may be present such as the liver or spleen edges, kidneys, aorta, sigmoid colon, stool, or spine. A rectal examination and pelvic/vaginal examination may be indicated but should be performed only by an experienced practitioner and after obtaining laboratory studies (should not be neutropenic for a rectal examination). Care should be taken to palpate the mass gently and limit the number of examiners. Imaging will also help determine size and location. A careful general physical examination is vital as many tumors may have associated signs and symptoms or underlying syndromes. Aniridia, hemihypertrophy, and genitourinary abnormalities have been reported in association with Wilms tumor. Subcutaneous nodules (typically bluish), periorbital ecchymoses, opsoclonus-myoclonus, and presence of organomegaly are seen with neuroblastoma. Signs of precocious puberty may be seen with tumors involving the liver, adrenal glands, or gonads (i.e., germ cell tumors). The neurological examination may show evidence of a Horner's syndrome with apical tumors (often neuroblastoma) or spine compression with large abdominal masses. See Table 13.4 for the workup of a child with

---

Table 13.4 Evaluation of the child with an abdominal mass.

History and physical examination

Radiological studies

First steps
  Flat plate and upright views of the abdomen
  Abdominal ultrasound
Further assessment as needed
  Abdominal/pelvis CT or MRI
  Chest CT if with abdominal primary to assess extent of local disease and presence of metastatic
    disease
  Bone scan in suspected neuroblastoma, rhabdomyosarcoma, clear cell or rhabdoid tumor of the
    kidney
  MRI and plain radiography of the spine in tumors with neurologic impairment or other
    radiographic suggestion of spinal invasion
  MIBG scan for neuroblastoma

Laboratory studies

First steps
  CBC with differential, reticulocyte count (bleeding into mass may cause iron deficiency anemia;
    tumor may also involve the bone marrow and cause cytopenias), and review of peripheral
    smear
  Electrolytes, calcium, phosphorus, uric acid, LDH, BUN, creatinine, and liver transaminases
  Urinalysis
As indicated by history/examination/imaging:
  Urine for tumor markers: catecholamines (VMA and HVA)
  Serum markers: neuron-specific enolase, α-fetoprotein, β-HCG, ESR, copper, and ferritin
  Bone marrow aspirate/biopsy; if neuroblastoma, lymphoma, or rhabdomyosarcoma suspected
    or confirmed

Abbreviations: CT, computed tomography; MRI, magnetic resonance imaging; MIBG, metaiodobenzylguanidine; CBC, complete blood count; LDH, lactate dehydrogenase; BUN, blood urea nitrogen; VMA, vanillylmandelic acid; HVA, homovanillic acid; HCG, human chorionic gonadotrophin; ESR, erythrocyte sedimentation rate.

an abdominal mass. A **surgical consultation** should be obtained and the decision made whether to obtain a biopsy or perform a resection of the mass. Surgical staging is done by assessing tumor margins, nodal involvement, presence of locally invasive or distant disease, and for possible tumor spillage (see Chapters 18 and 19).

Suggested Reading

Neville KA, Steuber CP. Clinical assessment of the child with suspected cancer. In Basow DS (ed), UpToDate. Waltham, MA, 2011.

Wilne S, Koller K, Collier J, et al. The diagnosis of brain tumours in children: a guideline to assist healthcare professionals in the assessment of children who may have a brain tumour. Arch Dis Child 95:534–539, 2010.

14 Oncologic Emergencies

The prognosis for children diagnosed with cancer has steadily improved over the past 50 years, and it is now estimated that more than 80% of children newly diagnosed with cancer will ultimately be cured of their disease. Given this positive outlook, it becomes even more important that life-threatening complications arising either as a result of the patient's cancer diagnosis or the treatment being provided be promptly recognized and appropriately treated.

Oncologic emergencies can be categorized based on their pathogenesis, including emergencies caused by space-occupying lesions, those caused by abnormalities of blood and blood vessels, and metabolic emergencies.

Emergencies caused by space-occupying lesions

Superior vena cava syndrome and superior mediastinal syndrome

Superior vena cava syndrome (SVCS) refers to the signs and symptoms resulting from the compression or obstruction of the SVC caused by an anterior mediastinal mass. These include orthopnea, headache, facial swelling, dizziness or fainting, sudden pallor, and exacerbation of symptoms with the Valsalva maneuver. The physical examination often reveals a plethoric, edematous face and neck, jugular venous distension, papilledema, and pulsus paradoxus. Blood pressure changes, pallor, and even cardiac arrest can result from postural changes. Superior mediastinal syndrome is the combination of SVCS and tracheal compression that leads to symptoms of cough, dyspnea, air hunger, and wheezing. Examination often reveals decreased breath sounds, wheezing, stridor, or cyanosis. Affected children are often incredibly anxious as well.

Malignant tumors are the most common primary cause of SVCS. The most common cause is non-Hodgkin lymphoma (NHL; usually lymphoblastic lymphoma or diffuse large B-cell lymphoma). Other malignant causes include Hodgkin lymphoma, T-cell acute lymphoblastic leukemia (T-ALL), malignant teratoma, thymoma, neuroblastoma, rhabdomyosarcoma, or Ewing sarcoma. A secondary cause can be thrombosis of the major vessels caused by the presence of a central venous catheter. Nonmalignant causes include mediastinal granulomas (histoplasmosis), aortic aneurysms, vascular thrombosis complicating cardiovascular surgery for congenital heart disease, shunting for hydrocephalus, catheterizations, and infections (e.g., tuberculosis and syphilis).

Handbook of Pediatric Hematology and Oncology: Children's Hospital & Research Center Oakland,
Second Edition. Caroline A. Hastings, Joseph C. Torkildson, and Anurag K. Agrawal.
© 2012 John Wiley & Sons, Ltd. Published 2012 by John Wiley & Sons, Ltd.

The SVC is a thin-walled vessel with low intraluminal pressure, prone to thrombosis, and surrounded by thymus and nodes that drain the right side and lower left side of the chest. Part of the SVC is also in the pericardial reflection. Lymph nodes, thymus, and the pericardium may become enlarged from infection or tumor involvement and compress the SVC. Adjacent coronary and collateral vessels can become clotted. Compression, clotting, and edema lead to diminished air flow and blood flow. Additionally, the trachea and right mainstem bronchus are less rigid in children as compared to adults.

Evaluation

1. *History and physical examination.* The history is nonspecific, with a typically short period of progressively worsening symptoms. Patients with ALL may have a short history of fever, bone pain, bruising, petechiae, or other signs of marrow dysfunction. Presenting symptoms and signs include cough and dyspnea (commonest), closely followed by dysphagia, orthopnea, hoarseness, chest pain, facial edema, wheezing, pleural effusion, pericardial effusion, features of carbon dioxide retention like anxiety, confusion, lethargy, headache, distorted vision, and syncope, and occasionally other symptoms like conjunctival suffusion and cyanosis.

2. *Chest radiography including a lateral view.* This usually shows mediastinal widening, tracheal deviation or compression, and possibly pleural effusions.

3. *CT scan of the chest.* This helps delineate distortion of normal anatomy, identify tracheal compression, and allow assessment of mediastinal mass width. This may be done in the prone position if the patient is unable to lie supine.

4. *Tissue diagnosis with least invasive procedures, with no sedation, and local anesthesia only.* A biopsy is essential for diagnosis, but must be able to be performed safely.

General anesthesia may cause cardiovascular and/or respiratory compromise by increasing abdominal tone and decreasing respiratory muscle tone and lung volume. Sedatives can also decrease venous return and should be used cautiously.

5. *Bone marrow aspiration under local anesthesia.* If the bone marrow is involved, this test will allow the diagnosis to be made without a biopsy of the mass itself.

6. *Examination of pleural fluid/pericardial fluid/ascitic fluid.* In addition to relieving distress, removal of fluid and subsequent cytological examination may allow a definitive diagnosis to be made, especially in the case of NHL.

7. *Echocardiography.* This is necessary to look for pericardial effusion and cardiac tamponade and to evaluate myocardial function.

8. *Pulmonary function tests.* The patient's peak expiratory flow rate and the shape of the flow volume loop can reliably predict the patient's ability to tolerate various diagnostic and therapeutic procedures.

9. *Measurement of β-HCG (β-subunit of human chorionic gonadotrophin) and AFP (α-fetoprotein).* Elevations in these markers are diagnostic of a malignant germ cell tumor, but they are generally not available urgently.

Management

1. Children should be under close observation in the intensive care unit with elevation of the head, continuous cardiovascular and respiratory monitoring, and pulse oximetry.

2. Children with impending or actual airway obstruction should receive emergent radiation therapy, given in 1 to 2 Gy fractions for 1 to 4 days. A small area of the tumor should be shielded to prevent radiation-induced changes if a biopsy still needs to be performed to establish the diagnosis. The surgeon and radiation oncologist should communicate to ensure that the most easily accessible area is shielded.

Tracheal swelling and further airway compromise can occur as a result of the radiation.

3. Empiric therapy for suspected malignancy may need to be initiated due to the life-threatening situation. Steroids, cyclophosphamide, vincristine, or anthracyclines have been given in this situation to children with suspected leukemia or lymphoma. Prednisone is commonly used as most of these children are ultimately diagnosed with lymphoma or leukemia, especially if other clues to the diagnosis are apparent (e.g., organomegaly, generalized adenopathy, evidence of tumor lysis syndrome [TLS], elevated WBC [white blood cell] counts). Intravenous methylprednisolone is started at a dose of $50 \, mg/m^2$/day divided BD. Hydration should be given and the child monitored for tumor lysis syndrome that may be exacerbated by the initiation of therapy and is discussed later.

Spinal cord compression

Acute spinal cord compression occurs in about 5% of children with cancer. Prolonged cord compression leads to irreversible neurological injury with paralysis, sensory loss, and loss of bowel and bladder control. Once a neurological deficit occurs, it often progresses to paraplegia within days or even hours. The most frequent cause of cord compression is external compression caused by extension of a paravertebral tumor through an intervertebral foramen into the epidural space. The tumor compresses the vertebral venous plexus leading to cord edema, venous hemorrhage, myelopathy, and ischemia. The most common tumors leading to spinal cord compression include neuroblastoma, Ewing sarcoma, NHL, and Hodgkin lymphoma. Intraspinous chloromas in patients with acute myelogenous leukemia (AML) are a less common cause. Spinal cord astrocytomas and ependymomas can also cause cord

compression, more commonly from an intramedullary location.

Evaluation

1. Localized back pain or radicular pain extending down the leg occurs in up to 80% of children with cord compression. The duration is variable but generally short; one series reported a range of 5 days to 4 weeks. Characteristically, straight leg raising, neck flexion, or the Valsalva maneuver aggravates the pain. Pain is almost always the first presenting symptom, with weakness and bowel or bladder dysfunction occurring later. Sensory loss may occur but is often difficult to identify, especially in young children. Any objective neurological deficit requires further evaluation.

2. Plain radiographs are generally not helpful in identifying abnormalities in children, as cord compression typically occurs via extension of tumor through the intervertebral foramina without bony erosion or injury. MRI is the best study for demonstrating intraspinous extension, but is not always immediate available. While CT is less sensitive in identifying extension of disease into the spinal canal, it will effectively identify paraspinous disease.

3. Examination of the cerebrospinal fluid (CSF) is rarely helpful, and patients may experience rapid neurological deterioration following a lumbar puncture (spinal coning).

Management

1. Patients with rapidly progressing spinal cord dysfunction require immediate intervention. Dexamethasone 1 mg/kg should be given IV even before imaging is performed, and an MRI should be obtained immediately. Patients with suspicious findings who are stable should be started on a lower dose of oral dexamethasone (0.25 to 0.5 mg/kg every 6 hours) with imaging performed within 24 hours.

2. If imaging reveals a tumor with spinal cord compression, this must be promptly relieved. Surgical decompression with a laminectomy quickly relieves pressure and allows tumor to be removed for diagnosis. It should be performed if the diagnosis is unknown. If the diagnosis is known and the tumor is radiosensitive, emergent radiation therapy should be promptly initiated. Chemotherapy is an alternative for chemotherapy-responsive tumors such as neuroblastoma, Ewing sarcoma, Hodgkin lymphoma, and NHL; the onset of action in these tumors is similar to radiation therapy.

The prognosis for recovery of function is directly related to the degree of disability at diagnosis. This is associated with the duration of symptoms and the length of time required to make the diagnosis. Patients who are ambulatory at diagnosis typically remain ambulatory; approximately 50% of children who are nonambulatory at diagnosis regain the ability to ambulate.

Increased intracranial pressure and brain herniation

Brain tumors are the most common solid tumor in childhood, and the majority of patients present with signs and symptoms of increased intracranial pressure (ICP). Fortunately, few of these patients progress to actual brain herniation. Most pediatric brain tumors are infratentorial and cause increased ICP by obstructing the third or fourth ventricle with resultant obstructive hydrocephalus. They can also cause increased ICP simply by mass effect. This most commonly occurs with astrocytomas, as well as with primitive neuroectodermal tumors including medulloblastoma.

The presentation can vary significantly depending on patient age. Common symptoms in infants include vomiting, lethargy, personality changes, loss of developmental milestones, and increased head circumference. Older children commonly complain of headache. This is frequently intermittent at first, and then becomes more frequent and severe. It characteristically occurs in the morning, and is often but not always accompanied by vomiting without diarrhea. Other signs and symptoms include diplopia, ataxia, hemiparesis, speech disturbance, neck stiffness, dizziness, lethargy, and coma.

Some tumors may also cause focal neurological changes. Cerebellar astrocytomas may lead to ipsilateral weakness, hypotonia, and ataxia. Herniation of a cerebellar tonsil often causes head tilt and neck stiffness. Tumors near the third ventricle (craniopharyngiomas, germ cell tumors, optic gliomas, and hypothalamic and pituitary tumors) may cause visual loss, increased intracranial pressure, and hydrocephalus. A pineal tumor may lead to Parinaud's syndrome (impairment of upward gaze, convergence nystagmus, and alterations in pupillary response).

Evaluation

1. Assessment of vital signs is critical. Increased ICP will often result in Cushing's triad: bradycardia, hypertension, and apnea.
2. A careful physical examination looking for signs of increased ICP or impending herniation must be done quickly. In addition to the findings mentioned above, impending brain herniation may cause changes in respiratory pattern, pupil size and reactivity, extraocular movements, spontaneous motor function, and responsiveness to verbal and physical stimuli.

Management

If increased ICP or impending brain herniation is suspected, appropriate management must be initiated prior to more definitive testing to hopefully avoid death or permanent neurological injury. The following steps should be initiated:
1. Fluid intake should be limited to no more than 75% maintenance.

2. A loading dose of dexamethasone 0.5 to 1 mg/kg should be given IV followed by 0.25 to 0.5 mg/kg every 6 hours.

3. An emergent CT scan of the head should be performed. A noncontrast scan will effectively identify bleeding, most tumors, cerebral edema, and hydrocephalus.

4. If the diagnosis of increased ICP is confirmed, the patient should be admitted to the ICU. Neurosurgical consultation should be immediately obtained if a tumor is identified or the patient has hydrocephalus.

5. Acetazolamide 5 mg/kg/dose every 6 hours can be given to decrease CSF production.

6. Intubation and hyperventilation to decrease the pCO_2 to 20 to 25 mmHg will decrease cerebral perfusion. Care must be taken not to cause cerebral ischemia.

7. Surgical options (external ventricular drainage, third ventriculostomy) should be considered.

8. Prophylaxis with antiseizure medication should also be considered.

9. Intracranial pressure monitoring may be beneficial.

10. An MRI should be obtained as soon as possible to look for or confirm the presence of a tumor.

Massive hepatomegaly

Massive hepatomegaly is the most emergent complication of stage 4S neuroblastoma in infants, especially those under 4 weeks of age. While 4S neuroblastoma often regresses spontaneously, when it occurs during early infancy the resulting hepatomegaly can cause death due to respiratory insufficiency or hepatic failure.

Evaluation

1. The patient should be examined for evidence of gastrointestinal dysfunction, respiratory compromise (respiratory rate >60/min or oxygen requirement), poor venous return (leg edema), renal dysfunction (poor

urine output and azotemia), or disseminated intravascular coagulation.

2. A biopsy and staging evaluation including CT scan of the chest, abdomen, and pelvis, bone scan, bilateral bone marrow aspiration and biopsy, and other imaging such as MRI of the brain and spine should be performed quickly if the patient is able to tolerate these procedures. This will allow prompt initiation of appropriate therapy.

Treatment

1. If the patient is stable and does not exhibit any of the findings above, careful observation and supportive care should be provided.

2. If the patient is unstable, treatment with chemotherapy or radiation therapy should be considered. Cyclophosphamide 5 mg/kg/day for 5 days has been shown to be effective, as has radiation therapy at a dose of 150 cGy/day × 3 days.

Emergencies caused by abnormalities of blood and blood vessels

Hyperleukocytosis

Hyperleukocytosis is defined as a peripheral WBC count exceeding 100×10^9/L. It is most commonly seen at presentation or relapse of AML, ALL, or chronic myelogenous leukemia (CML). Using this definition, the incidence of hyperleukocytosis at presentation is 9% to 13% of children with ALL, 5% to 22% with AML, and almost all children in chronic phase of CML. However, clinically significant hyperleukocytosis occurs with WBC counts $>200 \times 10^9$/L in AML and $>300 \times 10^9$/L in ALL and CML. Using these criteria, the incidence is lower. The most common complication of hyperleukocytosis in AML and CML is stroke, whereas in ALL it is TLS. It is more common in infantile ALL and AML, T-cell ALL, and in any phase of CML.

Hyperleukocytosis leads to occlusion of small veins in the brain, lung, and other organs through the formation of WBC aggregates (white thrombi). The excessive leukocytes also cause local hypoxia by competing for available oxygen, leading to blood vessel damage and bleeding. The degree of obstruction is related to the whole blood viscosity, which is related to the deformability of the cells present and the sum of the packed erythrocyte and packed leukocyte volumes. As myeloblasts and monoblasts are less deformable than lymphoblasts or granulocytes, leukostasis is more likely to occur in AML than in ALL or CML. Other factors that can increase the risk of leukostasis include dehydration and an elevated hemoglobin level.

Poor perfusion and anaerobic metabolism in the microcirculation lead to lactic acidosis. When the WBC count is $>300 \times 10^9$/L, local proliferation of cells occurs within the cerebral vasculature and brain and vessel damage occurs, leading to secondary hemorrhage. Vessel damage can occur anywhere in the body, though the most clinically significant is in the brain and lungs.

Evaluation

1. Signs and symptoms of leukemia are usually present (pallor, fatigue, fever, bleeding, bone pain, adenopathy, organomegaly, anemia, thrombocytopenia).
2. Possible signs and symptoms of leukostasis in the lungs or brain include hypoxia, acidosis, dyspnea, cyanosis, blurred vision, papilledema, stupor, coma, or ataxia. Priapism may also occur in this setting.
3. The laboratory assessment should include frequent monitoring (q6 to 8 hours) of the WBC count to follow the rate of rise or the response to therapy. Metabolic studies also need close monitoring as the child may have evidence of tumor lysis and renal dysfunction. Evaluate electrolytes, BUN, creatinine, uric acid, calcium, phosphorus,

magnesium, liver function studies, and LDH at presentation, and then follow the electrolytes, BUN, creatinine, calcium, phosphorus, and uric acid frequently to assess response to therapy.

Treatment

1. Therapeutic intervention should be immediate.
2. If the child is being transported, these simple measures should be initiated prior to transport. The mainstay of therapy is aggressive hydration, typically two to three times maintenance intravenous fluids. The fluids should be alkalinized to promote excretion of uric acid by converting it to a more soluble urate salt. A fluid such as D_5W 1/4NS with 40 mEq/L $NaHCO_3$ is quite suitable. Allopurinol or urate oxidase (rasburicase) should also be started to prevent or decrease the severity of hyperuricemia. If urate oxidase is given, alkalinization is not required as the uric acid level falls precipitously and uric acid solubility is no longer an issue. This topic is discussed more fully in the section on TLS.
3. If aggressive hydration does not bring the WBC count down quickly to 100 to 200×10^9/L or the WBC count is rapidly rising due to rapid tumor growth, cytoreduction may be necessary. Two techniques that have been used previously to acutely decrease the number of circulating WBCs are leukapheresis and exchange transfusion. Because of the infectious disease concerns with exchange transfusion, leukapheresis is used almost exclusively where it is available and technically feasible. The purpose of leukapheresis is to decrease tumor bulk, decrease the risk of TLS, and correct the anemia and hyperviscosity (goal of >30% leukocyte reduction with leukapheresis). If used, single volume exchange transfusion should be performed with repeat laboratory analysis to determine effectiveness. Further exchanges can be

performed to reach the goal of a total WBC count $<200 \times 10^9$/L.

4. Therapy for the underlying malignancy should begin as soon as possible and is the only permanent therapy for hyperleukocytosis. In general, it is safer from a metabolic viewpoint to initiate chemotherapy with a lower WBC.

5. Emergency cranial radiation therapy has not been demonstrated to improve outcome and is not recommended.

6. Platelet transfusions can be given safely in small volumes, as platelets have not been shown to increase viscosity or worsen leukostasis. Platelets should be given if the child is bleeding or the platelet count is $<20 \times 10^9$/L. Red cell transfusions should be given with extreme caution due to the potential to increase total blood viscosity and worsen leukostasis. The only indication is cardiovascular compromise caused by anemia. The hemoglobin level should be kept below 10 g/dL.

Anemia

Anemia is a common finding in children presenting with malignancy. Up to 80% of children presenting with ALL will be anemic at diagnosis. This can result from bleeding, inflammation, or marrow infiltration by tumor. It is rarely an emergency; children can tolerate a hemoglobin level as low as 2 to 3 g/dL if it develops slowly from decreased production. Conversely, levels as low as 5 g/dL can be life threatening if they occur as a result of sudden hemorrhage.

Treatment

1. Anemia in this situation is treated with packed red blood cell (PRBC) transfusions. As a general rule, 10 mL/kg of PRBCs will increase the hemoglobin level by 2 to 3 g/dL. In practice, children with acute anemia due to blood loss may need 15 to 20 mL/kg to reach this level.

2. Several authors of textbooks on pediatric oncology recommend that children with profound anemia (hemoglobin <5 g/dL) that has developed over an extended period of time be transfused more slowly (1 vs. 3 mL/kg/h) to avoid causing congestive heart failure. This concern is based on an extrapolation of the Starling law of cardiac physiology, but there are few data supporting this concern. Two published studies as well as experience in our own institution suggest that this practice is unnecessary, especially if these children are being cared for in the ICU where more careful monitoring is being performed. This can avoid potentially exposing patients to additional donor units unnecessarily.

3. All blood products given to known or potential oncology patients should be irradiated to prevent transfusion-associated graft-versus-host disease (TA-GVHD). They should also be leukoreduced to decrease the risk of CMV transmission.

4. Erythropoietin is not used in children at this time to increase the hemoglobin and decrease the need for transfusion due to data from adult studies that suggest patients receiving erythropoietin have inferior outcomes compared to those who do not.

Leukopenia

Leukopenia is commonly found in newly diagnosed oncology patients as well as during therapy. This predisposes them to a variety of infections with bacteria, viruses, fungi, and protozoa. The evaluation and management of this is discussed in Chapter 27.

Coagulopathy

Coagulopathy in children with cancer results from a variety of mechanisms. The most common is thrombocytopenia, which can result from decreased platelet production (marrow infiltration or adverse effect of therapy) or from increased consumption (infection/DIC, splenomegaly, and sinusoidal obstruction syndrome). Abnormal platelet function is seen in patients with uremia. Reduced levels of coagulation factors are seen in patients with liver disease or in DIC when coagulation factors are abnormally consumed. It is important to remember that consumption can deplete anticoagulant proteins as well, potentially making the patient hypercoagulable.

Evaluation

1. The CBC will reveal thrombocytopenia, and the prothrombin time (PT), partial thromboplastin time (PTT), fibrinogen, and D-dimers will provide evidence of a clotting disorder.
2. Patients presenting with a stroke-like syndrome should have measurements of protein C, protein S, and antithrombin III, especially if they have recently received asparaginase therapy.
3. A patient with an alteration in consciousness or neurological abnormalities associated with symptoms or signs suggestive of a coagulopathy should have a noncontrast CT scan of the brain performed emergently looking for evidence of bleeding or thrombosis.

Management

1. The short-term therapy for thrombocytopenia is platelet transfusion. Patients who are ill or unstable should be transfused to keep their platelet count $>20 \times 10^9/L$. Patients who are actively bleeding should be transfused if their platelet count is $<50 \times 10^9/L$ in case they have a component of platelet dysfunction. Patients undergoing invasive procedures (intubation, central venous catheter placement, or biopsy) should be transfused to a platelet count of 50 to $100 \times 10^9/L$ depending on the procedure.
2. One pheresed unit of platelets/m^2 will typically increase the platelet count by 50 to $60 \times 10^9/L$, although the increase in platelet count is less predictable than the increase in hemoglobin following PRBC transfusion.
3. As with PRBCs, platelets should be irradiated and leukoreduced to decrease the risk of TA-GVHD and CMV transmission, respectively.
4. Patients with bleeding and an abnormal PT/PTT should receive fresh frozen plasma (FFP) at a dose of 10 mL/kg. This will correct most clotting factor deficiencies with the exception of Factor VIII and fibrinogen. Patients with a fibrinogen level <100 mg/dL or a persistently prolonged PTT despite FFP replacement should receive cryoprecipitate at a dose of 5 mL/kg; a typical unit of cryoprecipitate has a volume of 20 to 50 mL. FFP and cryoprecipitate do not need to be irradiated or leukoreduced as they are acellular products and have no risk of causing TA-GVHD or transmitting CMV.

Metabolic emergencies

Tumor lysis syndrome

TLS is a pattern of specific metabolic abnormalities that occurs as a result of extremely rapid cellular turnover. It is almost always encountered in the context of malignant tumors that either have a rapid rate of apoptosis or after initiation of therapy in bulky tumors that are exquisitely sensitive to the therapy being provided. The rapid lysis of tumor cells in either situation causes large amounts of potassium, phosphate, and nucleic acids to be released into the circulation, resulting in hyperuricemia, hyperphosphatemia, and hyperkalemia. When the uric acid concentration in the renal tubule exceeds its solubility coefficient, urate crystals form in the tubule causing obstruction. Lactic acidosis, secondary to poor tissue oxygenation in patients with high WBC counts, may contribute to uric acid deposition. In addition, phosphates are released when tumor cells lyse. When the calcium– phosphorus product exceeds 60, precipitation occurs in the microvasculature, particularly in an alkaline environment, further obstructing the renal tubules and resulting in hypocalcemia. Lymphoblasts are particularly rich in phosphate, containing up to four times the amount found in normal lymphocytes. Potassium is also released from tumor cells, is secondarily elevated in poor renal function, and can lead to fatal arrhythmia. The complete syndrome includes all these components, with progressively worsening renal failure. Tumor infiltration of the kidney and dehydration can further impair renal function and accelerate the development of TLS.

In children, TLS develops most frequently in association with Burkitt lymphoma or T-ALL. These malignancies typically present with a large tumor mass, short doubling time (38 to 116 hours in Burkitt lymphoma), poor urine output, and elevated uric acid and LDH. TLS has also been reported in children with hepatoblastoma and advanced stage neuroblastoma.

Evaluation

1. Evaluate for signs and symptoms of metabolic abnormalities. These include lethargy, nausea, vomiting, hypotension, muscle spasm, and cardiac dysrhythmia.
2. Perform a metabolic panel in all children with suspected malignancy to assess for TLS. Frequent reassessments should be performed early in therapy as well, particularly in patients with high tumor burdens and those expected to respond rapidly to treatment. The timing of this will depend on the underlying disease, evidence of preexisting renal dysfunction, timing of initiation of therapy, and the risk of TLS.

3. Carefully monitor vital signs, intake and output for evidence of renal insufficiency, and possible symptoms of hypocalcemia (anorexia, vomiting, cramps, spasms, tetany, and seizures). A renal ultrasound may be indicated in suspected renal dysfunction.

Therapy

1. Aggressive hydration should be provided at a rate of two to three times maintenance. If alkalinization of serum and urine is desired, an appropriate starting fluid is D_5W 1/4NS+ 40 mEq/L $NaHCO_3$. The bicarbonate should then be titrated to keep the urine pH between 7 and 7.5, which will optimize the excretion of both uric acid and calcium phosphate.
2. An agent to prevent or reverse hyperuricemia should also be initiated immediately. Allopurinol is the most commonly used agent for this purpose, and it can be given at presentation and as needed during the early phase of therapy for the prevention or treatment of TLS. The urine is typically alkalinized when allopurinol is used, as it often does not cause a significant decrease in the uric acid level until the rate of tumor lysis slows. It is given at a dose of $300 \, mg/m^2/day$ divided every 8 hours (800 mg/day maximum). Another agent, rasburicase (urate oxidase), is a recombinant enzyme that acts as a catalyst in the degradation of uric acid into allantoin, a highly soluble product compared with uric acid. It works quickly (within 30 minutes of IV infusion) and keeps the uric acid level low for 12 to 24 hours or longer, depending on the underlying rate of cell turnover. Rasburicase has been studied in children with cancer who have hyperuricemia as a result of tumor lysis and has been found to be safe and effective. However, it is quite expensive compared to allopurinol. Many hospital pharmacies have practice guidelines that specify the conditions where

rasburicase should be prescribed to avoid overuse. It is given at a dose of 0.15 to 0.2 mg/kg/day in 50 mL preservative-free normal saline IV over 30 minutes. While the package insert states that this dose should be repeated daily for up to 5 days, in practice a single dose will often keep the uric acid level low for 48 hours or more, and may be sufficient to prevent TLS for the entire course. Patients treated with rasburicase do not require alkalinization, which is an advantage when managing other electrolyte abnormalities. It will precipitate hemolysis in patients with G6PD deficiency and has caused methemoglobinemia in susceptible individuals. Routine screening for G6PD deficiency is not recommended before use, but families should be asked about this possibility. It also has rarely caused anaphylaxis.

3. Potassium should not be added to IV fluids until it is clear that the potassium is stable and not increasing due to TLS or renal insufficiency.

4. The patient's intake and output must be closely monitored to ensure it remains balanced, taking into account insensible losses.

5. Careful metabolic monitoring should be performed.

6. An ECG should be obtained if the potassium is 7 mEq/L or higher. This may show widened QRS complexes and peaked T waves in hyperkalemia. Symptomatic hyperkalemia requires immediate therapy with calcium gluconate, albuterol, and glucose and insulin, along with kayexalate to remove excess potassium from the body. If this is ineffective, continuous renal replacement therapy or dialysis may be required.

7. If hyperphosphatemia is present, treatment is forced saline diuresis with furosemide and dietary phosphate restriction. Oral phosphate binders are typically not effective, as they do nothing to remove phosphate from the circulation. Persistent hyperphosphatemia may require dialysis.

Hypercalcemia

Malignancy-associated hypercalcemia (MAH) is a rare complication of childhood cancer, occurring in 0.4% to 1.3% of newly diagnosed cases. It is seen most frequently in ALL and alveolar rhabdomyosarcoma, but has also been reported in children diagnosed with rhabdoid tumor, hepatoblastoma, Hodgkin lymphoma, NHL, AML, brain tumors, and neuroblastoma. The cause of MAH can be increased bone resorption from skeletal metastases or production of calcium-mobilizing substances such as parathyroid hormone (PTH)-related peptide or osteoclast-activating factor by the tumor. MAH in turn adversely affects the ability of the kidney to concentrate the urine, leading to dehydration, decreased glomerular filtration rate (GFR), a further reduction in calcium excretion, and worsening hypercalcemia.

Evaluation

1. Symptoms of mild hypercalcemia (12 to 15 mg/dL) include generalized weakness, poor appetite, nausea, vomiting, constipation, abdominal or back pain, polyuria, and drowsiness. More severe hypercalcemia (>15 mg/dL) results in profound muscle weakness, severe nausea and vomiting, coma, and bradydysrhythmias with broad T waves and prolonged PR interval on the ECG.

2. Patients exhibiting any of these symptoms should have a serum Ca^{2+} level measured immediately. Measurement of an ionized Ca^{2+} should be done if there is any question about the validity of the total calcium measurement or to rule out primary hyperparathyroidism or pseudohypercalcemia due to increased plasma protein binding capacity.

3. Measurement of the intact parathyroid hormone (PTH) level should be performed to exclude concomitant hyperparathyroidism. PTH levels are usually low, normal, or suppressed in MAH. The serum concentration of calcitriol should be measured when the hypercalcemia is suspected to be due to Hodgkin lymphoma or NHL, as it has been implicated as a key mediator of hypercalcemia in almost all cases of Hodgkin lymphoma and 30% to 40% of cases of NHL.

Treatment

1. The goals of treatment are to increase renal clearance of calcium and decrease bone resorption.

2. Aggressive hydration will help increase renal excretion of calcium. Forced diuresis with normal saline at two to three times maintenance and furosemide 2 to 3 mg/kg every 2 hours was previously recommended. Furosemide blocks calcium reabsorption by the kidney, and can decrease the calcium level in 24 to 48 hours. However, a recent meta-analysis suggests the data to support this approach are limited, and it can also cause severe loss of sodium, potassium, and magnesium. At present, the use of furosemide is recommended only for patients experiencing fluid overload following aggressive saline diuresis.

3. If the patient is hypophosphatemic, phosphate replacement at a dose of 10 mg/kg/dose 2 to 3 times/day may inhibit osteoclastic activity and promote calcium deposition into bone.

4. Bisphosphonates have become the treatment of choice for adults with MAH, but these have not been widely studied in children. The most published experience is with pamidronate at a dose of 0.5 to 2 mg/kg given IV over 2 to 24 hours. This has been highly successful in correcting MAH within 1 to 4 days of treatment. When MAH is associated with ALL, rapid initiation of induction therapy has been shown to be very important in reversing the hypercalcemia.

Suggested Reading

Coiffier B, Altman A, Pui CH, et al. Guidelines for the management of pediatric and adult tumor lysis syndrome: an evidence based review. J Clin Oncol 26:2767–2778, 2008.

Kelly KM, Lang B. Oncologic emergencies. Pediatr Clin N Am 44:809–830, 1997.

Seth R, Bhat AS. Management of common oncologic emergencies. Indian J Pediatr 78: 709–717, 2011.

15 Acute Leukemias

Acute leukemia is the most common type of malignancy in children, accounting for approximately 25% of newly diagnosed cancers in patients less than 15 years of age. Approximately 2500 to 3000 new cases are diagnosed each year in the United States. The peak incidence is between 2 and 5 years of age. Acute lymphoblastic leukemia (ALL) accounts for 75% of cases of leukemia, followed by acute myelogenous leukemia (AML) in 20%, with the remainder being other, rarer forms. The acute leukemias are biologically classified by blast morphology, surface proteins, cytogenetic abnormalities, and cytochemical staining. This information, in addition to clinical features, is utilized for risk stratification into treatment groups. Risk-based therapy optimizes curative potential while minimizing risks and side effects.

A number of hypotheses regarding the etiology and pathogenesis of acute leukemia have been described, including Knudson's two-hit hypothesis that entails an initial early event (possibly prior to birth), followed by a second, environmentally-mediated (possibly infectious) event. Ionizing radiation and exposure to benzene have been associated with an increased risk of developing leukemia. Certain syndromes and chromosomal abnormalities have also been associated with a high incidence of developing leukemia (e.g., Down syndrome [DS], Fanconi anemia, Bloom syndrome, ataxia telangiectasia). Siblings, in particular identical twins, have an increased risk of developing leukemia as children. Most cases of leukemia stem from somatic genetic alterations, as opposed to an inherited genetic predisposition. Though unclear at this time, inciting events in the development of leukemia in children and adolescents involve complex relationships between host genetic polymorphisms, environmental exposures, and infections.

Acute lymphoblastic leukemia

The majority of ALL cases arise from B-cell committed progenitors. T-cell ALL represents approximately 15% of ALL cases. Cytogenetic abnormalities are common and provide important prognostic information. Hyperdiploidy (an excess of chromosomes; e.g., >50) is seen in approximately one-third of children with B-precursor ALL, and the TEL-AML translocation t(12;21)(p13; q22) is present in another 25% of cases. Both of these cytogenetic findings are associated with a favorable outcome, whereas hypodiploidy ($\leq$44 chromosomes), and the presence of certain translocations such as the Philadelphia chromosome t(9;22)

Handbook of Pediatric Hematology and Oncology: Children's Hospital & Research Center Oakland, Second Edition. Caroline A. Hastings, Joseph C. Torkildson, and Anurag K. Agrawal.
© 2012 John Wiley & Sons, Ltd. Published 2012 by John Wiley & Sons, Ltd.

and the mixed lineage leukemia (MLL) rearrangement t(4;11) or t(1;19) have traditionally been associated with poorer outcomes. The addition of tyrosine kinase inhibitors in therapy may be significantly altering the outcome of patients with the Philadelphia chromosome translocation. It is important to note that conventional cytogenetics may not detect these common translocations seen in ALL and therefore FISH (fluorescent in situ hybridization) is necessary for detection.

Clinical presentation

The clinical manifestations of leukemia are a direct result of marrow invasion with resultant cytopenias (anemia, thrombocytopenia, leukopenia, and/or neutropenia) and rarely extramedullary involvement (see Table 15.1). Children typically present with nonspecific symptoms related to anemia

such as fatigue, irritability, and anorexia as well as clinical signs such as pallor, tachycardia, and more rarely evidence of congestive heart failure. Low-grade fever of unknown etiology may be a presenting manifestation due to presumed cytokine release or may be related to infection secondary to neutropenia and immunosuppression. Bleeding secondary to thrombocytopenia is usually mild and manifests as petechiae, bruising, gingival oozing, and/or epistaxis. Life-threatening hemorrhage may occur, but is very rare. Bone pain (typically long bones) is common and may result in refusal to walk or irritability in young children. This may result from direct leukemic infiltration of the periosteum or expansion of the marrow cavity by leukemic cells. Pathologic fractures may also be present at diagnosis and cause significant pain (see Table 15.2). Patients with T-cell ALL present

Table 15.1 Common clinical and laboratory features of acute lymphoblastic leukemia (ALL) at presentation.

Finding	Percentage of patients (%)
Fever	60
Pallor	40
Bleeding	50
Bone pain	25
Lymphadenopathy	50
Splenomegaly	60
Hepatosplenomegaly	70
White blood cell count ($\times 10^9$/L)	
<10	50
10–49	30
≥50	20
Hemoglobin (g/dL)	
<7.0	40
7.0–11.0	45
>11.0	15
Platelet count ($\times 10^9$/L)	
<20	30
20–99	45
≥100	25

Table 15.2 Radiographic changes of the bones in leukemia.

Osteolytic lesions involving the medullary
cavity or cortex
Subperiosteal new bone formation;
pathologic fracture
Transverse metaphyseal radiolucent bands
Transverse metaphyseal lines of increased
density (growth arrest lines)

with some distinctive features. It more frequently occurs in males, and the incidence of central nervous system (CNS) leukemia at diagnosis is higher than for B-cell ALL (10% to 15% vs. 2% to 5%). Patients are more likely to present with a mediastinal mass (nearly 50%) or a white blood cell (WBC) count above $100 \times 10^9/L$ (30% to 50%). The presence of an anterior mediastinal mass may cause airway or cardiovascular compromise (see Chapter 14).

Frequently seen laboratory abnormalities include elevated liver enzymes and lactate dehydrogenase (LDH). Evidence of tumor lysis related to a large tumor burden and rapid cell turnover may result in hyperuricemia, hyperkalemia, and hyperphosphatemia (with resultant hypocalcemia due to precipitation of calcium phosphate).

CNS involvement occurs in less than 5% of children at presentation, but is more common in children with T-cell disease. It is usually detected in an asymptomatic child with analysis of the cerebrospinal fluid (CSF). Rarely, a patient may present with signs or symptoms of increased intracranial pressure (e.g., cranial nerve VI palsy with resultant esotropia and diplopia, papilledema, visual changes, morning headache, vomiting, lethargy, irritability, possible seizures) or evidence of parenchymal involvement, hypothalamic syndrome, or diabetes insipidus. Other rare complications such as chloromas causing compression of the spinal cord or CNS hemorrhage (related to leukostasis and coagulopathy) are rare and more likely to be associated with AML.

Leukemic involvement of the testes occurs in 2% to 5% of boys at diagnosis and presents as painless enlargement, either unilaterally or bilaterally. Early testicular involvement is also associated with T-cell disease, elevated WBC count, and lymphomatous features.

Diagnostic evaluation

Children presenting with more than one cytopenia and clinical symptomatology suggestive of bone marrow infiltration should undergo a diagnostic evaluation to investigate for the possibility of acute leukemia.

Laboratory and imaging studies indicated are:

• Complete blood count (CBC), differential, review of peripheral blood smear by an experienced individual
• Bone marrow aspirate (consider biopsy for dry tap or inadequate specimen) for morphology, blast count, immunophenotyping, cytogenetics, cytochemistry
• Metabolic panel, to include liver function studies, electrolytes, lactate dehydrogenase (LDH), uric acid, phosphorus, calcium, blood urea nitrogen, and creatinine
• Blood culture if febrile; cultures of other suspected sites of infection
• Chest radiography to evaluate for the presence of a mediastinal mass
• Plain films of the long bones for patients presenting with pain to evaluate for pathologic fracture or evidence of leukemic changes

Typically the bone marrow is 80% to 100% replaced with lymphoblasts at diagnosis. At times, due to the packed condition of the marrow, it may be difficult to aspirate a sample (dry tap) and a bone marrow biopsy may provide diagnostic samples. The diagnosis of acute leukemia requires the presence of 25% or more blasts (M3 bone marrow); however, the diagnosis is suspected when the marrow contains 5% to 25% blasts (M2 bone marrow with M1 being a normal bone marrow with <5% blasts) (Table 15.3). Lymphoblasts have a typical morphology with a high nuclear to cytoplasmic ratio, fine nuclear chromatin, and the presence of nucleoli. In addition, the cells tend to have a uniform size and appearance. Immunophenotyping and cytochemistry are used to differentiate ALL and AML and identify T- and B-cell ALL. Lymphoid malignancies should lack myeloid cell surface markers (CD13 and CD33; CD [cluster of differentiation]). B-cell ALL should have B-cell surface markers such as CD10, CD19, kappa, and lambda, whereas T-cell ALL should have T-cell surface markers including CD2, CD5, and CD7. T-cell ALL cells should also stain for terminal deoxynucleotidyl transferase, an immature lymphoid marker.

After the diagnosis is confirmed, evaluation of the CSF should be done prior to therapy (this is frequently done at the time of the diagnostic bone marrow aspirate if the clinical suspicion is high). A lumbar puncture is done to assess possible involvement of the CSF and to assist with therapeutic decision-making and risk stratification. Many patients require a platelet transfusion prior to the initial lumbar puncture, which should be performed by an experienced clinician to decrease the chance of a traumatic tap. There is some evidence that a platelet count of $100 \times 10^9/L$ is desired to decrease this risk. In addition, evidence exists that a traumatic tap at diagnosis (with peripheral blasts) can theoretically seed the CSF space increasing the risk of later CNS relapse. Subsequent procedures may be done with platelet counts of 20 to $50 \times 10^9/L$, per institutional and provider preference. A cell count and cytocentrifuge examination for cell morphology is done on the fresh CSF. The diagnosis of CNS leukemia requires the presence of 5 or more WBCs/μL and identification of blasts on the CSF cytocentrifuge examination. CNS leukemia is classified as follows:

- CNS1: no detectable blasts
- CNS2: <5 WBCs/μL, blasts present
- CNS3: $\geq$5 WBCs/μL and blasts present or signs of CNS leukemia (i.e., facial nerve palsy, hypothalamic syndrome, or brain/eye involvement)

A traumatic lumbar puncture is defined as the presence of $\geq$10 red blood cells/μL. Formulas are available to assist with interpretation of CNS status in the event of traumatic initial taps with blasts on cytospin (Steinherz/Bleyer algorithm).

Other assessments prior to initiation of therapy

An echocardiogram and electrocardiogram are done as baseline studies in all patients who will be receiving anthracyclines. These drugs are frequently given in induction for high risk patients and in the delayed intensification phase for all patients. Acute and delayed cardiotoxicity may occur, though

---

Table 15.3 Differential diagnosis of acute lymphoblastic leukemia (ALL).

Nonmalignant disorders
  Aplastic anemia
  Immune thrombocytopenia
  Infections: EBV, CMV, pertussis,
    parapertussis
**Malignant disorders (round blue cell
  tumors with marrow involvement)**
  Lymphoma
  Neuroblastoma
  Retinoblastoma
  Medulloblastoma
  Rhabdomyosarcoma

Abbreviations: EBV, Epstein-Barr virus; CMV, cytomegalovirus.

late complications are more often related to high cumulative doses (i.e., $>300\,mg/m^2$) given at a young age (<4 years) and associated with other risk factors for cardiac disease such as mediastinal radiation, obesity, family history of early cardiovascular disease, and abnormal lipid profiles.

Viral serologies for hepatitis B and C, cytomegalovirus (CMV), herpes simplex virus (HSV), and varicella zoster virus (VZV) are obtained as baseline information (see Chapter 25). This aids in determining if later infection with one of these viral agents could be related to transfusion (potentially in the case of hepatitis B and C), and whether the infection is primary or reactivation (in the case of CMV, HSV, and VZV). Baseline knowledge of previous exposure may impact later treatment choices.

Risk group classification

The concept of risk stratification allows patients at comparatively high risk of relapse to be treated with more intensive and potentially more toxic therapies, whereas patients at lower risk of relapse are given lower intensity regimens that maintain the same low risk of recurrence while minimizing exposure to unnecessary agents and decreasing toxicity. Classification into risk groups is generally based on clinically apparent prognostic factors identified by retrospective analysis and then verified by prospective studies. Many risk factors have been utilized in risk classification for acute leukemia, but only age, WBC, and immunophenotype (i.e., AML vs. ALL, T- vs. B-cell ALL) at diagnosis continue to be the most significant factors for initial classification.

The commonly used National Cancer Institute criteria classify standard risk (SR) ALL as children 1 to 10 years of age with a WBC $<50 \times 10^9$/L and high risk (HR) ALL as children with age ≥ 10 years or WBC $\geq 50 \times 10^9$/L. Utilizing these criteria, approximately two-thirds of pre-B and one-third of T-cell ALL patients are classified as SR. Better outcomes are observed in younger children, B-cell phenotype, those with more favorable cytogenetic features, and females.

Further stratification into treatment groups is done within the first few weeks of therapy based on early morphologic response to therapy (as measured by day 7 and/or day 14 bone marrow aspirate), cytogenetic abnormalities identified on the diagnostic marrow, and remission status at the end of induction (morphologic and as measured by minimal residual disease [MRD] detection). Other considerations include presence of extramedullary disease such as testicular or CNS disease. Infants have a special category as they are a particularly high risk group, especially the very young.

Treatment

Treatment of childhood leukemia is one of the success stories in pediatric oncology, though much remains to be accomplished. Remarkable advances have occurred by the identification of more effective drug combinations, recognition of drug sanctuary sites and routine presymptomatic CNS directed therapy, intensification of therapy in early phases, and identification of clinical and biologic variables predictive of outcome for use in risk stratification.

Most children with cancer in the United States are treated at pediatric oncology centers and have access to participation in clinical trials. These studies have accelerated the advances made in the diagnosis and treatment of pediatric cancer and clearly are a major reason for many of the successes. The Children's Oncology Group is a national collaborative group of professionals involved in the treatment of children with cancer. Most pediatric cancer centers register patients on these trials. Families are asked to give informed consent to participate in these trials, which may include clinical and biologic questions. For families not wishing to participate, the standard of care is offered (best published clinical regimen). Many centers may also participate in smaller pilot studies or have their own clinical protocols.

The purpose of therapy in ALL is to induce a permanent biologic and clinical remission (no evidence of disease on laboratory and physical assessment). Overall, approximately 85% of children with ALL will be cured of their disease. Treatment regimens are classically divided into phases of therapy:

- **Induction:** refers to the first 28 to 35 days of therapy, after which the child should be in a morphologic remission. Remission induction rate in SR ALL is 98%.
- **Consolidation:** further systemic chemotherapy is given, in addition to a focus on CNS prophylaxis.
- **Interim Maintenance:** similar drugs as maintenance, but in a more intensified manner.
- **Delayed Intensification:** refers to reinduction and reconsolidation; may be given once or twice, depending on the protocol.
- **Maintenance:** continuation of therapy; this phase lasts 2 to 3 years (longer in males due to theoretical increased risk for testicular relapse).
- **CNS directed therapy:** intrathecal methotrexate; cranial radiation in select groups (CNS3, T-cell).

Open clinical trials will likely alter some aspect of therapy for certain risk groups in an attempt to improve outcomes and diminish acute and late toxicity. Some examples may include adding a new agent in certain phases, altering chemotherapy dosing or timing in specific phases, or possibly asking a radiation-related question.

Conventional induction therapy includes prednisone or dexamethasone, asparaginase, and vincristine in addition to intrathecal cytarabine (Ara-C) and methotrexate. Patients with HR ALL also receive daunorubicin. Consolidation for HR patients incorporates cyclophosphamide, cytarabine, asparaginase, 6-mercaptopurine, and intensified therapy directed toward the CNS (either intrathecal methotrexate alone or with radiation for patients with CNS disease). SR patients receive intensified CNS therapy with minimal systemic chemotherapy. The delayed intensification (DI) phase has led to significantly improved outcomes as has further intensification of the interim maintenance phase (intensified vincristine and methotrexate compared to standard maintenance). DI is a concept in which reintensification of therapy following attainment of remission can be achieved with some alteration in drugs utilized previously in the induction and consolidation phases. Maintenance classically consists of pulses of steroid (prednisone or dexamethasone) and vincristine in addition to oral methotrexate and 6-mercaptopurine. Individualized drug dosing is required to maintain certain hematologic levels and differences in metabolism and tolerability are likely related to individual polymorphisms. This aspect of management in addition to the length of maintenance makes it a unique cancer therapy for children.

CNS prophylaxis continues with periodic intrathecal methotrexate throughout therapy. Children with CNS3 disease receive augmented therapy with 1800 cGy cranial radiation, in addition to intrathecal methotrexate. Treatment of children with CNS2 disease is controversial although recent Children's Oncology Group studies have showed no difference between CNS1 and CNS2 patients receiving equivalent therapy. This is due to the addition of medications with improved penetration through the blood–brain barrier, including dexamethasone instead of prednisone and high-dose methotrexate. Without CNS prophylaxis, it is estimated that 60% to 70% of children would relapse in the CNS (based on historical data). T-cell patients are at higher risk for CNS relapse and augmented CNS-directed therapy is given to all patients (even without overt CNS involvement) with prophylactic 1200 cGy cranial radiation.

Complications of therapy

Because of the myelosuppressive nature of therapy and the underlying disease state, children undergoing chemotherapy and/or radiation may expect to experience complications during the course of their treatment. Many of these complications can be anticipated and prevented (see Chapter 25). Most patients will require transfusion support with packed red blood cells and/or platelets (see Chapter 5). Children with neutropenia are instructed to take special precautions to decrease the risk of infection exposure. Any child receiving chemotherapy who develops a fever should have emergent medical attention, especially during phases of anticipated neutropenia (i.e., induction, consolidation, delayed intensification; see Chapter 27). Certain therapies are associated with specific toxicities: anthracyclines with cardiotoxicity, vincristine with peripheral neurotoxicity, intrathecal methotrexate with central neurotoxicity, steroids (especially dexamethasone) with avascular necrosis of bone, and radiation with acute and late effects (see Chapter 30). These anticipated side effects should also be discussed in detail with the patient and family to help with earlier recognition and supportive care should be initiated as needed. Potential late toxicities are monitored throughout the course of treatment and in the off-therapy phase of follow-up.

Relapse

Despite the dramatic improvements in our knowledge about the biology of ALL, prognostic factors, and more tailored therapy, 20% of children with ALL will relapse, with only about one-third of those patients going on to have a long-term remission with intensified therapy. Due to the frequency of ALL as compared to other pediatric malignancies, relapsed ALL is the fourth most common oncologic diagnosis in children. Timing and site of relapse are prognostic and important determinants for future therapy. Sites of relapse include the bone marrow or an extramedullary site, such as the CNS or testes, or some combination of sites. Early relapse (<18 months since therapy initiation) is associated with a particularly grim prognosis. Concepts of therapy include systemic retreatment and radiation therapy to sites of extramedullary relapse. Allogeneic hematopoietic stem cell transplantation (HSCT) may improve the outcome of patients with marrow or combined relapse. Overall survival after relapse is also impacted by cumulative toxicity from prior therapy and high infection rates due to the increased intensity of therapy. In general, children with late, isolated extramedullary relapse fare better.

New agents

New agents are currently under investigation to improve outcomes for high-risk and relapsed patients. Such agents include the tyrosine kinase inhibitors (imatinib, dasatinib) in Philadelphia chromosome positive ALL and nelarabine in T-cell disease. Finding agents with favorable toxicity profiles for use in highly treated relapse patients is a challenge. Monoclonal antibodies such as inotuzumab and epratuzumab (anti-CD22 antibodies) may be part of the solution. Clofarabine, a new generation nucleoside analog that inhibits DNA synthesis, is currently being investigated in relapsed and refractory ALL. Other drugs are being explored utilizing newly acquired knowledge of novel signaling pathways such as mTOR inhibitors. It is anticipated that the next generation of clinical trials will be utilizing a combination of conventional chemotherapy and immunomodulator therapy.

Acute myelogenous leukemia

Approximately 20% of acute childhood leukemia is myelogenous. Unlike ALL, AML does not have a peak incidence in children as there are only subtle increases in incidence from infancy to adolescence. On the other hand, there appears to be a steady increase with age in adults, in whom the incidence of AML is approximately four times that of ALL. AML is associated with a poorer prognosis than ALL, with long-term survival expected to be 50% to 60%. Additionally, therapy for AML, which includes multiagent chemotherapy and HSCT, is one of the most toxic therapies in childhood cancer. Hispanic children are noted to have a higher incidence of AML, mostly accounted for by the acute promyelocytic leukemia subtype (APL; M3). The incidence of secondary AML following treatment of childhood cancer is rising, due in part to increased survival after primary malignancy as well as increased use of agents that cause direct DNA damage (e.g., alkalytors [cyclophosphamide, ifosfamide], anthracyclines [doxorubicin, daunorubicin], radiation therapy), and those that inhibit topoisomerase II (e.g., epidophyllotoxins [etoposide] and anthracyclines).

The etiology of AML is likely sporadic although several inherited and acquired risk factors may predispose to this disease. The most common inherited predisposition to develop leukemia is DS. Children with DS have a 10- to 20-fold increased risk of developing acute leukemia compared to other children. In early life, children with DS have a particularly high risk of the megakaryoblastic subtype of AML (AMKL; M7). Overall, children with DS constitute approximately 10% of children with AML. In addition, approximately 10% of neonates with DS may develop a transient myeloproliferative disorder that mimics congenital AML but typically improves spontaneously by 4 to 6 weeks of age. However, these children have a 20% to 30% risk of developing AML before 3 years of age. Children with transient myeloproliferative disorder or presumed congenital AML who do not display phenotypic features of DS should have a karyotype performed to look for possible trisomy 21 mosaicism.

Patients with inherited bone marrow failure syndromes such as Fanconi anemia, Kostmann syndrome, Bloom syndrome, dyskeratosis congenita, Shwachman–Diamond syndrome, congenital amegakaryocytic thrombocytopenia, and Diamond-Blackfan anemia have a predisposition to malignancy, including AML. Other conditions such as Li-Fraumeni syndrome, Noonan syndrome, acquired paroxysmal nocturnal hemoglobinuria, and myelodysplastic syndrome confer an increased risk. Twins and siblings of AML patients have an increased risk of AML, though this is much more significant in monozygotic twins within 6 years of initial diagnosis. Exposure to ionizing radiation has also been convincingly implicated, especially following the atomic bombs in World War II.

Clinical presentation

AML and ALL are indistinguishable at presentation, with the majority of signs and symptoms being related to infiltration of the marrow and other body organs. Dependent on the number of circulating myeloblasts and total WBC, some of the presenting manifestations may be life threatening. Children with extreme leukocytosis (WBC $> 200 \times 10^9$/L) may present with metabolic abnormalities and tumor lysis syndrome (see Chapter 14). Clinically, they are at risk for hypoxia in the small vessels of the brain and lungs as a result of increased blood viscosity related to the rheology of the myeloblasts (large, adherent, and nondeformable cells). This may translate to sludging in the small vasculature of the retinal, pulmonary, and central nervous systems with resultant decreased oxygen delivery, hypoxia, and stroke.

Patients typically present with signs and symptoms related to pancytopenia with pallor, fatigue, anorexia, and bleeding. Fever is very common at presentation, often with no apparent infectious etiology. Bone pain is also common, though not typically associated with fractures. Some unique and suggestive features of AML at presentation include leukemia cutis in infants (blueberry muffin rash thought secondary to extramedullary hematopoiesis) and chloromas (extramedullary collections of myeloblasts). Chloromas may occur in up to 10% of children with AML and present most commonly in the bones, skin, soft tissues, and lymph nodes, but may occur anywhere in the body. Gingival hypertrophy is a unique finding in AML secondary to chloroma of the gums. A particularly rare yet important presentation is spinal cord compression from a chloroma in the paraspinal/epidural region.

Life-threatening bleeding is another complication somewhat unique to AML. Although the majority of patients will be thrombocytopenic secondary to marrow infiltration with myeloblasts, patients with concomitant coagulopathy due to disseminated intravascular coagulation are at particularly high risk, a finding seen most commonly in APL (M3 AML). This association is thought to be secondary to the release of thromboplastin from cytoplasmic granules in the promyelocytic blasts.

Children with AML and hyperleukocytosis (WBC $>100 \times 10^9$/L) are at risk for tumor lysis syndrome at presentation and with the initiation of therapy. Risk factors include the presence of bulky disease with lymphadenopathy and/or hepatosplenomegaly as well as a rapidly escalating WBC count suggesting a high mitotic index (see Table 15.4).

Diagnostic evaluation

The same studies suggested for the evaluation of ALL should be obtained in the evaluation of the child with suspected AML. It is common to see severe anemia and thrombocytopenia in association with an elevated total WBC count. The definitive diagnosis is made with the evaluation of the bone marrow, with at least 25% to 30% of the cellular elements identified as myeloblasts based on immunophenotyping and cytochemistry. Morphologic review may also reveal Auer rods (clumps of azurophilic granules shaped into elongated needles and located in the cytoplasm), classically only seen in some subtypes of AML (i.e., M2 and M3). A lumbar puncture should be done as up to 5% of children will have overt CNS involvement at presentation. A coagulation evaluation should be performed in these patients including PT, INR, PTT, fibrinogen, and D-dimers to evaluate for the possibility of disseminated intravascular coagulation (most typically seen in M3).

Table 15.4 Clinical manifestations of hyperleukocytosis in acute myelogenous leukemia (AML).

Organ at risk	Consequence
Lungs	Hypoxia, respiratory distress, pulmonary infiltrates
CNS	Alteration of mental status, stroke, intracranial bleeding
Eyes	Decreased visual acuity
Kidneys	Renal insufficiency (exacerbated by tumor lysis syndrome)

Abbreviation: CNS, central nervous system.

Several morphologic classification systems are available for AML, including the classic French-American-British (FAB) classification of M0 to M7 and the World Health Organization (WHO) categorization into four major subgroups (Table 15.5). Additionally, chromosome analyses are performed to obtain important diagnostic and prognostic markers. Approximately 60% of children with primary AML demonstrate clonal abnormalities in the blast lineage prior to therapy initiation. The t(8;21) translocation is the most common chromosome translocation and is associated with the M2 subgroup and a more favorable prognosis. The t(15;17) translocation is classically seen in APL (AML M3). Inversion of chromosome 16 (inv(16)) is associated with acute myelomonoblastic leukemia (AML M4) and also portends a favorable

prognosis. Finally, chromosomal aberrations including monosomy 7 or 7q deletion, monosomy 5 or 5q deletion, and complex abnormalities (≥ 3 or more unrelated changes) all impart a worse prognosis. Monosomy 5 and 7 are also highly associated with cases of secondary myeloproliferative disorders and AML that develop after chemotherapy for a primary malignancy.

See *Other assessments prior to initiation of therapy* in the ALL section for further information.

Risk group classification

Historically AML has been classified utilizing the FAB morphologic classification system (Table 15.5). The WHO classification system was subsequently developed to also include cytogenetics, disease biology, and clinical history. Host factors such as age,

Table 15.5 Morphologic classification for acute myelogenous leukemia (AML).

AML	Subtype	Clinical/biologic features
M0	Undifferentiated leukemia	Similar to ALL, requires CD13, CD33, CD117, and absence of lymphoid markers
M1	Acute myeloblastic leukemia without differentiation	MPO + by special stains/flow cytometry
M2	Acute myeloblastic leukemia with differentiation	Auer rods, t(8;21) common, chloromas, good prognosis
M3	Acute promyeloblastic leukemia	Auer rods, DIC/bleeding, t(15;17), good prognosis with ATRA therapy
M4	Acute myelomonoblastic leukemia	Mixed myeloblasts (20%) and monoblasts, peripheral monocytosis
M5	Acute monocytic leukemia	$\geq 80\%$ marrow nonerythroid cells are monocytic, MLL (11q23) rearrangements in infants, CNS disease more common, chloromas (e.g., gingival hyperplasia)
M6	Erythroleukemia	Rare in children
M7	Acute megakaryoblastic leukemia	Classically seen in Down syndrome with GATA1 mutation, good prognosis; rare in non-DS with t(1;22), poor prognosis

Abbreviations: ALL, acute lymphoblastic leukemia; MPO, myeloperoxidase; DIC, disseminated intravascular coagulation; ATRA, all-trans retinoic acid; MLL, mixed lineage leukemia; CNS, central nervous system; DS, Down syndrome.

gender, race, and constitutional abnormalities all have some prognostic influence on outcome. Females do slightly better than males, older children do better than infants (though outcomes in infants are improving with current therapies), and Caucasians fare better than non-white patents. Children with DS, particularly those under the age of 4 years at diagnosis, have an improved outcome with less intensive therapy (overall survival 80%) but also show increased toxicity with therapy. Children with an initial WBC $< 20 \times 10^9$/L have an improved outcome and those with hyperleukocytosis (WBC $>100 \times 10^9$/L) have a worse outcome. A number of recurring cytogenetic abnormalities are associated with AML and confer prognostic significance. Overall, poor risk features include WBC count $>100 \times 10^9$/L, monosomy 7, and secondary AML. Good risk features include certain FAB subtypes (M1/M2 with Auer rods, M3, M4 with eosinophilia), rapid response to initial therapy, and favorable chromosomal features such as t(8;21), t(15;17), and inversion 16. As with ALL, assessment of MRD is becoming an important marker of outcome with chemotherapy and transplant.

Treatment

As with ALL, the goal of induction therapy is to induce a clinical and biologic remission by rapidly reducing the number of malignant cells. Approximately 80% of children achieve remission with induction therapy. The most effective induction regimens use a combination of cytarabine and an anthracycline, typically daunorubicin. Individual trials have built upon this backbone with changes in dosing and timing, alternative anthracyclines, or introduction of new supportive care strategies to better manage potential adverse effects of therapy. Other agents utilized in continuation therapy include etoposide, dexamethasone, 6-thioguanine, and asparaginase. Prior studies

have shown no added benefit for a maintenance phase following intensification. Allogeneic HSCT is recommended for patients with high risk cytogenetics (i.e., monosomy 7, FLT3/ITD [internal tandem duplication], monosomy 5, or 5q-) or those who have not attained a remission following two courses of induction therapy. Patients with favorable risk cytogenetics and good early responses to induction therapy receive allogeneic HSCT only in the case of relapse and if a second remission has been achieved. It remains unclear if HSCT has benefit for those AML patients with intermediate risk features (usually defined as neither high risk features nor low risk features) and decisions must be made on an individual basis assessing the clinical status of the patient, availability of an appropriate match, and family preference.

The morphologic subtypes of AML with highest involvement of the CNS are FAB M4 and M5. Overall, the frequency of CNS involvement is between 15% and 20% at diagnosis. All patients receive CNS consolidative therapy with intrathecal cytarabine in addition to high-dose cytarabine, which has good CSF penetration. AML patients with myeloblasts in the CNS can usually be cleared with intrathecal cytarabine. Cranial irradiation is reserved for those children with refractory CNS involvement. Children with Down syndrome rarely have CNS involvement, and due to their increased risk of toxicity, CNS prophylaxis has been greatly reduced without negative consequence in these patients.

APL is distinctly different from the other AML subtypes and has a particularly good prognosis due to the development of targeted therapies. Approximately 3% of patients with APL die in the early phases of therapy as a result of the unique hemorrhagic complications of this disease. Patients receive treatment with differentiating agents such as all-trans retinoic acid

(ATRA) and arsenic trioxide (ATO). The t(15;17) translocation is present in the majority of cases and leads to the production of a fusion protein involving the retinoic acid receptor alpha and promyelocyte gene leading to arrest of differentiation at the promyelocyte stage. ATRA induces the differentiation of immature promyelocytes into mature granulocytes, followed by restoration of normal hematopoiesis. ATRA does not cross the blood–brain barrier and is therefore ineffective in treating CNS involvement with APL. A WBC $\geq 10 \times 10^9$/L is associated with a higher risk of relapse. Higher WBC count is also associated with the microgranular variant (M3v), presence of the FLT3/ITD mutation, and the bcr3 isoform. Treatment includes induction with ATRA and anthracycline therapy (i.e., idarubicin or daunorubicin) followed by anthracycline consolidation and maintenance with intermittent ATRA and low dose 6-mercaptopurine. The use of arsenic trioxide in the initial treatment of patients with APL remains controversial and is currently under investigation. Similarly, the length and use of a consolidation phase as well as the need for intrathecal chemotherapy are yet to be answered questions. Patients can expect an event-free overall survival of 70% to 80%. Toxicities with ATRA may be significant; specifically, ATRA may lead to a differentiation syndrome in 2% to 6% of patients and present with fever, respiratory distress, weight gain, edema, and, importantly, hyperleukocytosis. The incidence of ATRA syndrome has decreased due to the addition of anthracycline therapy in induction and can be treated with IV dexamethasone. ATRA may cause other side effects including dryness of the lips and mucosa, fever, transaminitis, and headache associated with pseudotumor cerebri. Due to the rarity of APL in pediatric patients, the role of arsenic trioxide and transplant after relapse is still poorly defined.

Complications of therapy

Given the intensity of therapy for AML, children can expect to experience a number of complications that include cytopenias requiring frequent blood product support, mucositis, liver toxicity, need for parenteral hyperalimentation, and severe, prolonged marrow suppression. Infection is common and should be anticipated. Once neutropenic, these children are at particularly high risk for the development of sepsis with Gram-negative organisms in addition to invasive fungal disease. Routine antifungal prophylaxis with fluconazole is recommended in addition to PCP prophylaxis. *Streptococcus viridans* sepsis is associated with the use of high-dose cytarabine and resultant altered integrity of the gastrointestinal mucosa. Sepsis with this organism can be rapidly fatal. Empiric therapy for fever and neutropenia should include coverage for *S. viridans* and be started immediately with the first fever. Prolonged hospitalization is expected during the course of treatment for AML and these patients should be in protective environments.

Coagulopathy at diagnosis is not uncommon, especially in the child with APL. Coagulation studies should be done routinely. In general, platelet counts should be maintained above 10×10^9/L ($>50 \times 10^9$/L for the APL patient at diagnosis). The use of fresh frozen plasma, cryoprecipitate, and platelets are important supportive care measures due to the frequently observed coagulopathy, hypofibrinogenemia (fibrinogen <150 mg/dL), and thrombocytopenia, respectively. This will help prevent bleeding complications, especially in the APL patient (in addition to the early initiation of ATRA therapy).

Relapse

Even with current intensive therapies, only about half of children diagnosed with AML are expected to be long-term survivors. As mentioned, patients with DS and APL have an improved prognosis. Some patients succumb to early mortality related to progressive disease, infection, bleeding, and other complications of therapy. After relapse, chemotherapy alone results in <10% 1-year disease-free survival (DFS). For those patients that can again obtain a morphologic remission after reinduction chemotherapy, HSCT improves survival to 30% to 50%. MRD after reinduction therapy for AML relapse has been shown to be a vital prognostic factor in DFS after HSCT. Newer modalities of therapy are needed and are under investigation. These include targeted immunotherapy (gemtuzumab targeted against CD33), tyrosine kinase inhibitors (lestaurtinib and sorafenib for patients with FLT3 mutations), nucleoside analogues (clofarabine), farnesyltransferase inhibitors (tipifarnib), histone deacetylase inhibitors (vorinostat), proteasome inhibitors (bortezomib), and demethylating agents (decitabine and azacitidine).

Suggested Reading

Pui CH, Carroll WL, Meshinchi S, Arceci RJ. Biology, risk stratification, and treatment of pediatric acute leukemias: an update. J Clin Oncol 29:551–565, 2011.

Seibel NL. Treatment of acute lymphoblastic leukemia in children and adolescents: peaks and pitfalls. Am Soc Hematol Educ Prog 374–380, 2008.

16 Central Nervous System Tumors

Central nervous system (CNS) tumors are the most common cancer diagnosed in children after leukemia, accounting for 20% of all pediatric malignancies. The most common location is infratentorial in children up to 14 years of age, while supratentorial tumors are more common in adolescents. Spinal cord tumors are also more common in adolescents than in younger children (9% vs. 3%).

The cause of most pediatric CNS tumors is unknown. The majority of them are sporadic, although a small percentage is associated with genetic disorders such as neurofibromatosis, tuberous sclerosis, von Hippel–Lindau syndrome, and Li-Fraumeni syndrome (germ line mutation of p53, a suppressor oncogene). Radiation therapy is the most frequently identified cause of pediatric CNS tumors; these occur as second malignancies in children who have previously received radiation therapy for the treatment of leukemia or primary CNS tumors.

In general, brain tumor classification is based on embryonic derivation and histologic cell of origin, and occasionally on tumor location. The World Health Organization Classification System for brain tumors contains more than 100 entries, making it difficult for pathologists to agree on a diagnosis in specific cases. Microscopic criteria useful in grading of tumors include cellular pleomorphism, mitotic rate, degree of anaplasia, and presence or absence of necrosis. A growing number of chromosomal abnormalities and specific genomic signatures have been identified in pediatric brain tumors, and the use of these is becoming increasingly important for accurate pathologic classification.

Clinical presentation

It is often difficult to make the diagnosis of a CNS tumor in a child. The presenting symptoms of CNS tumors can be quite variable, depending on the location of the tumor, its rate of growth, and the age of the child. Additionally, most of the symptoms are nonspecific, and occur more commonly in children with a variety of benign conditions. Prompt diagnosis of a CNS tumor requires an appropriate index of suspicion and a good understanding of the duration of symptoms that is expected with other disorders. Due to the frequent association of hydrocephalus with infratentorial tumors, 50% of children with brain tumors will present with signs of **increased intracranial pressure (ICP)**, including lethargy, vomiting, and irritability. These symptoms may

Handbook of Pediatric Hematology and Oncology: Children's Hospital & Research Center Oakland, Second Edition. Caroline A. Hastings, Joseph C. Torkildson, and Anurag K. Agrawal.
© 2012 John Wiley & Sons, Ltd. Published 2012 by John Wiley & Sons, Ltd.

be less prominent in infants because the cranial sutures remain open and the skull can accommodate the increase in ventricular size. For this reason, accurate measurement of the head size should be part of every well-baby examination. Headache is a presenting symptom in 70% of children with posterior fossa tumors and 50% of central tumors. Features that are helpful in distinguishing tumor-related headache from a primary headache syndrome include nausea and vomiting (particularly in the morning), increasing frequency and/ or severity over a few weeks, and abnormalities on neurologic examination. Neurologic deficits such as ataxia, visual changes, and hemiparesis occur in about 25% of cases. Weakness is sometimes subtle, but parents often relate a loss of physical function or developmental milestones. Visual changes include diplopia caused by cranial nerve dysfunction and loss of visual acuity caused by optic nerve involvement or papilledema.

Two specific clinical syndromes are frequently associated with childhood brain tumors. **Parinaud's syndrome** consists of paralysis of upward gaze, accommodative paresis, nystagmus during attempts at upward gaze, eyelid retraction (Collier's sign), and "setting-sun sign" (conjugate downward gaze). It is most commonly associated with pineal region tumors, but can also be caused by obstructive hydrocephalus from any cause, posterior fossa tumors, or a number of infectious or vascular abnormalities leading to ischemia or damage to the dorsal midbrain. **Diencephalic syndrome** is a rare cause of failure to thrive in infants and young children. Characteristic features include profound emaciation with normal caloric intake, absence of subcutaneous fat, locomotor hyperactivity, euphoria, and alertness. It is almost always associated with hypothalamic/ suprasellar tumors, most commonly optic pathway gliomas.

Seizures are relatively rare in younger children but occur twice as often in adolescents (13% vs. 25%). They can be focal or generalized. When focal they may provide a clue as to the location of the tumor. An often-overlooked symptom in school-age children is deterioration in school performance and behavioral changes. It is not uncommon for these children to be referred by a psychologist or psychiatrist after many months of unsuccessful therapy for these symptoms.

Symptoms of spinal cord tumors are caused by **compression of the spinal cord** or nerve roots by the mass. The most common symptom in children with spinal cord tumors is back pain. Unlike adults, the complaint of back pain is very rare in childhood. "Benign" causes of back pain include trauma, medical conditions such as sickle cell disease, or involvement in aggressive sports such as football, gymnastics, skateboarding, or motocross bicycling. In the absence of such a history, there should be concern that a tumor might be the cause. Tumor-related pain is often described as being worse in the supine position or with Valsalva's maneuver. Other symptoms associated with spinal cord tumors include sciatica, weakness, numbness, problems with or loss of bowel and/or bladder control, and spinal deformity.

Tumors within the spinal canal are either intramedullary (within the spinal cord or nerve roots) or extramedullary. Intramedullary spinal cord tumors are almost always glial in origin, the most common histologies being astrocytoma, myxopapillary ependymoma, and oligodendroglioma. Extramedullary tumors are either intradural or extradural. Extramedullary intradural tumors are most commonly neurofibromas, Schwannomas, or more rarely meningiomas. Extradural tumors are usually not CNS tumors at all, but metastatic tumors from other locations such as neuroblastoma, lymphoma, or Ewing sarcoma. Tumors within the vertebral bodies such as primary bone tumors, tumors metastatic to bone, and histiocytosis can also extend into the spinal canal and cause the above symptoms.

Diagnostic evaluation

Imaging studies

The first step in evaluating a child with a suspected CNS tumor is neuroimaging. A variety of imaging techniques can be useful in this assessment.

Computerized tomography

Computerized tomography (CT) was the first imaging modality to revolutionize the diagnosis of CNS tumors both in children and in adults. It is often still the first imaging study obtained when evaluating patients suspected of having a tumor. However, magnetic resonance imaging (MRI) has largely replaced it as the definitive neuroimaging study. Advantages of CT include widespread availability, rapid acquisition time, superior resolution of bone and vascular structures including lesions of the skull base, and utility in patients with contraindications to MRI (e.g., ferrous metal implants). Its limitations include inferior resolution of the brain itself, particularly within the posterior fossa, and significant radiation exposure, especially with regular monitoring.

Magnetic resonance imaging

An MRI with and without gadolinium enhancement is the single best study for evaluating the majority of tumors within the brain and spine. It provides greater sensitivity in areas that may be obscured by proximity to bone, such as the temporal lobe and posterior fossa. It also provides multiplanar images. Contrast MRI allows for identification of tumor within areas of surrounding edema, detects focal areas of blood–brain barrier (BBB) breakdown, and improves delineation of cysts from solid tumor.

Recent advances include MR spectroscopy, tractography, and functional MRI scanning. MR spectroscopy allows the determination of the chemical makeup of tissue within a predefined region of interest. Different types of tumors have characteristic spectroscopic signatures, allowing the identification of the most likely tumor type before surgery takes place. Tractography is a software technique that allows identification of the location of white matter tracts and their associated nuclei. This has become very useful as a preoperative planning tool that allows the neurosurgeon to avoid disruption of eloquent nuclei and fiber tracts during surgery. Functional MRI is another technique that precisely identifies specific motor regions, speech and language centers, and other eloquent areas for preoperative planning purposes.

Positron emission tomography

Positron emission tomography (PET) imaging is a relatively new modality for evaluating a variety of tumors including those of the CNS. It detects the relatively higher rate of metabolism present in many neoplasms by measuring the rate of metabolism of one of a growing number of radioactively labeled compounds. It has been used to distinguish between recurrent tumor and necrotic tissue, scar, or edema, each of which can develop following the treatment of a malignant brain tumor. It is used to determine the most appropriate site for a biopsy. Its utility in young children is limited due to the need for a 30- to 60-minute period of limited mental activity between injection and scanning to optimize the distinction between normal and abnormal structures.

Single-photon emission CT

Single-photon emission CT is a three-dimensional imaging technique introduced in the early 1980s for the investigation of regional cerebral blood flow that often correlates with tumor metabolic activity. In this technique, radioactive thallium and radiolabeled tyrosine have been used to localize brain tumors as well as distinguish viable tumor from radiation necrosis. It is much less expensive than PET scanning, but the resolution is less and the 20- to 30-minute acquisition times needed for high-quality pictures again limit the utility in young children.

Other studies

Lumbar puncture

Certain primary CNS tumors such as medulloblastoma, primitive neuroectodermal tumor (PNET), ependymoma, malignant germ cell tumors (GCTs), and, to a lesser extent, malignant gliomas have a propensity to metastasize throughout the subarachnoid space. As with other malignant tumors, the presence of metastatic disease alters both treatment and prognosis. For this reason, a lumbar puncture (LP) is a routine part of the diagnostic workup of these patients. Spinal fluid is collected and sent for cell count and differential, glucose, protein, and cytological examination to look for malignant cells. Measurements of α-fetoprotein (AFP) and the beta subunit of human chorionic gonadotropin (β-HCG) should also be performed on patients with suprasellar and pineal region tumors to identify malignant germ cell tumors. These markers can, if present, also be used to measure response to therapy. The diagnostic LP should be delayed for at least 7 days following tumor resection to allow any nonviable tumor cells present in the CSF as a result of the surgery itself to be cleared.

Bone marrow aspiration

In the past it was recommended that patients with medulloblastoma undergo a bone marrow aspiration at the time of diagnosis to rule out metastatic disease prior to starting therapy. However, more recent studies have indicated that fewer than 3% of patients diagnosed with medulloblastoma have extraneural metastases at diagnosis, with fewer than 25% of these having disease in the marrow. Therefore, recent clinical trials have no longer recommended routine examination of the bone marrow, but have instead recommended this only for patients with unexplained cytopenias. Extraneural metastases are almost unheard of in other types of pediatric CNS tumors, making bone marrow aspiration at diagnosis unnecessary.

Bone scan

While 90% of extraneural metastases in patients with medulloblastoma are to bone, this remains an unlikely presenting finding since, as mentioned above, fewer than 3% of patients have extraneural metastases at diagnosis. Therefore, bone scan should be reserved for brain tumor patients who present with bone pain with the underlying diagnosis of medulloblastoma.

Treatment

Children with CNS tumors are typically treated with some combination of neurosurgery, radiation therapy, and chemotherapy. The specific treatment chosen is dependent on the histology, location, resectability, and prognosis of the patient's tumor.

Neurosurgery

Initial neurosurgical intervention is indicated in the majority of patients. Exceptions include diffuse intrinsic pontine gliomas due to the infiltrative nature of the tumor throughout the pons and tumors that are radiographically consistent with germ cell tumors and present with elevation of both AFP and β-HCG. This combination confirms the diagnosis of nongermanomatous germ cell tumor (NGGCT) without a biopsy, and aggressive surgery at diagnosis has not been shown to improve survival. The role of surgery in children with functioning pituitary adenomas is also limited.

The goals of neurosurgical intervention are to achieve the maximum tumor removal possible while minimizing morbidity and mortality and to obtain tissue for a histologic diagnosis. In the case of medulloblastoma, PNET, ependymoma, and high-grade gliomas, extent of surgical resection is one of the major predictors of outcome.

Children with increased ICP caused by obstructive hydrocephalus will likely have a CSF diversion procedure performed as well, either before their definitive surgery if they are unstable or at the time of resection. An external ventricular drain will often be placed initially and will be clamped at some point after surgery to determine if normal CSF flow has been restored. Children who redevelop symptoms of increased ICP will likely require placement of a permanent shunt.

Radiation therapy

Radiation therapy has played a pivotal role in the management of children with malignant brain tumors for decades. It has been used to destroy remaining tumor in cases of incomplete surgical resection and to treat microscopic residual disease and metastatic disease in children who have malignant tumors with a high likelihood of tumor regrowth. The dose of radiation used is dependent on the type of tumor and the location and volume to be irradiated.

Unfortunately, the use of radiation therapy is associated with significant adverse late effects, particularly in young children. Those children receiving radiation before 6 years of age can be expected to suffer significant impairment of intellectual and physical development as a result of this therapy. A group of young Canadian children with medulloblastoma who received "curative" doses of radiation therapy were followed longitudinally into adulthood; none of the survivors were capable of independent living. Another concern is the development of secondary malignancies in the radiation field. Children receiving prophylactic craniospinal radiation for leukemia have been shown to have a >20-fold increase in the risk of secondary CNS tumors; more than 80% of these tumors occurred in children who were radiated before 5 years of age. Children with standard risk medulloblastoma who survive >5 years following conventional treatment including radiation without a relapse are more likely to die from a secondary radiation-induced cancer than from a recurrence of their primary tumor.

A variety of innovations in radiation therapy delivery have been developed recently to minimize the side effects of radiation. These include 3D conformal planning techniques and intensity-modulated radiation therapy, which minimize the dose of radiation delivered to adjacent normal tissue. Another innovation is proton beam therapy, which takes advantage of the shorter decay path of high-energy protons compared with gamma rays (photons). This minimizes the exit dose delivered beyond the site of the tumor. These innovations have proven very valuable in decreasing the radiation exposure to heart, lung, bowel, and reproductive organs in children receiving whole spine radiation. Nevertheless, the use of radiation therapy continues to carry the risk of significant morbidity. Work continues to develop novel strategies that will allow the avoidance of radiation therapy completely in children with CNS tumors, or at least to delay it in very young children.

Chemotherapy

The utility of chemotherapy in the treatment of CNS tumors was recognized more recently than in other tumors. It was initially felt that the BBB would prevent the delivery of effective concentrations of chemotherapeutic agents to the tumor. However, it became apparent that many drugs do adequately cross the BBB, or that this barrier is abnormally permeable in many malignant brain tumors. Other factors such as tumor heterogeneity, cell kinetics, drug distribution, and drug excretion may also have a significant impact on effectiveness of chemotherapy. Lower grade tumors are characterized by a low mitotic index and relatively slow growth rate; it was long felt that these tumors would be less sensitive to chemotherapy, while more malignant tumors would be more sensitive. However, several studies over the last two decades have demonstrated that many low-grade tumors are sensitive to chemotherapy. Commonly used drugs for the treatment of brain tumors include vincristine, methotrexate, temozolomide, procarbazine, lomustine (CCNU), cisplatin, carboplatin, cyclophosphamide, and etoposide.

Specific tumor types

Primitive neuroectodermal tumor

PNETs are the most common malignant brain tumors in children. They are comprised primarily of small cells with hypochromatic nuclei and can occur throughout the CNS. There has been controversy regarding whether these tumors should be classified as a single entity or divided by location. The WHO has chosen the latter approach, and divided these tumors into medulloblastoma (occurring in the cerebellum), pinealoblastoma (occurring in the pineal gland), and supratentorial PNET (occurring elsewhere in the supratentorial region).

Medulloblastoma is the most common malignant CNS tumor in children, accounting for up to 20% of all childhood brain tumors. Supratentorial PNET is much less common, comprising about 2.5% of cases when pinealoblastoma is included. It has a propensity to metastasize early; in up to 40% of cases, widespread seeding of the subarachnoid space is present. Extraneural spread is unusual at diagnosis, but may develop later if tumor recurrence occurs.

The initial mode of therapy is surgery, and extent of surgical resection directly affects prognosis and treatment. Patients with $<1.5\,\text{cm}^3$ of residual tumor after surgery and no evidence of metastatic disease are defined as standard risk, while patients with $>1.5\,\text{cm}^3$ of residual disease or metastatic disease are considered high risk. Once the diagnosis is confirmed, patients should be staged with an MRI of the spine and an LP for cell count, glucose, protein, and cytology. Additional studies looking for extraneural metastases are no longer considered necessary.

PNETs including medulloblastoma are very sensitive to radiation therapy, and as a result this has traditionally been considered the mainstay of postsurgical therapy. Due to the high likelihood of metastases throughout the CNS, it has been considered necessary to deliver a dose of radiation to the entire brain and spine (craniospinal irradiation; CSI) to these patients, with a higher (boost) dose delivered to the region of their tumor. As the long-term consequences of radiation have become more apparent, especially for young children, strategies to delay or avoid radiation in young children have become more widely used and attempts have been made to decrease the doses of radiation given to older children.

The value of chemotherapy both in improving survival among patients with PNETs and in allowing a reduction in the dose of radiation therapy required for cure has become increasingly evident over the past three decades. For the past several years a combination of cisplatin, vincristine, CCNU, and cyclophosphamide has been used following completion of radiation therapy with good effect. Vincristine is also used during radiation therapy, and the Children's Oncology Group is evaluating whether the addition of carboplatin during radiation therapy will improve outcomes further in children with high risk disease.

Due to the devastating effects that CSI can have in children less than 6 years of age at the time of treatment, an alternative strategy was developed in the early 1990s that substituted very intensive chemotherapy followed by consolidative myeloablative chemotherapy and hematopoietic stem cell rescue without radiation therapy for these young children. Known as the Head Start regimen, this strategy proved fairly effective for children with standard risk embryonal tumors, but results were suboptimal for patients with high risk medulloblastoma or supratentorial PNET, including pinealoblastoma. In 1995, the second Head Start study added high-dose methotrexate to the existing chemotherapy; results from this modification were very encouraging. Patients with standard risk medulloblastoma had 5-year event-free survival (EFS) rates of 50% and overall survival rates of 75%. Children who relapsed following chemotherapy alone were effectively salvaged with reoperation and radiation therapy in half of the cases. This strategy led to more than 70% of children with standard risk disease treated on Head Start II being cured without radiation therapy. The Children's Oncology Group is investigating a similar strategy for children <3 years of age with high risk medulloblastoma and supratentorial PNET.

The outlook for children >3 years of age with standard risk medulloblastoma is quite good; 5-year EFS with current multimodality therapy is >80%. Children with high risk medulloblastoma and supratentorial PNET do less well; the most recently published 5-year EFS rates are 50% to 60%.

Gliomas

Gliomas account for just over 50% of all CNS tumors in childhood. They are a heterogeneous collection of tumors including astrocytoma (60%), ependymoma (15%), oligodendroglioma (15%), mixed gliomas (5%), and other unspecified glial tumors (5%). They can occur anywhere in the CNS, although certain subtypes have a propensity to occur in specific locations.

Gliomas are classified histologically into grades 1 to 4 based on cellular pleomorphism, cell density, mitotic index, and necrosis. Grade 1 and 2 tumors are defined as low grade gliomas (LGG); they are considered by some to be "benign," but many neuro-oncologists disagree with this definition. Grade 3 and 4 gliomas are defined as high grade gliomas (HGG) and are clearly malignant. For most gliomas, the histologic classification is the most important factor in choosing therapy and predicting long-term outcome.

Surgical resection is a key component of therapy for most gliomas that are amenable to this approach. This includes cerebellar gliomas and supratentorial gliomas that are not centrally located or within the optic pathway. Gliomas occurring in the tectal region of the midbrain are an exception to this rule; these are very indolent tumors that typically require no intervention. LGG that are completely resected do not require adjuvant therapy and are simply observed. If they recur, re-resection is generally curative. Surgery should be used judiciously, however. Most LGG can be controlled successfully with chemotherapy, so surgery that leaves the patient with significant postoperative morbidity should be avoided. HGG always require adjuvant therapy, but the likelihood of cure is related to the degree of surgical resection.

Radiation therapy was a key part of the treatment of all gliomas for many years, but it is used very rarely now to treat children with LGG due to the frequency of long-term consequences of this therapy and the realization that these tumors can be managed successfully with chemotherapy. It remains an essential component of therapy for HGG, however. Since these tumors metastasize much less frequently than PNETs, children do not require CSI, but they do require doses of 50 to 60 Gy to their tumor sites to achieve local control.

The value of chemotherapy in the management of children with LGG has become increasingly apparent over the past ten years. This is especially true for children with neurofibromatosis-associated LGG, as the frequency of secondary malignant tumors in these children after treatment with radiation therapy is alarmingly high. The goal of therapy in this situation is different than with other tumors. Chemotherapy rarely leads to total disappearance of the tumor, but rather produces a state of stable disease that is hopefully maintained after therapy is discontinued. In this regard, management of incompletely resected LGG is similar to managing a chronic illness like asthma, with periods of stability, occasional flares of disease, and a hope that the child will eventually "grow out" of their condition.

Gliomas arising in the brain stem deserve special mention. These comprise about 15% of brain tumors in children. About 70% of these arise in the pons and are diffusely infiltrative, and are termed diffuse intrinsic pontine gliomas. These are the most deadly of all childhood brain tumors; median survival of children with this diagnosis is 8 to 9 months, and 90% of affected children are dead within 2 years of diagnosis regardless of the treatment provided. Radiation

therapy has been estimated to prolong survival for a median of 2 months; since the therapy takes 6 weeks to deliver, the impact of this treatment on improving quality of life may be minimal, especially for children requiring anesthesia for their radiation. Many trials have been conducted over the past 25 years trying to improve the survival of children with this tumor, all with disappointing results.

Although ependymomas are traditionally classified with other glial tumors, their behavior and management is quite different. They represent about 5% to 10% of childhood primary brain tumors. About 60% of intracranial ependymomas occur in the posterior fossa and 40% are supratentorial. Grade 1 ependymomas are rare and almost never occur in the brain, although Grade 1 (myxopapillary) ependymomas of the spine comprise about 10% of childhood ependymomas. Grade 4 ependymoma does not exist.

The extent of surgical resection is the most important prognostic factor in children with ependymoma. The 5-year EFS for patients having a complete resection is 80%, versus 40% for those patients having a near-total or subtotal resection. Unfortunately, ependymomas are often difficult to completely resect, especially in the posterior fossa due to their predilection to surround cranial nerves and other vital structures. It remains unclear that postoperative chemotherapy improves survival in patients with ependymoma, but it may improve outcome when given before second look surgery to improve the likelihood that a complete resection can be achieved. Radiation therapy remains an important component of therapy for this tumor; the doses required are similar to those needed to achieve local control of other glial tumors. Ependymomas are more likely to metastasize within the CNS than other gliomas, especially if they originate in the posterior fossa or are Grade 3. Assessment of the spinal fluid postoperatively is important, although negative spinal fluid cytology does not reliably identify patients less likely to recur away from their primary tumor site.

Germ cell tumors

CNS GCTs are relatively uncommon. Their management shares many similarities with GCTs occurring outside the CNS. They are discussed in Chapter 21.

Summary

In summary, although brain tumors occur relatively commonly in children, the variations in histologic appearance, presentation, treatment, and prognosis make their management quite challenging. The best outcomes for these children occur when they are diagnosed early and treated at a center with a multidisciplinary neuro-oncology program. Therefore, every effort should be made to ensure that potential signs of a brain tumor are not missed and that early referral to such a multidisciplinary center occurs.

Suggested Reading

Robertson PL. Advances in treatment of pediatric brain tumors. NeuroRx 3:276–291, 2006.

Wen PY, Schiff D, Kesari S, et al. Medical management of patients with brain tumors. J Neurooncol 80:313–332, 2006.

17 Hodgkin and Non-Hodgkin Lymphoma

Hodgkin and non-Hodgkin lymphoma together account for approximately 10% to 12% of malignancies in children; they are third in relative frequency after acute leukemias and brain tumors. Non-Hodgkin lymphoma (NHL) comprises approximately 60% of all lymphomas.

Hodgkin lymphoma

Hodgkin lymphoma (HL) is rare among children <5 years of age and relatively rare in the adult population, but is the most commonly diagnosed cancer among adolescents aged 15 to 19. HL is classified into two general groups: **classical HL** (95% of cases) and **nodular lymphocyte predominant HL** (NLPHL, 5% of cases). Classical HL is further subdivided into nodular sclerosis, mixed cellularity, lymphocyte-depleted, and lymphocyte-rich forms. The tumor cells in classical HL are designated Hodgkin and Reed–Sternberg (HRS) cells, whereas in NLPHL they are designated lymphocyte-predominant (LP) cells. HRS cells are now felt to derive from germinal center B-cells that have acquired unfavorable immunoglobulin V gene mutations and that normally would have undergone apoptosis, whereas LP cells derive from antigen-selected germinal center B-cells. In both forms of the disease, the tumor cells comprise only 0.1% to 10% of the cells within the tumor.

Epidemiologic studies suggest that two different forms of pediatric HL exist: childhood and adolescent/young adult (AYA). The childhood form is defined as occurring in those ≤14 years of age, and is characterized by a male predominance and a histologic subtype that is more likely to be mixed cellularity (30% to 35%) or nodular lymphocyte predominant (10% to 20%). An increased proportion of childhood HL is associated with Epstein–Barr virus (EBV) infection, and studies suggest that early exposure to EBV is a risk factor for developing HL in childhood. AYA HL occurs in patients between 15 and 35 years of age. There is no gender predilection. The most common histologic subtype is nodular sclerosis (70% to 80%). EBV infection appears to play a role in AYA HL also. Other infectious agents that have been associated with HL include human herpesvirus 6 and cytomegalovirus. There is clearly an association between HL and alterations in immune function. HL is seen more commonly in patients with HIV disease, acquired immunodeficiency (e.g., hematopoietic stem cell or solid organ transplant), and autoimmune disease.

Handbook of Pediatric Hematology and Oncology: Children's Hospital & Research Center Oakland, Second Edition. Caroline A. Hastings, Joseph C. Torkildson, and Anurag K. Agrawal.
© 2012 John Wiley & Sons, Ltd. Published 2012 by John Wiley & Sons, Ltd.

Clinical presentation

The most common presentation of HL is painless cervical or supraclavicular adenopathy. The nodes are typically described as rubbery or firm and nontender, although may be sensitive to touch with rapid growth. As the disease progresses, the nodes enlarge and often aggregate into larger masses that may become fixed to the underlying tissue. As children often have reactive or infectious adenopathy, it is common to have received treatment with several courses of antibiotics before ultimately coming to biopsy. This is more common with cervical than with supraclavicular adenopathy, as the latter is less frequently associated with infection or inflammation and leads more quickly to referral for possible malignancy. At least two-thirds of patients with cervical or supraclavicular adenopathy have mediastinal involvement as well. This is frequently asymptomatic, but may be associated with cough (usually nonproductive), shortness of breath, chest pain, or superior vena cava syndrome. HL limited to infradiaphragmatic sites occurs in <5% of pediatric cases, occurring most commonly in femoral, superficial iliac, or inguinal nodes.

Constitutional symptoms commonly occur in patients with HL. They are caused by cytokines produced by the HRS cells within the tumor. Certain specific symptoms known as "B symptoms" have been demonstrated to have a negative prognostic significance. These are unplanned weight loss of >10% of body weight over the 6 months preceding diagnosis, drenching night sweats, or fever >38°C for at least three consecutive days. Other common constitutional symptoms include generalized pruritus and alcohol-induced pain.

Evaluation

1. A careful history and physical examination is imperative. The presence of B symptoms and any other unusual symptoms should be identified, as patients with HL can present with a variety of paraneoplastic syndromes. All superficial nodal groups should be carefully examined, and the size of any enlarged nodes and their character should be documented.

2. The laboratory evaluation should include a complete blood count (CBC) with differential, erythrocyte sedimentation rate (ESR), C-reactive protein (CRP), complete metabolic panel (including transaminases, lactate dehydrogenase [LDH], and alkaline phosphatase), serum copper, and serum ferritin. One or more of these nonspecific inflammatory markers may be elevated and thus be useful initially to monitor response to therapy and later to identify possible recurrence.

3. A posterior-anterior (PA) and lateral chest radiograph will identify bulky mediastinal disease, if present. This is important, as it will influence the approach used to obtain diagnostic material since patients with bulky mediastinal disease are more likely to experience complications with general anesthesia. Other important imaging studies include a CT scan of the neck, chest, abdomen, and pelvis. The radiologist should be reminded to include the Waldeyer ring in the scan as this nodal area can be involved with disease as well, especially in patients with upper cervical node involvement. Oral and intravenous contrast are required for accurate identification of intra-abdominal adenopathy. Splenic involvement occurs in 30% to 40% of children at diagnosis. Positron emission tomography (PET)-CT is now commonly used at diagnosis as a very sensitive tool for identifying sites of involvement, when it is available. A gallium scan should be performed if PET is not available.

4. Bone marrow involvement at initial presentation of pediatric HL is uncommon and rarely occurs as an isolated site of extranodal disease. However, it is seen more commonly in patients with advanced stage (stage III

or IV) disease or patients with B symptoms. These patients should undergo bone marrow aspiration and biopsy from at least two sites as part of their diagnostic evaluation. All patients experiencing a recurrence of their disease should have their bone marrow examined.

5. Skeletal metastases are also rare at diagnosis, and bone scans have typically been performed only in patients with bone pain, unexplained elevations in the alkaline phosphatase, or other sites of extranodal disease. PET-CT is a sensitive test for identifying bone metastases and ultimately may replace bone scanning all together. It is important to remember that typical PET-CT imaging stops at the knee; patients with distal lower extremity pain will need to have the exam carried further or have alternative imaging of these areas.

Staging

The most widely used staging system for pediatric HL is the Ann Arbor staging system. This system divides lymph node regions into nodal sites (e.g., neck, axilla, and mediastinum), and the number of involved sites then determines the stage. Stage I disease involves only a single nodal site, whereas stage II involves two or more sites that lie together on one side of the diaphragm. Stage III disease spans the diaphragm and stage IV is disseminated systemic disease. Additional modifiers include A or B, to describe the absence or presence of systemic symptoms respectively, and E, involvement of a single extranodal site that is contiguous or proximal to a known nodal site. The presence of bulky mediastinal disease, described as greater than one-third of the intrathoracic diameter, is also considered.

Treatment

The first successful treatment strategy for HL was based solely on the use of radiation therapy (RT). While this approach was fairly effective in curing the disease in low risk patients, it resulted in unacceptable musculoskeletal hypoplasia, cardiovascular and pulmonary dysfunction, and the development of subsequent secondary cancers. This led to the development of combined modality therapy with the goal of improving event-free and overall survival, especially in higher risk patients, and decreasing the long-term adverse effects of a radiation only approach. Current research efforts in HL treatment seek to maintain the excellent survival rates presently achieved while continuing to decrease the frequency of later adverse events. Today, patients with favorable disease presentations receive fewer cycles of multiagent chemotherapy than those with advanced and unfavorable clinical presentations, either alone or combined with low-dose, involved-field radiation. With current therapy, more than 80% of children diagnosed with classical HL are expected to be long-term disease-free survivors, regardless of stage at diagnosis.

For treatment purposes, patients with HL are typically divided into low, intermediate, and high risk disease groups. These groups are defined by clinical stage, presence of bulky disease, and presence of B symptoms. The current approach to therapy also includes the adaptation of treatment based on the patient's response to early therapy, a so-called response-based approach.

A variety of chemotherapy agents have been shown to be effective in treating HL. However, many early regimens such as nitrogen mustard, vincristine, procarbazine, and prednisone (MOPP) resulted in a very high rate of secondary malignancy. Newer regimens have replaced nitrogen mustard with cyclophosphamide (COPP) and added other agents such as doxorubicin, bleomycin, vinblastine, and etoposide.

Classical HL—low risk disease

A number of studies have attempted to eliminate the use of RT completely in children with low risk disease. This approach has resulted in an increased rate of relapse in patients not receiving RT, but many of these patients were successfully salvaged with combination chemotherapy and RT, thus long-term survival was not affected. The most recent Children's Oncology Group study treated patients with three cycles of doxorubicin, vincristine, prednisone, and cyclophosphamide. Those having a complete response by PET-CT or gallium scan were observed; those having a partial response received involved-field radiation therapy (IFRT).

Classical HL—intermediate and high risk disease

The majority of patients with intermediate risk disease either have stage I/II disease with one or more unfavorable features (B symptoms, lymph node bulk, hilar lymph node involvement, involvement of three or more lymph node regions, and extranodal extension to contiguous structures) or have stage IIIA disease. High risk patients typically include those with stage IIIB or IV disease. Due to their more advanced stage, these patients are treated with more aggressive chemotherapy followed by IFRT. Current therapy includes doxorubicin, bleomycin, vincristine, etoposide, prednisone, and cyclophosphamide (ABVE-PC); slow responders may also receive additional chemotherapy. The role of IFRT continues to be investigated in the treatment of intermediate risk patients, whereas high risk patients all receive consolidation with IFRT.

Nodular lymphocyte predominant HL

Several studies have demonstrated that patients with NLPHL who present with stage I disease and a single involved lymph node can be successfully treated with surgery alone. Stage I patients with more than one involved node and stage II patients, which represent more than 80% of patients with NLPHL, are successfully treated with similar protocols used in low risk classical HL patients. Current studies are investigating whether therapy can be reduced even further in this group of very low risk patients.

Complications of treatment

Short term

The chemotherapy regimens used for the treatment of HL are moderately emetogenic. The nausea and vomiting can usually be controlled with serotonin receptor antagonist antiemetics such as ondansetron. It is not uncommon for patients to develop anticipatory nausea and vomiting with repeated cycles; this can be managed with benzodiazepines such as lorazepam. Myelosuppression occurs very commonly, especially with the more intensive regimens, and patients occasionally require hospitalization for fever and neutropenia. Varicella zoster occurs frequently both during and after therapy, with a frequency that correlates with the intensity of therapy. Appropriate preventive and therapeutic steps should be taken quickly in the event of exposure or infection (see Chapter 25). Peripheral neuropathy can result from vincristine and vinblastine therapy, as can constipation. Pulmonary toxicity can result from bleomycin, with development of restrictive lung disease and reductions in diffusion capacity. Anthracycline-induced cardiac toxicity is unusual with the decreased doses used in current regimens, but is more common when combined with mediastinal RT.

Long term

The most significant long-term complication of HL therapy is the development of a second malignant neoplasm. The frequency has decreased with recent modifications in chemotherapy and reductions in RT dose and volume, but it remains a concern during long-term follow-up. One specific issue is the risk of development of early breast cancer in female patients treated during adolescence, especially those treated with mediastinal radiation. Other potential long-term consequences of therapy include sterility/infertility (most common in males treated with alkylating agents), secondary acute myelogenous leukemia (etoposide, alkylating agents), pulmonary fibrosis (bleomycin), and atherosclerotic heart disease (anthracyclines + RT). Comprehensive long-term follow-up is essential for survivors of HL due to their increased risk of late complications of therapy.

Non-Hodgkin lymphoma

NHL is about 1.5 times as common as Hodgkin lymphoma. The incidence is low in children less than 5 year of age, but from that point it increases steadily with age throughout life. In all age groups, there is a significant male predominance, particularly among patients with Burkitt lymphoma (BL). During childhood, the disease is more common among non-Hispanic whites and Asians/Pacific Islanders; after age twenty, it occurs more commonly in African-Americans. The incidence of different histologic subtypes is very different in children and adults.

Children with congenital or acquired immune system dysfunction have a high risk of developing lymphoma. Congenital conditions include ataxia-telangiectasia, as well as Bloom, Wiskott-Aldrich, and Chédiak–Higashi syndromes; acquired conditions include HIV and prolonged immunosuppressive therapy following bone marrow or solid organ transplant. EBV is clearly associated with BL in underdeveloped countries,

and has been linked to several subtypes of NHL in the developed world. Other identified risk factors include *Helicobacter pylori* infection, tobacco exposure, and chemical or other environmental exposures. It is likely that there is not a single etiology responsible for the development of all cases of NHL.

The histologic classification of NHL has changed frequently over time and has become more precise as our understanding of the development of lymphoma has improved and better diagnostic tools (immunophenotyping, cytogenetics, molecular biology, and gene profiling) have been developed. The current World Health Organization classification is now widely used. There are four major histologic subtypes of NHL that occur commonly in children (in order of frequency): diffuse, large B-cell lymphoma (DLBCL), lymphoblastic lymphoma (LL), BL, and anaplastic large cell lymphoma (ALCL).

DLBCL and ALCL tend to be heterogeneous immunologically. Most are B-cell derived, although some are T-cell derived or arise from the macrophage–histiocyte lineage. Burkitt and Burkitt-like subtypes are virtually all B-cell tumors, distinguished only by the amount of cellular heterogeneity. The most common site of occurrence of LL is the mediastinum, and these tumors are virtually all of T-cell origin. Less commonly LL occurs in bone or subcutaneously; these tumors are typically of B-cell origin. All of these subtypes can invade the bone marrow and undergo leukemic transformation.

Clinical presentation

The clinical presentation of NHL varies and depends on the primary site of disease, histologic subtype, and extent of disease. NHL can arise anywhere in the body, but occurs most frequently in the lymph nodes, thymus, Waldeyer's ring, Peyer's patches, and bone marrow. In the United States, BL typically presents in the intestine, resulting in obstruction. These children usually present with nausea, vomiting, and abdominal distention. It is not unusual for NHL to be confused with a surgical abdomen, such as appendicitis. BL also presents in Waldeyer's ring or in the facial bones. T-cell LL most commonly arises from the thymus; these children typically present with respiratory symptoms, cervical or supraclavicular adenopathy, or superior vena cava syndrome. Children may have very limited disease affecting the tonsils, nasopharynx, or Waldeyer's ring, and the diagnosis has resulted from the pathologic examination following a tonsillectomy and adenoidectomy. Lymphomas arising in less common sites such as superficial lymph nodes, bone, skin, thyroid, orbit, eyelid, kidney, and the epidural space can be caused by any subtype of lymphoma.

Diagnostic evaluation

It is not unusual to begin with a surgical procedure for excision or biopsy of a node or laparotomy in the case of an acute abdominal presentation. Many times the diagnosis is not suspected prior to these procedures. In any event, histologic confirmation is necessary for diagnosis. The diagnosis of NHL is usually made using biopsy material but it can also be confirmed by cytological examination of effusion fluids or review of bone marrow smears. In this way, major surgical procedures can often be avoided in patients presenting with BL and LL, who are frequently unstable at presentation. If possible, sufficient material should be obtained for immunologic and cytogenetic or molecular biology studies. Many therapeutic trials now have requirements for submission of material for central pathology review or biology studies; these requirements should be taken into consideration when planning a diagnostic procedure.

The laboratory studies that should be obtained include:

- A CBC with differential and review of the peripheral smear to assess for possible bone marrow involvement or leukemia.
- Serum chemistries to include liver transaminases, blood urea nitrogen, creatinine, LDH, uric acid, electrolytes, calcium, and phosphorus. Lymphomas, particularly LL and BL, can present with overt tumor lysis syndrome (TLS) and/or renal dysfunction. The LDH can be useful prognostically, especially in patients with advanced stage disease.
- Bilateral bone marrow aspirations and biopsies as the child may actually have leukemia, defined as a marrow with >25% replacement by lymphoblasts.
- A lumbar puncture to assess the cerebrospinal fluid for involvement by NHL.

Radiologic procedures that should be performed will vary depending on the location of the mass and associated symptoms, but should include:

- A prompt PA and lateral chest radiograph to evaluate for mediastinal involvement.
- CT scan of the neck, chest, abdomen, and pelvis if the patient is sufficiently stable.
- MRI of the brain for patients with immunodeficiency-related NHL as these patients more commonly present with parenchymal brain disease.
- MRI of the brain and spine for patients with focal neurologic symptoms.
- PET-CT to include all identified sites of disease. Ideally, this should be performed following the diagnostic procedure, as these patients frequently have residual abnormalities in their surgical bed on plain CT that are discovered on PET-CT to not represent active disease.

Staging

NHL is staged using the St. Jude (Murphy) staging system that is presented in Table 17.1.

Table 17.1 St. Jude staging system for non-Hodgkin lymphoma.

Stage	Description
I	A single tumor (extranodal) or single anatomic area (nodal), excluding mediastinum or abdomen
II	A single tumor (extranodal) with regional node involvement On same side of diaphragm: • Two or more nodal areas • Two single (extranodal) tumors ± regional node involvement • A primary gastrointestinal tract tumor (usually ileocecal) with or without associated mesenteric node involvement, grossly completely resected
III	On both sides of the diaphragm: • Two single tumors (extranodal) • Two or more nodal areas All primary intrathoracic tumors (mediastinal, pleural, thymic) All extensive primary intra-abdominal disease; unresectable All primary paraspinal or epidural tumors regardless of other sites
IV	Any of the above with central nervous system or bone marrow involvement (<25%) at diagnosis

Treatment

Therapy is based on clinical staging, localized versus disseminated disease, and histologic subtype. In general, children with localized NHL have an excellent prognosis, with a 90% long-term survival. Therapy may begin with surgical resection in the case of primary gastrointestinal tumors that are amenable to complete resection, but this is not a necessary part of therapy for treatment of other sites (unless a life-threatening complication is present).

These tumors are exquisitely sensitive to chemotherapy, and multidrug regimens, similar to those used for leukemia, are frequently recommended. Radiotherapy is generally reserved for some patients with CNS+ lymphoblastic lymphoma, relapsed patients, or oncologic emergencies due to tumor compression. In general, B-cell lymphomas require intensive short-course therapy ranging from 2 to 8 months in duration depending on initial tumor burden. Rituximab is now frequently added to treatment regimens for patients with B-cell lymphoma, although clear evidence that it significantly improves pediatric outcomes is lacking. Patients with LL have superior outcomes with longer acute lymphoblastic leukemia-type therapy. CNS prophylaxis in either type is indicated in advanced stages and in those patients with parameningeal or overt CNS disease at diagnosis. The optimal treatment of ALCL is not yet well defined. Patients with stage I and II disease do well with brief, multiagent intensive chemotherapy and CNS prophylaxis. Patients with advanced stage disease who express the fusion protein generated by the anaplastic lymphoma kinase (ALK) gene have superior outcomes compared to patients who are ALK negative. The latter patients typically require a more intensive, anthracycline-containing regimen.

With the initiation of therapy, the child must be closely monitored for the development of TLS and resultant metabolic abnormalities. Some therapeutic regimens begin with a "reduction phase" of treatment, using minimal therapy until the time of massive lysis has passed, then proceeding to the induction phase with institution of multidrug therapy.

Suggested Reading

Hudson MM, Schwartz C, Constine LS. Treatment of pediatric Hodgkin lymphoma. In: Bleyer WA, Barr RD (eds), Cancer in Adolescents and Young Adults. New York: Springer, 2007, pp 35–66.

Patte C, Bleyer A, Cairo M. Non-Hodgkin lymphoma. In: Bleyer WA, Barr RD (eds), Cancer in Adolescents and Young Adults. New York: Springer, 2007, pp 127–149.

Punnett A, Tsang RW, Hodgson DC. Hodgkin lymphoma across the age spectrum: epidemiology, therapy, and late effects. Semin Radiat Oncol 20:30–44, 2010.

Shukla NN, Trippet TN. Non-Hodgkin's lymphoma in children and adolescents. Curr Oncol Rep 8: 387–394, 2006.

18 Wilms Tumor

Wilms tumor is the second most common retroperitoneal tumor in children, accounting for approximately 6% of childhood malignancies. A tumor of the developing kidney, it typically occurs in young children between the ages of 1 and 5 years, with equal incidence among boys and girls (though interestingly occurs at earlier ages in boys). Most cases of Wilms tumor are sporadic, with approximately 1% being familial and 2% to 4% associated with rare congenital syndromes. Familial cases are more likely to present with bilateral tumors and occur at a younger age.

Genetics

Congenital anomalies occur in 12% to 15% of cases, the most common being hemihypertrophy, aniridia, and genitourinary tract (GU) anomalies such as cryptorchidism, hypospadias, horseshoe kidney, ureteral duplication, and polycystic kidney. Most children with Wilms tumor have a normal karyotype; however, a chromosomal deletion in the short arm of chromosome 11 (11p13 deletion) is seen in association with congenital aniridia. The Wilms tumor 1 (WT1) gene encodes a transcription factor important in normal kidney development. Mutations within the WT1 gene have been identified in two syndromes associated with Wilms tumor: WAGR syndrome (*Wilms* tumor, *Aniridia*, *GU* anomalies, and mental *Retardation*) and Denys–Drash syndrome (Wilms tumor, nephropathy, and GU anomalies including pseudohermaphroditism). Beckwith–Wiedemann syndrome (macroglossia, omphalocele, visceromegaly, with or without hemihypertrophy) is associated with imprinting defects at several genes at chromosome 11p15.5, a locus referred to as the WT2 gene. Patients with this syndrome have a genetic predisposition to develop Wilms tumor, with an incidence as high as 5% to 10%.

Clinical presentation

Most children with Wilms tumor are generally in good health at presentation and come to medical attention due to abdominal enlargement or when a family member has felt a mass. Associated signs and symptoms include abdominal pain, malaise, fever, hypertension, and microscopic hematuria. Bleeding within the tumor may occur and result in anemia, pallor, and fatigue. Tumor thrombus may extend into the vena cava, causing partial obstruction, hypertension, and distention of abdominal veins. Polycythemia may be seen in Wilms

Handbook of Pediatric Hematology and Oncology: Children's Hospital & Research Center Oakland, Second Edition. Caroline A. Hastings, Joseph C. Torkildson, and Anurag K. Agrawal.
© 2012 John Wiley & Sons, Ltd. Published 2012 by John Wiley & Sons, Ltd.

tumor and may or may not be related to elevated erythropoietin levels. Acquired von Willebrand disease with reduced von Willebrand factor (VWF), factor VIII coagulant, and ristocetin cofactor levels has been reported in approximately 8% of patients newly diagnosed with Wilms tumor and typically resolves with therapy initiation. Its occurrence in Wilms tumor is thought secondary to binding of VWF to the tumor with subsequent degradation as well as hyaluronic acid secretion by nephroblastoma cells leading to decreased efficacy of VWF.

Evaluation of suspected Wilms tumor

- **History:** include family history of malignancies, congenital anomalies, or syndromes
- **Physical examination:** assess gently for abdominal/flank mass (usually distinct and not crossing the midline), congenital anomalies (hemihypertrophy, GU malformations, aniridia), hypertension, abdominal venous distention, and liver enlargement
- **Laboratory studies:** urinalysis with microscopic evaluation, complete blood count (polycythemia and anemia), serum chemistries (hypercalcemia in rhabdoid tumor or congenital mesoblastic nephroma), and coagulation studies including von Willebrand panel
- **Diagnostic imaging studies:**
  - Doppler abdominal ultrasound to evaluate the tumor, possible vena cava involvement, blood flow, and contralateral kidney
  - Abdominal CT or MRI with special attention to evidence of bilateral involvement, vessel involvement or extension to the inferior vena cava (IVC), lymph node involvement, and liver metastases
  - Chest radiography and chest CT to assess for lung metastases (most common site)
  - Bone scan to assess for metastases if the tumor is a clear cell sarcoma and for all

patients with Wilms tumor with lung or liver metastatic disease and bony symptoms
  - MRI of the brain for metastases if the tumor is a rhabdoid tumor or clear cell sarcoma
  - Echocardiogram for detecting tumor extension from the IVC to the right atrium and also indicated in the child receiving anthracycline chemotherapy

Pathologic diagnosis

Children with suspected Wilms tumor should have an immediate consultation with a pediatric surgeon. Surgical removal of the involved kidney and intact tumor is indicated at diagnosis if possible. Cases with tumor in the renal pelvis and IVC require a detailed imaging assessment to guide the surgeon. In some cases, complete removal of the primary tumor at diagnosis may not be possible. In these cases, open biopsy is indicated for pathologic confirmation and determination of histology.

Tumor pathology is critical in diagnosis as well as helping to determine the staging and therefore subsequent treatment. Classic Wilms tumor presents with three types of nephroblastoma tissue elements: blastema, stroma (mesenchyme), and epithelium. Additional assessment includes determination of histology as either favorable (well-differentiated components) or unfavorable (presence of anaplasia with poor differentiation and a worse prognosis). Other malignant tumors of the kidney need to be considered and ruled out including rhabdoid tumor of the kidney, clear cell sarcoma of the kidney, and renal cell carcinoma. Chromosome analysis is performed on the tumor and may prove to be especially useful in association with congenital anomalies and familial cases. Loss of heterozygosity (LOH) of chromosomes 1p and 16q has also recently been confirmed to be a negative prognostic indicator.

Staging

Staging is done postoperatively and is determined based on the extent of disease, ability to perform a total resection, and the pathologic findings. Patients unable to undergo a radical nephrectomy at diagnosis due to excessive risk receive preliminary staging and preoperative chemotherapy with delayed resection. A careful pathologic evaluation at the time of excision should be performed regardless of whether this occurs at diagnosis or later following preoperative chemotherapy, as the histology may be different than that seen on initial biopsy. This evaluation includes identifying tumor histology and looking for extension of disease outside the kidney, including penetrance of the tumor through the renal capsule into the renal pelvis and vessels and presence of nodal involvement.

Clinicopathologic staging is as follows:
- **Stage I:** tumor limited to the kidney and completed excised without tumor rupture or biopsy prior to resection
- **Stage II:** tumor extends through the renal capsule, has been biopsied, or ruptured prior to excision with spillage confined to the flank; tumor may involve the perirenal soft tissue and/or infiltrate vessels outside the kidney but is completely excised
- **Stage III:** residual nonhematogenous dissemination of tumor confined to the abdomen; tumor may extend beyond surgical margin at resection, may involve local lymph nodes, or have tumor spillage with peritoneal implants
- **Stage IV:** hematogenous dissemination of tumor to lungs, liver, bone, brain, or distant lymph nodes
- **Stage V:** bilateral renal involvement

Patients with bilateral involvement of tumor (stage V) should have each side independently staged with treatment based on the side with the highest stage.

Treatment

The prognosis of Wilms tumor is excellent, with more than 85% of children being cured of their disease. Histology is more prognostic for outcome than staging; for example, patients with stage IV disease but with favorable histology still have a 4-year survival of more than 85%, compared to children with diffuse anaplasia and advanced disease who have very poor outcomes. Children with stage I and II favorable histology tumors have an event-free survival rate exceeding 95%.

Many tumors are low stage at presentation and are able to be fully resected. Additionally, these tumors are very sensitive to chemotherapy and radiation. Based on the exceedingly good outcomes, contemporary studies have looked to decrease therapy in the lower risk stratum. This includes the elimination of chemotherapy in patients younger than 2 years with stage I disease and tumor mass of <550 g without LOH at 1p and 16q. For patients receiving chemotherapy, the backbone of therapy is based on previous studies by the National Wilms Tumor Study Group and includes vincristine, doxorubicin, and dactinomycin. Higher stage patients may require radiation therapy in addition to this chemotherapeutic backbone. Patients with stage IV disease or patients with advanced stage and LOH at 1p and 16q receive more aggressive therapy with the addition of cyclophosphamide and etoposide. In general, patients with pulmonary metastasis will require lung irradiation although newer protocols are studying whether this can be eliminated in patients with a rapid response to chemotherapy and no additional risk factors. Finally, patients with higher stage anaplastic disease as well as patients with rhabdoid tumor of the kidney or metastatic clear cell sarcoma receive a similar regimen with the addition of carboplatin.

Relapse is uncommon in Wilms tumor; patients may be salvaged with aggressive multiagent chemotherapy, radiation if previously not given, and possibly may benefit from high-dose chemotherapy with autologous stem cell rescue. As survival is excellent, much attention has focused on late effects related to therapy and limiting potential toxicities. Patients are at risk for hypertension and renal insufficiency, as most children will have a solitary remaining kidney. Patients with bilateral disease, partial resection, and radiation exposure are particularly at risk for developing proteinuria and renal compromise in addition to hypertension. Cardiac complications may be seen in those patients who receive anthracyclines and lung irradiation. Additionally, patients with right-sided tumors who receive flank irradiation and those receiving whole abdomen irradiation have an increased risk of developing a secondary liver cancer. These potential issues must all be taken into account in the patient's long-term follow-up plan.

Suggested Reading

Davidoff AM. Wilms tumor. Curr Opin Pediatr 21:357–364, 2009.

Nakamura L, Ritchey M. Current management of Wilms tumor. Curr Urol Rep 11:58–65, 2010.

Pritchard-Jones K. Nephrectomy only for Wilms tumor: negotiating the tangled web requires multiprofessional input. Pediatr Blood Cancer 54:865–866, 2010.

19 Neuroblastoma

Neuroblastoma is a neoplasm of the sympathetic nervous system and the most common solid tumor of early childhood, with a peak incidence around 2 years of age. Neuroblastoma is a disease of developing neural crest tissue and has an extremely heterogeneous prognosis based on multiple factors such as the age of the patient, differentiation and biology of the tumor, and extent of disease spread. Screening in the Japanese infant population found a high incidence of neuroblastoma, although the majority of these cases matured or involuted spontaneously, again implying the heterogeneous prognosis based on patient age. Although survival rates for neuroblastoma have improved over the last 30 years, the majority of these gains have been observed in patients with lower risk disease. Recent breakthroughs hold promise to increase survival in those with high risk disease as well.

Familial cases of neuroblastoma are quite rare. However, genetic risk factors for neuroblastoma have been identified including the anaplastic lymphoma kinase 1 and PHOX2B homeobox genes. Patients with Hirschsprung's disease, neurofibromatosis type I, and congenital hypoventilation syndrome may have genetic alterations in PHOX2B and an increased risk of developing neuroblastoma, although clear genetic links have not as yet been identified. More commonly, amplification of the oncogene N-myc in tumor tissue has been found to have a profound negative impact on prognosis. Similarly, a near diploid (low DNA index, DNA index = 1) chromosome number in the tumor has also been found to be a negative prognostic indicator as compared to patients with a DNA index >1. Based on these factors, in addition to age, stage, and histology (favorable or unfavorable based on mitosis-karyorrhexis index and maturity of the tumor), a complicated risk-stratified treatment regimen has been created.

Clinical presentation

As neuroblastoma originates from primordial neural crest cells that normally give rise to the adrenal medulla and the sympathetic ganglia, tumors present in the abdomen and along the sympathetic neural pathway. The most common presentation is an **abdominal mass** with primary tumor in the adrenal gland, often with metastatic disease via lymphatic and hematogenous spread. Tumors are often seen along the paraspinal ganglion and may be found in the neck, thorax, and pelvis. Infants are more likely to have thoracic and cervical tumors. Common sites of metastasis are the lymph nodes, bone marrow, bone, liver, and skin.

Handbook of Pediatric Hematology and Oncology: Children's Hospital & Research Center Oakland,
Second Edition. Caroline A. Hastings, Joseph C. Torkildson, and Anurag K. Agrawal.
© 2012 John Wiley & Sons, Ltd. Published 2012 by John Wiley & Sons, Ltd.

The **signs and symptoms** at presentation depend on the site of the tumor, size, and the degree of spread. Patients with locoregional disease may be relatively asymptomatic, whereas patients with widely metastatic disease are often ill-appearing with fever, pain, weight loss, and irritability. Abdominal tumors are usually palpable, hard, fixed masses. The liver may be enlarged, leading to respiratory compromise, especially in the infant. There may be evidence of anemia (pallor, weakness, and fatigue), coagulopathy (bruising and bleeding), and bone pain or limping with bone or bone marrow involvement. Thoracic masses are usually picked up in the posterior mediastinum incidentally by imaging studies done for other reasons. Cervical masses may initially be treated as cervical adenopathy related to infection. The presence of Horner's syndrome (miosis [contracted pupil], ptosis, enophthalmos [posterior eye displacement], and anhidrosis) or heterochromia iridis should prompt an evaluation for cervicothoracic neuroblastoma. Pelvic masses may cause bowel or bladder symptoms and tumors along the sympathetic ganglia may cause spinal cord compression. Skin lesions tend to be limited to infants and appear as bluish, nontender subcutaneous nodules. Sphenoid or retro-orbital bone involvement may occur and appear clinically as "raccoon eyes" secondary to periorbital hemorrhage.

In addition to Horner's syndrome, the clinician should be aware of potential **paraneoplastic syndromes** with neuroblastoma. One unusual presentation is opsoclonus-myoclonus-ataxia syndrome (OMAS), also referred to as "dancing eyes/dancing feet." These children have cerebellar and truncal ataxia as well as myoclonus (muscle jerks) and opsoclonus (rapid, involuntary, uncoordinated eye movements). Developmental delay, language deficits, and behavioral abnormalities (e.g., irritability) may also be present. Children with OMAS should be carefully evaluated for the presence of an occult neuroblastoma. Children with OMAS tend to have a low-stage, highly curable neuroblastoma. Unfortunately, this cure often has little impact on the OMAS, and these children are frequently left with severe, chronic neurologic deficits. The pathophysiology of this syndrome is not well defined but is likely due to formation of an antibody directed against the neuroblastoma cells also targeting cerebellar neurons. In addition to treatment of the neuroblastoma, these children may benefit from immunosuppressive therapy with agents such as dexamethasone, cyclophosphamide, intravenous immune globulin (IVIG), and adrenocorticotropic hormone (ACTH). Neuroblastoma patients may also present with hypersecretory diarrhea secondary to hypersecretion of vasoactive intestinal peptide (VIP) from the neuroblastoma cells. In most cases, treatment of the underlying disease will eliminate the VIP hypersecretion.

Diagnostic evaluation

History
Assess for constitutional symptoms, abdominal pain, bowel or bladder control problems, bleeding, bone pain, and limping.

Physical examination
Assess vital signs (fever and hypertension) and evaluate for abdominal mass, spinal cord compression, unusual signs/symptoms associated with neuroblastoma (heterochromia, raccoon eyes, Horner's syndrome), subcutaneous nodules in infants, enlarged liver or lymph nodes, and evidence of anemia or coagulopathy.

Laboratory studies
Obtain complete blood count with differential, serum chemistries (liver function

studies and lactate dehydrogenase), ferritin (may be a tumor marker and elevated in neuroblastoma, though also an acute-phase reactant), and urine for catecholamines including homovanillic acid (HVA) and vanillylmandelic acid (VMA). These urine metabolites are elevated in more than 90% of children with neuroblastoma, especially in the higher stages of disease. In patients with clinical suspicion for neuroblastoma and negative urine markers, urine dopamine can be measured in addition to 24-hour urine collections for HVA and VMA. Neuron-specific enolase (NSE), a serum marker specific to the sympathetic nervous system, is relatively specific to neuroblastoma although it can be elevated after brain injury and seizures.

Diagnostic studies

Patients with confirmed neuroblastoma should have bilateral bone marrow aspiration and biopsy performed to assess for bone marrow involvement. Special stains (S100, synaptophysin, and NSE) are used to differentiate this tumor from other small, round blue cell tumors of childhood such as rhabdomyosarcoma, Ewing sarcoma, lymphoma, and primitive neuroectodermal tumor. Lumbar puncture should be avoided as this procedure may increase the incidence of central nervous system metastases.

Imaging studies should include:

• CT or MRI of the primary site (MRI is preferred due to the radiation exposure associated with repeated CT imaging). Calcifications and hemorrhage are commonly seen, especially in large abdominal masses. The tumors tend to be large and displace adjacent organs; however, the tumor can wrap around major structures, causing obstruction and dysfunction. If there is suspicion of paraspinal or intraspinal involvement, MRI and plain films of the spine should be done.

• Bone scan (technetium-99m).

• MIBG (metaiodobenzylguanidine) scan (^{123}I-MIBG scan preferred over ^{131}I-MIBG due to decreased risk to thyroid function). Prior to MIBG scanning, the patient must receive thyroid protection with potassium iodide (SSKI) drops and should have baseline thyroid function (FT4/TSH) checked. MIBG, a functional analog of norepinephrine, is taken up by sympathetic neurons and is a sensitive test for neuroblastoma cells. It is also positive in pheochromocytoma.

• Due to the high radiation doses with both bone scan and MIBG scanning, patients can be followed solely with MIBG if results of baseline imaging are concordant.

Localized tumors should be surgically removed if it deemed safe and feasible. Many tumors are initially unresectable. These tumors should be surgically biopsied, with sampling of local lymph nodes. Diagnosis is generally established by pathologic assessment of the resected or biopsied mass and can be confirmed by diagnostic features such as bone marrow involvement with appropriate immunohistochemical markers, MIBG avidity, and positive urine catecholamines and serum NSE.

Staging

The International Neuroblastoma Staging System as shown in Table 19.1 was most recently revised in 1993 and provides a basic prognostic model that has been more recently complemented by biologic and pathologic assessments including N-myc amplication, DNA ploidy, and histology. A new risk-stratified staging system by the International Neuroblastoma Risk Group is currently being prospectively evaluated in clinical trials.

Table 19.1 International Neuroblastoma Staging System.

Stage I	Localized tumor confined to the area of origin; complete gross resection, with or without microscopic residual disease; negative lymph nodes
Stage IIA	Unilateral tumor with incomplete gross resection; negative lymph nodes
Stage IIB	Unilateral tumor with complete or incomplete gross resection; positive ipsilateral lymph nodes, negative contralateral lymph nodes
Stage III	Tumor infiltrating across midline with or without regional lymph node involvement, unilateral tumor with contralateral lymph node involvement, or midline tumor with bilateral regional lymph node involvement
Stage IV	Tumor disseminated to distant lymph nodes, bone, bone marrow, liver, or other organs (except as defined by stage IVS)
Stage IVS	Localized primary tumor as defined for stage I or II with dissemination limited to liver, skin, and/or bone marrow (under 1 year of age and <10% bone marrow involvement)

Treatment

Risk stratification divides patients into multiple potential treatment categories that are continually evaluated through clinical studies. For simplicity, we divide treatment strategies into three main groups: (1) observation, (2) chemotherapy, and (3) high-dose chemotherapy with autologous stem cell rescue and adjuvant therapy with immunomodulators (described below).

Observation
1. All Stage I patients (after surgical resection)
2. Stage IIA/B patients with >60% tumor resection and N-myc nonamplification
3. Stage IVS patients with N-myc nonamplification, favorable histology, and DNA ploidy >1

Chemotherapy
1. Stage IIA/B patients with <60% resection
2. Stage III patients with N-myc nonamplification, not including patients >18 months of age with unfavorable histology
3. Stage IV patients with N-myc nonamplification, not including patients >12 months

of age with unfavorable histology and/or DNA ploidy = 1 and all patients >18 months of age
4. Stage IVS patients with N-myc nonamplification who have unfavorable histology and/or DNA ploidy = 1

High-dose chemotherapy with autologous transplant
• Stage III, IV, and IVS patients not included above and all patients >12 years of age with stage III or greater disease

As mentioned, clinical studies are ongoing to refine treatment groups. Specifically, attempts are being made to reduce treatment in some of the lower risk subgroups that still require therapy but have an excellent overall prognosis (>90% survival). Novel therapeutic agents are being utilized in addition to the current backbone of therapy that includes drugs such as carboplatin, cyclophosphamide, doxorubicin, and etoposide. The majority of work is centered on high risk patients who continue to have an extremely poor prognosis (30% to 40% survival). Multiple efforts are currently being evaluated in clinical trials including the benefit of myeloablative chemotherapy with autologous stem cell rescue as well as tandem transplantation. Therapy with isotretinoin (cis-retinoic acid; cis-RA) has been shown beneficial as a maturing agent in neuroblastoma patients after cytotoxic therapy with minimal residual disease and is being evaluated in combination with monoclonal antibodies directed at neuroblastoma-specific antigens, specifically gangliosidase (GD2). Pilot studies with anti-GD2 antibodies and concomitant use of cis-RA and cytokine therapy (interleukin-2 and GM-CSF) have shown promising results in the high risk, poor prognosis subgroup of neuroblastoma patients, potentially increasing survival in this population to as high as 60%.

Suggested Reading

Maris JM. Recent advances in neuroblastoma. N Engl J Med 362:2202–2211, 2010.

Park JR, Eggert A, Caron H. Neuroblastoma: biology, prognosis, and treatment. Hematol Oncol Clin N Am 24:65–86, 2010.

Yu AL, Gilman AL, Ozkaynak MF, et al. Anti-GD2 antibody with GM-CSF, interleukin-2, and isotretinoin for neuroblastoma. N Engl J Med 363:1324–1334, 2010.

20 Sarcomas of the Soft Tissues and Bone

Sarcomas comprise a heterogeneous group of malignant tumors that arise in the soft tissues or bone. Soft tissue sarcomas (STS) are derived from primitive mesenchymal cells such as muscle, connective tissue (tendons and synovial tissue), supportive tissue (fat and nerves), and vascular tissue (lymph and blood vessels). Rhabdomyosarcoma (RMS) is the most common STS in younger children, comprising more than half of these tumors in children up to 9 years of age. Other nonrhabdomyomatous soft tissue sarcomas (NRSTS) include synovial sarcoma, liposarcoma, fibrosarcoma, alveolar soft part sarcoma, leiomyosarcoma, and malignant peripheral nerve sheath tumor. STS account for approximately 6% of cancer cases in those less than 19 years of age (annual incidence 11 cases per million in the United States). The relative incidence of various STS varies by age, gender, and race. For instance, NRSTS such as fibrosarcoma and malignant hemangiopericytoma are more common in infants (less than 1 year of age). NRSTS also account for the majority of STS in patients over 10 years of age.

The most common bone sarcomas in children are osteosarcoma and Ewing sarcoma (annual incidence 8.7 per million). Approximately two-thirds of cases are osteosarcoma and one-third Ewing sarcoma.

Osteosarcoma is believed to arise from osteoblasts and has a bimodal age distribution with an initial peak in the second decade of life and a second peak in older adulthood. Ewing sarcoma is thought to derive from neural crest and is also most frequently diagnosed in the second decade of life.

Genetics

The majority of soft tissue and bone sarcomas develop without a predisposing genetic risk factor, although there have been multiple reported associations: RMS in patients with neurofibromatosis type 1, Beckwith-Wiedemann syndrome, Costello syndrome, Li-Fraumeni familial cancer syndrome, and cardio-facial-cutaneous syndrome. There has also been an association with maternal use of marijuana and cocaine as well as first-trimester exposure to radiation, including diagnostic radiographs. Children with hereditary retinoblastoma (who harbor the Rb germ line mutation) are at increased risk of developing sarcoma. Alveolar RMS (ARMS) has a characteristic translocation of the FKHR gene at 13q14 with PAX3 at 2q35 or less commonly PAX7 at 1p36, leading to a fusion transcription factor that is

Handbook of Pediatric Hematology and Oncology: Children's Hospital & Research Center Oakland,
Second Edition. Caroline A. Hastings, Joseph C. Torkildson, and Anurag K. Agrawal.
© 2012 John Wiley & Sons, Ltd. Published 2012 by John Wiley & Sons, Ltd.

thought to inappropriately activate gene transcription. Embryonal RMS (ERMS) displays a loss of heterozygosity in the short arm of chromosome 11, especially at 11p15. The allelic loss of 11p15 has also been seen in translocation negative, histologic ARMS. In general, patients with ERMS have a better prognosis than patients with ARMS, in large part due to the increased risk of metastatic disease at presentation with ARMS. DNA content or ploidy has also been implicated in prognosis with hyperdiploid tumors ($\geq$51 chromosomes) having a better outcome. NRSTS can occur in sites of prior radiation, and children with human immunodeficiency virus may develop leiomyosarcoma (often in association with Epstein–Barr virus). Interestingly, family members of children affected with Ewing sarcoma family of tumors (ESFT; also referred to as primitive neuroectodermal tumors) have an increased risk of neuroectodermal and stomach malignancies. The translocation t(11;22)(q24;q12) occurs in greater than 95% of ESFT and some consider this finding to be pathognomonic and sufficient to confirm the diagnosis. This translocation results in the EWS–FLI1 fusion transcript that acts as an aberrant transcription factor altering tumor suppressor gene pathways.

Osteosarcoma is characterized by complex unbalanced karyotypes with alterations in the Rb and p53 tumor suppressor pathways, linking this tumor to retinoblastoma and Li-Fraumeni syndrome, respectively. Osteosarcoma has long been thought to be associated with adolescent growth spurts and the higher incidence in large dog breeds and taller people support this correlation. Girls have a peak incidence younger than boys (12 vs. 16 years) correlating with the different average age for pubertal development. Well-documented risk factors include radiation exposure, Paget's disease, and other disorders associated with increased bone turnover. Soft tissue and bone sarcomas also occur as secondary malignancies.

Soft tissue sarcoma

Clinical presentation
STS may occur anywhere in the body and are not limited to muscle or connective tissues. The most common sites for RMS are head and neck (35%), genitourinary system (26%), and extremities (20%). Younger children less than 10 years of age tend to develop ERMS in head and neck or genitourinary locations, whereas adolescents tend to develop extremity, truncal, or paratesticular ARMS. The majority of RMS are localized, and, of the 15% to 20% of cases with metastatic disease at presentation, most involve the lungs, bone marrow, lymph nodes, or bone.

As RMS can arise from anywhere in the body, the presenting symptoms are highly variable. Typically, RMS presents as a painless growing mass. Depending on location, adjacent structures may be compressed and lead to symptoms such as airway obstruction or cranial nerve findings with nasopharyngeal tumors, proptosis with orbital tumors, and urinary obstruction with bladder or prostate tumors.

Diagnostic evaluation
Patients presenting with an enlarging mass suspected to be malignancy should have an open surgical biopsy for confirmation of diagnosis. Sufficient tissue should be obtained for pathologic evaluation and staining in addition to cytogenetic and molecular biologic studies. Patients may be eligible to participate in a clinical therapeutic or biologic trial that also mandates submission of tissue. A complete assessment of extent of disease with meticulous attention to sites of metastatic disease is

mandated prior to initiating definitive therapy. Some protocols also mandate biopsy of regional nodes or a sentinel node in patients with primary extremity tumors. These evaluations include:

• Complete **history** and **physical examination** with careful assessment of the mass, adjacent structures, and regional lymph nodes.

• **Laboratory studies** including complete blood count, complete metabolic panel with renal and liver function studies, coagulation testing, and urinalysis.

• **Radiographic studies** including magnetic resonance imaging (**MRI**) and/or computed tomography (**CT**) scan of the primary lesion, depending on the location. **Chest CT** and **radioisotope bone scan** should also be conducted to evaluate for potential lung metastases and bone metastases, respectively. Site-dependent studies may include: brain MRI for parameningeal head and neck tumors, ultrasound and cystourethroscopy in bladder or prostate tumors, and spine MRI in patients with evidence of medullary compression. Fluorine-18-fluorodeoxyglucose positron emission tomography (**FDG-PET**) imaging may be helpful to determine initial extent of disease and to monitor response to therapy.

• **Bilateral bone marrow aspirate and biopsy** should be performed, especially in patients with metastatic disease or alveolar histologic subtype of RMS.

• **Lumbar puncture** in patients with parameningeal head and neck primary lesions.

Staging and classification

RMS are stratified into groups based on prognostic factors. The principal determinants of prognosis are primary site, tumor size, histologic subtype, degree of regional spread and nodal involvement, distant metastatic disease, and extent of prechemotherapy tumor resection. Risk stratification is

essential to tailoring of therapy to maximize outcome. A unique aspect of the RMS staging is the postoperative clinical grouping system that is based on extent of surgical resection and results of the lymph node evaluation. Risk group classification is then based on pretreatment stage, postoperative clinical group, and histology. Favorable sites include the orbit, genitourinary (nonbladder nonprostate), and nonparameningeal head and neck locations. Unfavorable sites are bladder/prostate, extremity, cranial parameningeal, trunk, and retroperitoneum.

Low risk group: patients with nonmetastatic favorable site ERMS (stage I, regardless of degree of initial resection) and completely resected (groups I and II) nonmetastatic unfavorable site ERMS

Intermediate risk group: patients with any nonmetastatic ARMS and all ERMS with unfavorable sites (stages 2 or 3) that have been incompletely resected (group III)

High risk group: patients with metastatic tumors, both ARMS and ERMS

NRSTS are generally staged using the same criteria above. The major determinants of outcome include tumor grade, size, extent of initial resection, and presence of metastatic disease. Extent of resection is strongly correlated with treatment stratification and prognosis.

Pathologic diagnosis and treatment

RMS is classified pathologically as embryonal (ERMS) with botryoid and spindle cell variants or alveolar (ARMS). Investigation for particular translocations (see Genetics section) should be done to assist with definitive tissue diagnosis in combination with histochemical studies.

A multidisciplinary approach to the treatment of STS is crucial. Basic principles of therapy include systemic treatment of micrometastatic disease with adjuvant chemotherapy and aggressive local control with definitive surgery and addition of radiation as necessary.

Local control is achieved with either complete surgical resection (with negative margins) or surgery and radiation (if microscopic or gross residual disease remains after surgical intervention). Primary re-excision may be indicated prior to initiation of chemotherapy in certain situations such as: if the diagnosis was not suspected and only a biopsy was performed; gross or microscopic residual disease is amenable to wide excision; or if there is uncertainty about residual disease or margins. Aggressive surgical debulking that would result in significant loss of function is not recommended. RMS often arise in sites in which complete or wide resection is not feasible (e.g., orbit, most genitourinary and parameningeal sites). STS are moderately sensitive to radiation therapy, and this treatment modality is critical for tumors that cannot be fully excised surgically with negative margins. Radiation is typically delayed until the completion of 10 to 20 weeks of systemic chemotherapy, but may be indicated earlier in patients with intracranial primary tumors or in those with compromise of function that may be debilitating or life threatening. Current studies are evaluating the optimal timing of irradiation.

Chemotherapy provides the backbone of treatment for patients with RMS and is initiated following the initial surgical procedure. After definitive local control surgery and/or radiation, chemotherapy continues due to the risk of microscopic residual or metastatic disease. The most active drugs in the treatment of RMS are vincristine, dactinomycin, and cyclophosphamide (VAC), doxorubicin, and ifosfamide and etoposide (IE). VAC is considered the standard of therapy in all risk groups.

Recent trials have not been able to show improvement in survival in patients with metastatic rhabdomyosarcoma and new drug therapies are being investigated. Such therapies include irinotecan, temozolomide, bevacizumab (anti-vascular endothelial growth factor monoclonal antibody), temsirolimus (mTOR inhibitor), vinorelbine (vinca alkaloid), and cixutumumab (monoclonal antibody to the insulin-like growth factor-1 receptor). High-dose chemotherapy with hematopoietic stem cell rescue has not shown benefit in patients with high risk and metastatic disease.

Prognosis

Overall, survival without relapse is greater than 70% in children and adolescents 5 years from diagnosis. Low risk groups, representing approximately 30% of RMS, can be expected to have an excellent outcome with long-term survival greater than 90%. Of the 55% of patients with intermediate risk disease, 5-year overall survival is approximately 55% to 65%. In patients with metastatic alveolar disease (15% to 20% of the population), survival is poor, at less than 30%. Several caveats are present that help determine prognosis:

• Site of the primary tumor has a major impact on survival and is associated with pathologic subtypes, ease of surgical resectability, timing to presentation, and involvement of regional nodes.

• Extent of disease is the most significant predictive factor for survival. Children with localized, completely resected disease do better than those with widespread or disseminated disease.

• Patients with smaller tumors (<5 cm) have improved survival compared to children with tumors >5 cm.

• The alveolar subtype of RMS has an adverse prognosis and is often associated with an aggressive clinical course and metastatic disease at diagnosis and relapse.

• Patients between 1 and 9 years of age have a better prognosis compared to infants and older children.

Children with recurrent RMS have a dismal prognosis with long-term survival of less than 15%, particularly if the disease recurs in a metastatic site or area of prior irradiation. The majority of relapses occur within 3 years of therapy completion. Metastatic recurrence is essentially incurable, though treatment may offer palliation. Treatment with surgical resection and adjuvant multiagent chemotherapy is recommended with new drug combinations such as ifosfamide/carboplatin/etoposide, docetaxel/gemcitabine, and irinotecan in combination with temozolomide or vinorelbine. Durable remissions for several years may be obtained with aggressive local retreatment and systemic therapy. High-dose chemotherapy followed by hematopoietic stem cell rescue has not been shown to be advantageous in this group.

Nonrhabdomyomatous soft tissue sarcomas

Few clinical trials and prospective studies have been conducted in this population of children. Surgery is the mainstay of effective therapy and every effort should be made to completely excise the tumor with clear tumor margins. Patients with completely excised low-grade tumors or high-grade tumors <5 cm have a favorable outcome with survival exceeding 85%. Patients with high-grade NRSTS larger than 5 cm and those with unresectable, localized disease have an intermediate prognosis with approximately 50% survival. Patients with high-grade tumors and positive tumor resection margins typically receive adjuvant irradiation. It is not clear if adjuvant chemotherapy confers a survival advantage in

this group of patients. Patients with metastatic NRSTS have a dismal long-term prognosis and fewer than 20% survive 5 years from diagnosis. Neoadjuvant chemoradiotherapy is being explored in this group but there continues to be a paucity of new potential therapeutic agents.

Bone sarcomas

Primary malignant bone tumors in children are the sixth most common malignant neoplasm in children and the third most common malignancy in adolescents and young adults. They constitute approximately 6% of all childhood malignancies. The two most common bone tumors are osteosarcoma and Ewing sarcoma. Other malignant bone tumors include chondrosarcoma and non-Hodgkin lymphoma of bone. Bone lesions may also represent Langerhans cell histiocytosis, benign tumors, or metastatic disease. Osteosarcoma is classified into three major subtypes: osteoblastic, chondroblastic, and fibroblastic, reflecting the predominant type of matrix in the tumor. Histologic variants include telangiectatic, small cell, periosteal, and parosteal.

Clinical presentation

Patients typically present with a mass in the involved area and pain, with symptoms preceding diagnosis often by several months. Patients frequently attribute the pain to a minor trauma and indeed may present with a pathologic fracture in the affected bone. A palpable mass or swelling of the involved site typically arises after the onset of pain. Systemic symptoms such as weight loss or shortness of breath may be late sequelae and secondary to metastatic disease. Fever is a common symptom of ESFT and may lead to confusion with osteomyelitis and a longer period of time from development of symptoms to diagnosis.

Diagnostic evaluation

Osteosarcoma may occur in any bone but primarily occurs in the metaphyses of the most rapidly growing bones. The most common primary sites are the distal femur, proximal tibia, and proximal humerus with approximately 50% of tumors originating around the knee. Approximately 10% of patients have primary tumors in the axial skeleton including the pelvis, and 15% to 20% present with metastatic disease (lung, bone, lymph nodes, and rarely brain).

Most ESFT occur in bones and their locations tend to differ from that of osteosarcoma. Flat bones of the axial skeleton are more commonly affected; in long bones, the diaphyseal portion is usually involved. The most common primary locations include the pelvic bones, the long bones of the lower extremities, and the bones of the chest wall. Metastatic disease is present in 25% of patients at diagnosis and is primarily located in the lungs, bones, or bone marrow. Site of primary disease is related to the incidence of metastases at diagnosis; central primaries are associated more frequently with distant disease (40%), whereas distal primary lesions have the lowest incidence (15%).

The requisite elements of evaluation include:

• A complete **history** and **physical examination**.

• Routine **laboratory** studies include a complete blood count, complete metabolic panel with renal and liver function tests, serum creatinine, creatinine clearance, and urinalysis. A measured or calculated glomerular filtration rate should be obtained prior to initiation of nephrotoxic chemotherapy. The alkaline phosphatase may be elevated and has been associated with an inferior outcome in osteosarcoma. The serum lactate dehydrogenase may also be elevated and may correlate with tumor burden.

• **Imaging** studies should begin with **plain radiographs** to visualize osseous changes and confirm suspicion of a malignant tumor. Osteosarcoma usually produces dense sclerosis in the metaphyses of long bones with soft tissue extension seen in 75% of tumors, radiating calcifications (sunburst pattern) in 60% of tumors, osteosclerotic lesions in 45% of cases, lytic lesions in 30% of cases, and mixed lesions in 25% of cases. A triangular area of periosteal calcification in the border region of the tumor and healthy tissue is known as a Codman triangle. ESFT are described as lytic with an "onion peel" periosteal reaction and typically occur in the diaphysis. Patients with soft tissue ESFT only may have normal radiographs. Additional assessment of the primary tumor site with **MRI** should be undertaken to view the soft tissue component, surrounding structures, vessels and nerves, and the intramedullary extension to assist with surgical planning. MRI should include the entire involved bone and neighboring joints to evaluate for skip lesions. Metastatic disease is typically in the lungs or bone and therefore imaging with **chest CT** and **technetium-99m bone scan** is essential in the initial workup for staging. **FDG-PET** imaging is a sensitive screening tool for the detection of bone metastases in ESFT but its role in evaluation of osteosarcoma has yet to be determined.

• Bilateral bone marrow aspirate and biopsy should be performed in patients with ESFT.

• Baseline audiogram and echocardiogram should be obtained prior to initiation of ototoxic and cardiotoxic chemotherapy, respectively.

Pathologic diagnosis

Patients presenting with a bone mass suspicious for malignancy should undergo a diagnostic incisional or core biopsy. It is strongly recommended that an experienced oncologic orthopedic surgeon who will also be performing the definitive procedure perform the biopsy so that the biopsy tract can be excised en bloc with the planned surgical resection. Sufficient tissue should be obtained for diagnostic histopathology as well as for any submissions required for participation in a clinical trial. Biopsy may be taken from an extraosseous component, if present, to prevent pathologic fracture.

As the histologic and immunophenotypic features of ESFT overlap to some degree with many other small, round blue cell tumors of childhood, an expanded immunohistochemical panel should include assessment for CD99 (a cell surface glycoprotein with strong expression in ESFT) as well as markers for neuroblastoma (neuron-specific enolase and S100), synovial sarcoma (Leu-7), and rhabdomyosarcoma (vimentin, desmin, and myogenin). Molecular genetic studies using fluorescent in situ hybridization or reverse transcriptase-polymerase chain reaction are valuable in diagnosis, specifically for the detection of characteristic translocations that allow for definitive diagnosis of ESFT, RMS, and synovial cell sarcoma.

Treatment

Systemic multiagent chemotherapy prior to and following definitive radical surgery is the standard of care for treatment of osteosarcoma. Complete resection of all disease sites including metastatic lesions is critical to long-term survival. An assessment of histologic response to initial induction chemotherapy at the time of definitive surgery may guide subsequent treatment and helps define prognosis. The orthopedic oncologic surgeon determines the type of surgical procedure performed and factors used in this determination include the location and size of the tumor, patient age and skeletal maturity, presence of metastatic disease, and patient lifestyle choices. Limb sparing procedures are feasible in the majority of patients and the development of expandable endoprostheses has allowed the use of these

techniques in younger children. Tumors of the pelvis or axial skeleton present a difficult situation, as resection with adequate margins may not be possible. Outcome is related to degree of resection and these patients as a group have inferior outcomes compared to patients with extremity tumors.

Radiation therapy has limited utility in patients with osteosarcoma, but is indicated for those unable to undergo complete resection. The most active chemotherapeutic agents are cisplatin, doxorubicin, high-dose methotrexate, ifosfamide, and etoposide. Patients can expect to be treated for approximately 1 year, with a definitive surgical procedure performed at approximately week 12, followed by continuation of multiagent chemotherapy.

Patients presenting with metastatic disease undergo the same therapeutic approach with systemic chemotherapy and definitive surgery of the primary site in addition to surgery of metastatic sites, as feasible. Approximately one-third of osteosarcoma patients with pulmonary metastases will have additional microscopic pulmonary nodules not visible on the current, highest resolution CT imaging. It is recommended that pulmonary nodules identified on CT imaging be surgically resected by open thoracotomy that will allow intraoperative lung palpation to potentially identify additional sites of metastatic disease. Patients with unilateral lung metastases on imaging should undergo bilateral thoracotomies for this reason.

As with osteosarcoma, cure in ESFT can be achieved only with a multimodal approach, using surgery and/or radiation therapy for local control of the primary lesion and chemotherapy for eradication of subclinical micrometastases. Definitive surgery follows a period of induction chemotherapy and many patients are candidates for complete surgical resection with limb salvage procedures. Induction chemotherapy may also render initially unresectable tumors resectable. ESFT are radiation responsive, although typically this therapeutic modality is reserved for surgically unresectable tumors or in tumors with positive margins after resection. Patients who receive radiation therapy as the only local control modality have an inferior outcome. Frequently, these patients have other adverse features including large tumor size, unfavorable locations (e.g., vertebral tumors), or both. Radiation is also utilized in the treatment of metastatic disease. Debulking procedures have not been shown to improve outcome and should not be part of local control therapy.

Active chemotherapy agents in ESFT include vincristine, dactinomycin, cyclophosphamide, doxorubicin, ifosfamide, and etoposide (similar to RMS). As with osteosarcoma, the length of systemic therapy is approximately one year. The current standard of care for localized pediatric ESFT is alternating cycles of vincristine, doxorubicin, and cyclophosphamide (VDC) with ifosfamide and etoposide (IE) given in a compressed, every 2-week schedule. This increased time–dose intensity schedule has shown benefit in pediatric patients though not for adults. Although still being investigated, high-dose chemotherapy with autologous stem cell rescue has not as yet shown benefit in the treatment of bone sarcoma.

Prognosis

Most patients with bone sarcomas have micrometastatic disease at diagnosis since, in the past, 80% to 90% developed lung metastases following local control therapy (i.e., surgery and/or radiation) alone. Therefore, prior to the use of systemic chemotherapy, survival rates at 2 years were 15% to 20%. Currently, patients with localized disease can expect a long-term survival of greater than 70%. Survival in patients with metastatic disease remains dismal,

estimated at 2 years as 10% to 30%. The degree of tumor necrosis following neoadjuvant (presurgery) chemotherapy is an independent predictor of event-free and overall survival, presumably reflecting tumor sensitivity to chemotherapy. Specifically, osteosarcoma patients with a good response, defined as greater than 95% tumor necrosis at the time of surgery, have a superior survival. A similar cutoff is yet to be defined for ESFT. To date, intensified treatment for those with less favorable tumor necrosis has not improved outcome.

The prognosis for patients with recurrence is quite poor. Most local recurrence is associated with concomitant distant disease. Time to relapse and tumor burden correlate with postrelapse outcome. Late recurrence (e.g., >5 to 10 years) has been reported in bone sarcoma. Surgical resection remains the mainstay of therapy for curative second-line therapy. Patients with osteosarcoma who develop pulmonary lesions after completion of therapy can be cured with surgery alone. The role of adjuvant chemotherapy in relapse is controversial, though patients are often offered such treatments including cyclophosphamide/topotecan, irinotecan/temozolomide, and gemcitabine/taxotere. Radiation has a role in the treatment of patients with ESFT who develop new metastatic sites and for palliation and pain control in either osteosarcoma or ESFT.

Targeted and biologically based therapies are being investigated in patients with poor response to initial chemotherapy, those with metastatic disease, and those with recurrent disease. Novel agents with potential therapeutic benefit include monoclonal antibodies to insulin growth factor-1 receptor, tyrosine kinase inhibitors, mTOR inhibitors, and monoclonal antibodies to vascular endothelial growth factor. Specific novel therapies for osteosarcoma include bisphosphonates (e.g., zoledronic acid) and RANK inhibitors (e.g., denosumab); for

ESFT, transcription inhibition of the EWS-FLI1 translocation is being studied.

Late effects

Site and extent of disease, as well as therapeutic interventions with chemotherapy, radiation, and surgery all contribute to late sequelae in sarcoma patients. A majority of first-line protocols utilize high cumulative doses of anthracyclines (i.e., doxorubicin) resulting in a lifelong risk of developing cardiomyopathy. Thus, lifelong cardiac monitoring with serial echocardiograms and periodic functional assessments is recommended. Alkylator therapy (e.g., ifosfamide) can lead to gonadal toxicity (primarily in males) and increased risk of secondary malignancy. Second malignant neoplasms occur in approximately 3% of patients within 10 years of therapy completion, likely related to both a genetic predisposition and treatment with mutagenic therapies. Platinum therapy (e.g., cisplatin) can lead to long-term oto- and nephrotoxicity. High-frequency hearing loss is common and some patients will require hearing aids. Renal dysfunction is rare but could result in chronic electrolyte wasting due to proximal tubular damage (see Chapter 30 for more details).

For osteosarcoma patients, contemporary orthopedic surgery techniques are aimed at preservation of function and improved limb salvage without compromising survival. Amputation may result in superior limb function in some cases. In a skeletally immature child, expandable prostheses may require subsequent revisions though some may benefit from newer self-expanding prostheses. Late prosthetic failures or infection can occur, requiring surgical revision or delayed amputation. Radiation therapy can lead to local effects including growth impairment, muscle fibrosis, and increased risk of secondary malignancy, in a dose-dependent manner.

Case study for review

A 9-year-old boy presents with a nontender 3 × 4 cm mass in the right inguinal region. He denies fever, weight loss, or pain elsewhere. The mass has been present and growing for several weeks.

1. What key elements should you obtain in the history?
2. What are you looking for on the physical examination?
3. What is your differential diagnosis for this boy?
4. How do you approach a diagnostic evaluation and staging?
5. What do you tell the child and his family?
6. Assuming you find out this is a localized undifferentiated sarcoma, what is the child's prognosis and what is the general treatment plan?

Key elements in the history include length of symptoms, possible relationship to infection (could this be a lymph node?), animal exposures and bites, travel, cuts or injuries to the affected leg, systemic symptoms such as malaise, fevers, unexplained weight loss, or discomfort that limits activities or necessitates medication.

The physical examination should be complete, head to toe. The mass should be measured and characterized for mobility, tenderness, warmth, and erythema. The mass may be hard and nontender if malignant disease is present. If the mass is suspected to be a node, it may be enlarged as a result of disease spread and therefore the distal extremity must be carefully examined. All other lymph node chains as well as the liver and spleen should also be carefully assessed.

The differential diagnosis of a mass in the inguinal area consists of lymphadenopathy secondary to an infectious or malignant etiology. Infections may be bacterial, protozoal, fungal, or viral and may be the result of introduction by a cut (which may have since healed), animal bite, or scratch. A mass that is hard, nontender, and nonmobile, without signs and symptoms of infection, is concerning for malignancy. Malignancies that can lead to regional spread in an extremity include sarcomas (bone and soft tissue).

Assuming you could find no lump or tender area on the extremity exam, it is prudent to begin a detailed investigation with imaging and biopsy. Imaging should consist of MRI of the inguinal area and leg (to the tips of the toes), bone scan, and plain films. An excisional biopsy should be performed as well given the concern for malignancy (and to prevent potential tumor tracking which can occur with an incisional biopsy). Once the mass is a biopsy-proven malignancy, further staging should evaluate for distant disease and include CT of the chest, abdomen, and pelvis.

Prior to initiation of the biopsy and imaging, it is best to be straightforward with the family and let them know your concern that this mass likely represents a malignancy. As the mass is in the inguinal area, it could represent regional spread of a distant tumor.

In this case, the child had a nonpalpable mass in the fifth distal toe found on MRI. The pathologic diagnosis of undifferentiated sarcoma was made on excisional biopsy of the inguinal mass. No other evidence of distant tumor was found on further imaging. Prognosis for undifferentiated sarcoma is generally similar to alveolar rhabdomyosarcoma, and patients with localized disease who receive systemic chemotherapy and aggressive local control (complete surgical excision and focal radiation) can expect to have approximately a 70% event-free survival. This is in stark contrast to patients with metastatic disease in which case survival is less than 20% despite aggressive therapy. Those patients with regional spread, similar to this case, have an intermediate prognosis. Such cases would be treated with aggressive multiagent chemotherapy in addition to aggressive local control. Future therapies may include novel biologic or targeted agents. In this child, local control would involve treatment of the toe and the inguinal mass. One should also consider treatment (i.e., radiation therapy) of the lymph nodes in between these regions in addition to nearby pelvic nodes.

Suggested Reading

Caudill JS, Arndt CA. Diagnosis and management of bone malignancy in adolescence. Adolesc Med State Art Rev 18:62–78, 2007.

Hayes-Jordan A, Andrassy R. Rhabdomyosarcoma in children. Curr Opin Pediatr 21:373–378, 2009.

Loeb DM, Thornton K, Shokek O. Pediatric soft tissue sarcomas. Surg Clin North Am 88:615–627, 2008.

McCarville MB. The child with bone pain: malignancies and mimickers. Cancer Imaging 9: S115–S121, 2009.

Spunt SL, Skapek SX, Coffin CM. Pediatric non-rhabdomyosarcoma soft tissue sarcomas. Oncologist 13:668–678, 2008.

Subbiah V, Anderson P, Lazar AJ, et al. Ewing's sarcoma: standard and experimental treatment options. Curr Treat Options Oncol 10:126–140, 2009.

21 Germ Cell Tumors

Germ cell tumors (GCT) arise from primordial cells involved in gametogenesis and occur primarily in the testes and ovaries. These tumors represent approximately 4% of pediatric cancers. Primordial germ cells (PGCs) are thought to originate in the yolk sac endoderm and migrate along the genital ridge and thus may also present in midline extragonadal sites such as the sacrococcygeal region, midline of the brain, mediastinum, and retroperitoneum. Due to the pluripotentiality of PGCs, GCT are an array of different histologic subtypes, adding to the complexity of the disease. In addition, GCT can occur due to tumorigenesis or as part of normal embryonal development, in part explaining the pediatric bimodal age of distribution (2 and 20 years). In addition, age of presentation and histologic subtype varies significantly between males and females. This is thought to be due in part to the differential timing of male and female development; female germ cells enter meiosis at 11 to 12 weeks of gestation while male germ cells begin meiosis with the onset of puberty.

Epidemiology

Due to the differential timing of germ cell maturation, GCT are more common in females until adolescence and then become more frequent in males. Testicular GCT have several known risk factors including infertility/testicular atrophy as well as cryptorchidism. Males with cryptorchidism have a higher incidence of testicular cancer in both the undescended testis and the normally descended contralateral testis despite surgical correction, hormonal therapy, or spontaneous descent. However, early correction may partially ameliorate this risk. The incidence of testicular GCT in the Caucasian population is increasing at a rate of 3% to 6% per year. Perinatal and environmental risk factors are thought to play a role although these are yet to be clearly elucidated. Young parental age at birth, low birth order, low birth weight, and breech birth have all been noted to be statistically significant risk factors in multiple studies. Maternal exposure to pesticides or hormones, parental smoking, and alcohol consumption may also be factors. Genetic risk factors also play a role, specifically in testicular GCT, as a family history of cancer, especially at a young age, has been associated with increased risk in pediatric patients. Additionally, there is a higher incidence in monozygotic twins and some familial clusters have been reported. A number of congenital genitourinary anomalies such as retrocaval ureter, bladder diverticulum, and inguinal hernia have been

Handbook of Pediatric Hematology and Oncology: Children's Hospital & Research Center Oakland, Second Edition. Caroline A. Hastings, Joseph C. Torkildson, and Anurag K. Agrawal.
© 2012 John Wiley & Sons, Ltd. Published 2012 by John Wiley & Sons, Ltd.

associated with increased risk, emphasizing that abnormalities in development likely play a role. Similarly, disorders of sexual development, especially in cases with excess Y chromosome material (e.g., gonadal dysgenesis), pose an increased risk in both males and females. Children with Down syndrome, who generally have a decreased risk of solid tumors, are at a predisposition to develop testicular GCT, whereas patients with Klinefelter syndrome have an increased risk of mediastinal GCT. Gain of chromosome 12p is also seen in the majority of testicular and malignant ovarian GCT. Approximately half of all pediatric GCT are extragonadal in origin, with about 15% of these being malignant.

Pathology and serum tumor markers

The main histologic variants of GCT include germinomas (dysgerminoma in the ovary and seminoma in the testis), embryonal carcinoma, yolk sac tumor (endodermal sinus tumor), choriocarcinoma, and teratoma (mature and immature). Mixed GCT are composed of two or more histologies. Teratomas contain tissues from all three germ layers (ectoderm, endoderm, and mesoderm). Mature teratomas contain no malignant germ cell elements and are most commonly located in the ovary or sacrococcygeal region. The vast majority of female GCT are teratomas. Teratomas in the prepubertal male are benign, whereas those occurring during or after the onset of puberty are always malignant, as they arise from other forms of testicular germ cell tumor (specifically embryonal carcinoma). Therefore, teratomatous elements in the testis largely occur as a component of a mixed GCT. In the female or prepubertal male, these tumors are thought to derive from a benign germ cell but may rarely develop malignant components (i.e., squamous cell carcinoma) and therefore are treated with complete surgical resection. Immature teratomas are tumors of intermediate malignant potential with less differentiated tissues.

Germinomas may be of pure histology or mixed. Syncytiotrophoblastic cells occur in about 5% of germinomas and secrete the beta subunit of human chorionic gonadotropin (β-HCG). Embryonal carcinoma is most often found as a component of testicular mixed GCT and is thought to be the driver for the development of other histologic subtypes including teratoma, yolk sac tumor, and choriocarcinoma. Yolk sac tumor is generally found as a part of testicular mixed GCT but can also be seen as a pure histologic variant in young children. Yolk sac tumor secretes α-fetoprotein (AFP).

Choriocarcinoma contains syncytiotrophoblastic cells and therefore also secretes β-HCG. Ovarian cases should be distinguished from metastatic gestational choriocarcinoma.

In the ovary and testis, GCT should be distinguished from sex cord stromal tumors, which arise from the nongerminative components of gonadal tissue and include tumors involving the Sertoli-Leydig cells of the testis and granulosa cells of the ovary. Sarcoma as well as gonadal infiltration by leukemia and non-Hodgkin lymphoma should also be considered in the differential diagnosis of gonadal tumors.

Due to the specific histologies that secrete AFP and β-HCG, these tumor markers can be quite helpful in distinguishing tumor type as well as following disease. Mature teratomas secrete neither marker; therefore, if a serum marker is present in the patient diagnosed with a mature teratoma, one must consider that the tumor contains one or more foci of yolk sac tumor if the AFP is positive, choriocarcinoma or germinoma if the β-HCG is positive, and that the patient in fact has a mixed malignant germ cell tumor. Due to physiologic changes in the secretion of fetal AFP, this marker can be difficult to utilize in young infants. AFP is made in the fetal liver and does not decline to adult levels until approximately 6 to 8 months of age. Age appropriate levels can be obtained from published tables. AFP can also be secreted by regenerating liver post-injury or by certain liver tumors such as hepatoblastoma. Degree of AFP elevation may be related to tumor volume. β-HCG is elevated in pregnancy and can also be seen in association with childhood hepatic tumors and other cancers involving the breast, stomach, and pancreas in adults. Nonspecific markers of GCT include lactate dehydrogenase isoenzyme 1, neuron-specific enolase, and placental alkaline phosphatase.

Clinical presentation

GCT should be considered in children who present with a pelvic, ovarian, or testicular mass, or a midline mass in the sacrococcygeal region, retroperitoneum, mediastinum, or pineal or suprasellar regions of the brain. GCT present with signs and symptoms related to the site and size of the primary tumor. Compression of internal structures can lead to pain, constipation, and urinary obstruction. Large ovarian tumors can additionally lead to decreased lung volumes and respiratory distress. GCT can metastasize, most commonly to the lungs, but patients rarely present with clinical symptoms referable to these metastases. Occasionally, patients may present with hormonal manifestations secondary to secretion of β-HCG. Specifically, peripheral conversion of androgen to estrogen can lead to gynecomastia or uterine bleeding.

Boys with gonadal GCT typically present with a slowly enlarging testicular mass, occasionally complicated by acute severe pain due to testicular torsion. The differential diagnosis of a testicular mass includes hydrocele, hematocele, varicocele, inguinal hernia, and torsion of a normal testis. Girls most frequently present with abdominal pain, distention, and weight gain. Torsion of an involved ovary, hemorrhage, or tumor rupture may occur and present as an acute surgical abdomen. Secretion of β-HCG may lead to isosexual precocity. Occasionally, the increasing abdominal girth and elevated urine and serum β-HCG have been confused with pregnancy.

The most common site of extragonadal tumors is the sacrococcygeal region. Although usually benign, patients can have malignant tumors of higher stage. Older age at diagnosis is associated with a greater risk of malignancy. Sacrococcygeal tumors are classified as four anatomic variants: type I (predominantly outside the body), type II (equally inside and outside the body), type III (largely intra-abdominal), and type IV (completely within the body). More than 90% of tumors present with some component of an externally visible mass. These tumors are often detected in utero with prenatal ultrasonography. They may also present later in children with constipation, urinary obstruction, urgency or frequency, lower back or pelvic pain, lower extremity weakness, or sensory changes, all signs and symptoms due to compression of normal structures by tumor.

Approximately 20% of children with GCT will present with metastatic disease, most commonly to the lung, liver, or lymph nodes, and rarely to the central nervous system, bone, or bone marrow. Regional spread resulting in surgically unresectable tumors occurs in approximately 25% of patients at presentation. Tumor dissemination occurs by local extension, intracavitary seeding, or hematogenous spread. Intracavitary seeding may involve the omentum, bowel, spleen, diaphragm, or pelvic organs.

Rarely, bone involvement can occur by direct extension.

Diagnostic evaluation and risk stratification

The following studies should be performed in a child with a suspected or confirmed GCT:
- Complete history
- Physical examination
- Baseline laboratory studies consisting of a complete blood count, transaminases, blood urea nitrogen, creatinine, and electrolytes
- Baseline **tumor markers** including AFP, β-HCG, and lactate dehydrogenase (LDH)
- Imaging studies to evaluate the extent of the mass and potential metastatic sites: ultrasound, CT, or MRI of the primary mass (testicular ultrasound in males, abdominal and pelvic ultrasound, CT, or MRI in females); abdominal and pelvic MRI or CT as well as baseline chest radiography with or without CT of the chest to evaluate for metastatic disease (all CTs should be done with contrast)

Determination of the extent of disease at diagnosis allows proper decision making regarding the safest and most reasonable place to biopsy. Localized tumors of the ovary or testis should be completely removed. Resection of ovarian tumors should include abdominal exploration and peritoneal washings for cytologic assessment. Risks and benefits of lymph node sampling and biopsy of the contralateral testis or ovary should be discussed with the surgeon, patient, and family.

GCT are known to grow rapidly and metastasize frequently. Diagnostic studies should be done expeditiously to allow initiation of therapy. Due to the potential underlying risk of contralateral testicular atrophy, infertility, or carcinoma in situ, sperm banking should be discussed with the patient and family prior to radical inguinal orchiectomy.

Treatment and prognosis

Staging is done postoperatively and is based on pathologic degree of tumor invasion, presence of lymph node involvement, continued positivity of tumor markers, positive peritoneal washings (in ovarian tumors), and presence of residual or metastatic disease. Factors known to affect prognosis include extreme tumor marker elevation and failure of these markers to appropriately decline following tumor resection, based on the appropriate half-life for each marker. Site of tumor is prognostic, with mediastinal tumors fairing more poorly. Histology is also important as pure germinomas are generally very chemotherapy sensitive and have a high response rate. Patients with higher stage, metastatic disease also fair more poorly.

In the patient with suspected GCT, every effort should be made to perform a complete resection with negative margins. In situations where the patient presents emergently with torsion, there may not be time to wait for a definitive diagnosis prior to surgery; every effort should be made in these cases to perform a gross total resection (GTR), assuming there is low operative risk, after sending the appropriate tumor markers. In the case of a large, invasive tumor, biopsy should be done followed by administration of chemotherapy and delayed surgical resection. Due to the location of some extragonadal tumors, especially those in the mediastinum and retroperitoneum, neoadjuvant chemotherapy is often required prior to surgery in order to help facilitate the chance of a safe GTR.

Depending on tumor location and histology, some GCT can be observed after GTR without additional therapy. Young patients with extragonadal tumors and a GTR can generally be observed after surgery, as these tumors rarely have malignant elements. Sacrococcygeal tumors must be removed with the coccyx in order to decrease the risk of local recurrence. Young patients are more likely to present with pure yolk sac tumors, and these patients can also be observed after GTR. Gonadal tumors that are histologically consistent with mature teratoma similarly require only observation after GTR. Localized testicular seminoma can be observed, although patients with continued elevation of tumor markers should undergo adjuvant radiotherapy. Patients with this pure histology are very chemotherapy sensitive and easily salvaged in the event of relapse. In general, patients with localized testicular mixed GCT can also be observed assuming that tumor markers normalize after surgery, again due to the high rate of salvage with potential relapse. Due to this risk of relapse, which is directly related to the amount of vascular tumor invasion, size of the primary tumor, and percent embryonal carcinoma, patients should be presented the options of observation versus chemotherapy. Due to the rarity of malignant ovarian GCT, recommendations for chemotherapy versus observation generally follow those presented for testicular tumors.

Higher stage, nonlocalized GCT are treated with chemotherapy and are generally very chemotherapy sensitive. Patients are treated with bleomycin, etoposide, and cisplatin (BEP) regimens for 3 to 4 cycles. These tumors exhibit a steep dose–response curve to platinum compounds, though the risk of toxicity (oto- and nephrotoxicity) must be considered. Due to the potential risk of long-term pulmonary fibrosis from bleomycin, etoposide/cisplatin (EP) and etoposide (VP-16), ifosfamide, and cisplatin (VIP) regimens have been developed as alternative therapies to BEP. Bilateral retroperitoneal lymph node dissection may also be recommended in patients with extensive disease at presentation. Patients with a poor response to therapy or recurrent disease may benefit from second-line therapies such as paclitaxel (Taxol), ifosfamide, cisplatin (TIP); vinblastine, ifosfamide, cisplatin (VeIP); or gemcitabine/oxaliplatin. GCT are also quite radiosensitive, although the high cure rates seen with chemotherapy alone have obviated the need for radiation in most cases. Radiation may be considered in refractory or recurrent disease, or for palliation. Additionally, high-dose chemotherapy with autologous stem cell rescue may be beneficial in a subset of refractory patients.

Patients treated with high-dose platinum agents may develop high-frequency hearing loss and require hearing assistive devices. Additionally, these drugs may lead to transient proximal tubule renal dysfunction and resultant electrolyte wasting. Patients who receive alkylator therapy (e.g., ifosfamide) are at risk for secondary malignancy and infertility (especially in males). Topoisomerase II inhibitors (etoposide) also increase risk for secondary neoplasms. Bleomycin may lead to pulmonary fibrosis, although the risk is poorly quantified.

Germ cell tumors of the central nervous system

Intracranial GCT comprise approximately 3% of primary childhood brain tumors with a peak incidence between the second and third decade of life. The majority of these tumors are germinomas, which account for 50% to 70% of cases. Nongerminomatous germ cell tumors (NGGCT) account for the remaining third and consist of multiple histologies including endodermal sinus (yolk sac) tumors, choriocarcinoma, mature and immature teratoma, and embryonal carcinoma. Most NGGCT are of mixed histology and may contain germinomatous elements but will not have this as a pure histology. Mature and immature teratomas predominate in the neonatal period. Patients typically present with symptoms depending on the location and size of the tumor, further influenced by the extent of pituitary dysfunction and the presence or absence of hydrocephalus. Midline pineal tumors are often associated with symptoms related to increased intracranial pressure due to obstruction of the cerebral aqueduct and Parinaud's syndrome (paralysis of upward gaze) due to involvement of the tectal plate. Tumors in the suprasellar area often lead to endocrinopathies such as diabetes insipidus (DI) and visual field defects. Occasionally DI is related to occult involvement of the infundibulum. In children with clinical symptoms of DI and consistent MRI findings (i.e., absence of a posterior pituitary bright spot, possibly in association with thickening of the pituitary stalk), the differential diagnosis should include GCT and Langerhans cell histiocytosis. The presence or absence of CSF tumor markers may assist with this diagnostic dilemma.

Children with midline brain tumors should be assessed for a GCT. CSF should be obtained for routine studies (glucose, protein, chamber count, and cytology) in addition to assessment of tumor markers (AFP and β-HCG). Patients with classic findings on MRI and elevated AFP with or without a significantly elevated β-HCG do not require a biopsy for diagnosis as they have chemical evidence of NGGCT. Patients with negative markers or a modest elevation in β-HCG only should have a biopsy performed. Central nervous system GCT often spread along the CSF pathways; thus, MRI of the spine should be obtained in addition to head imaging for diagnostic and staging purposes.

Patients with benign tumors such as mature teratoma should have a curative surgical GTR, as safely feasible. In other tumor types, the value of a surgical resection has not been clearly delineated and is recommended only in specific situations (i.e., persistence of tumor following induction chemotherapy). Pure germinomatous tumors are highly sensitive to both radio- and chemotherapy. In the past, radiotherapy was the modality of choice for these tumors due to the high cure rate (5-year survival >80%). Due to the recognized long-term risks from this therapy (neuropsychological and endocrine), adjuvant chemotherapy is now being used to allow a reduction in the dose and extent of radiotherapy without increasing relapse rate. Chemotherapeutic agents are similar to those used for systemic GCT and include platinum agents (cisplatin and carboplatin), alkylators (cyclophosphamide and ifosfamide), and topoisomerase II inhibitors (etoposide). Of note, patients with DI should be carefully monitored in an ICU setting while receiving alkylators or platinum therapy due to the increased risk of nephrotoxicity. Management during this therapy can be simplified by the use of IV vasopressin administered as a continuous infusion.

Patients with NGGCT have had a poorer outcome in the past as these tumors are generally less radiosensitive than pure germinoma. Outcome is related to tumor histology as those patients with pure embryonal carcinoma, endodermal sinus tumor, and choriocarcinoma fair much more poorly than those with mixed histology, especially those with a high proportion of teratoma or germinoma. Neoadjuvant platinum-based chemotherapeutic regimens have shown benefit in patients with NGGCT prior to radiation therapy. Second-look surgery is beneficial in those patients with an incomplete radiologic response or persistently elevated tumor markers following induction chemotherapy, prior to radiation therapy. High-dose chemotherapy with autologous stem cell rescue has been shown to be of benefit in patients with residual malignant disease after chemotherapy and surgery.

Patients with recurrent disease may be successfully treated, depending on initial therapy. Patients with pure germinoma treated solely with chemotherapy may benefit from additional chemotherapy followed by radiation therapy. Those that have previously received radiation may benefit from high-dose chemotherapy with autologous stem cell rescue. Patients with recurrent NGGCT have a much more dismal outcome though may benefit from additional chemotherapy, surgery, radiation, and/or high-dose chemotherapy with stem cell rescue.

Suggested Reading

Echevarria ME, Fangusaro J, Goldman S. Pediatric central nervous system germ cell tumors: a review. Oncologist; 13:690–699, 2008.

Horton Z, Schlatter M, Schultz S. Pediatric germ cell tumors. Surg Oncol 16:205–213, 2007.

Horwich A, Shipley J, Huddart R. Testicular germ-cell cancer. Lancet 367:754–765, 2006.

22 Rare Tumors of Childhood

The rarer tumors of childhood collectively comprise fewer than 20% of all pediatric cancers. The more frequently seen of these include retinoblastoma (2% to 3%), liver tumors (1%), and epithelial tumors of the adrenal or thyroid gland (2% to 3%), which are discussed herein. Many other rare pediatric malignancies also exist that are beyond the scope of this chapter.

Retinoblastoma

Retinoblastoma is the most common malignant ocular tumor in childhood, affecting 200 to 300 children per year in the United States. Retinoblastoma is rarely diagnosed after 5 years of age. This unique neoplasm has a strong genetic component related to mutation in the RB1 gene located on chromosome 13. It was the model for the development of Knudson's two-hit hypothesis after observation that children with bilateral retinoblastoma developed disease at an earlier age compared to those with unilateral disease. The genetic form of the disease is inherited in an autosomal dominant manner yet only 15% to 25% of children have a family history, suggesting the acquisition of a new germ line or somatic mutation in the majority. Genetic counseling is of utmost importance in affected families due to the risk of tumors in siblings as well as offspring of survivors, especially in those with bilateral retinoblastoma.

The RB1 gene is a tumor suppressor gene and individuals with loss of function of both allelic copies are predisposed to malignancy. Germline *de novo* mutations of the RB1 gene largely occur during spermatogenesis. Secondary mutations may then be germline or somatic depending on the timing of events. Those mutations that are germline are heritable for future generations.

Retinoblastoma arises from the photoreceptor cells of the innermost layer of the retina. The tumor frequently extends into the vitreous cavity, presenting with a fleshy nodular mass visible on ophthalmologic examination. Large tumors may occupy most of the posterior chamber. Less frequently, tumors may extend externally resulting in retinal detachment. The tumor tends to outgrow its blood supply and may develop areas of necrosis and calcification.

Due to the large mass or retinal detachment, the normal papillary red reflex is replaced by leukocoria (white papillary discoloration) and is often first noticed by the family. Strabismus is the second most common presenting sign and is due to visual impairment from the tumor. Other less

Handbook of Pediatric Hematology and Oncology: Children's Hospital & Research Center Oakland, Second Edition. Caroline A. Hastings, Joseph C. Torkildson, and Anurag K. Agrawal.
© 2012 John Wiley & Sons, Ltd. Published 2012 by John Wiley & Sons, Ltd.

common presenting signs include hetero-chromia, inflammatory changes, hyphema, and glaucoma. Familial cases are often detected early when the family is appropriately advised on the need for frequent and careful screening with ophthalmologic examinations under anesthesia. The differential diagnosis of leukocoria includes a number of rare nonmalignant conditions such as Coats disease, congenital cataracts, toxocariasis, retinopathy of prematurity, and persistent hyperplastic primary vitreous. Careful retinal examination by an ocular oncologist can rule out these other diseases and obviate the need for tissue biopsy. Patients with advanced disease may present with proptosis and swelling depending on the degree of extraocular invasion. Metastatic spread can occur through infiltration of the optic nerve, dissemination into the subarachnoid space, invasion into the choroid plexus, and anteriorly into the conjunctiva. Invasion through the optic nerve and subarachnoid can lead to involvement of the brain and spinal cord, invasion of the vascular choroid plexus can lead to vascular spread, and anterior invasion can lead to regional lymph node involvement.

Patients with bilateral retinoblastoma may present with a concurrent intracranial neuroblastic tumor, referred to as trilateral retinoblastoma. These patients tend to have a poor prognosis and usually present with a pinealoblastoma, although they may have a neuroblastic tumor in the suprasellar region as well. The intracranial tumor may present at the same time as the retinoblastomas, or after the identification and treatment of the original tumors, emphasizing the need for close follow up after initial treatment.

Ultrasound, CT, and MRI are typically used in addition to ophthalmologic examination to further characterize the tumor. CT is the most useful test as it effectively demonstrates intraocular calcifications that confirm the diagnosis, but it creates risk due to radiation that increases the likelihood of secondary malignancy. MRI is most useful for identification of extraocular extension and trilateral retinoblastoma. MRI of the spine and lumbar puncture for cerebrospinal fluid cytology should be done in patients with intracranial spread, involvement of the optic nerve, or evidence of tumor invasion beyond the lamina cribrosa on pathology after eye enucleation. In patients with delay in diagnosis and concern for metastatic disease, bone marrow studies and bone scan should be performed.

Treatment for retinoblastoma is individualized and dependent on multiple factors including unilaterality or bilaterality of disease, potential for preserving vision, and extent of intraocular and extraocular disease. Enucleation performed by an experienced ophthalmologist is indicated for large tumors filling the vitreous and in those with little or no likelihood of vision preservation. Enucleation is often indicated for unilateral localized retinoblastoma, and alone is effective therapy in these children. The eye must be removed intact to avoid seeding and care must be taken to resect enough optic nerve to ensure negative margins. After enucleation, patients are fitted with a prosthetic implant.

Focal treatments such as laser photocoagulation, cryotherapy, and thermotherapy may be utilized for very small tumors. Chemotherapy (usually vincristine, etoposide, and carboplatin) can be utilized for localized tumors in order to facilitate focal treatment for tumor eradication and prevent the need for enucleation.

Patients with bilateral disease may require enucleation of the more affected eye, but fortunately bilateral enucleation is rarely indicated. As with localized unilateral retinoblastoma, chemotherapy may be utilized prior to focal therapy to avoid enucleation in either eye or in the less-affected eye. External beam radiation therapy is generally reserved for patients with refractory or recurrent disease after these other treatment modalities have been exhausted due to the high incidence of side effects including risk of secondary malignancy.

Patients with regional extraocular disease and metastatic disease have historically faired very poorly. Newer studies have shown the potential benefit of chemotherapy (or high-dose chemotherapy with autologous stem cell rescue in those with metastatic disease) with external beam radiation therapy.

Children treated for retinoblastoma are at high risk for cosmetic and functional impairment related to either enucleation or radiation. Patients with a heritable muta-tion in the RB1 gene have an especially high rate of secondary malignancy after radiation therapy. Reported second malignancies include head and neck cancers, osteosar-coma, soft tissue sarcoma, and melanoma. Adult tumors also have an increased inci-dence in those with germline RB1 muta-tions, especially epithelial tumors such as lung cancer. Radiation therapy also may lead to decreased visual acuity, eye irrita-tion, and dry eye as well as growth abnor-malities in the orbital bones. After therapy, patients should be followed closely due to the risk of recurrent disease. Patients with bilateral retinoblastoma and those diag-nosed with unilateral retinoblastoma at a young age (i.e., <1 year of age) should be observed for the development of an intra-cranial mass and, in the case of unilateral disease, a contralateral retinal mass. Recur-rence or new disease rarely occurs after 5 years of age, although an ophthalmologist should examine these patients annually.

Liver tumors

Primary hepatic tumors in childhood and adolescence account for just more than 1% of malignancies in these age groups. Hepatoblastoma is the most common, representing more than 60% of hepatic tumors, and occurs almost exclusively during infancy and young childhood. The incidence of hepatoblastoma is increasing, possibly due to increased survival in very low birth weight infants. Hepatocellular carcinoma (HCC), approximately 20% to 25% of childhood primary liver tumors, is seen most often in children above 10 years of age. Although chronic hepatitis B infection is the leading cause of HCC in Asia, few American children with HCC have an apparent etiology. Benign hepatic tumors, such as hemangioendothelioma, hamartoma, mature teratoma, angiolipoma, and ade-noma, also occur in childhood and account for up to 20% of liver tumors in this age group. Other extremely rare malignant hepatic tumors include cholangiocarcinoma, rhabdoid tumor, yolk sac tumor, rhabdomyo-sarcoma, undifferentiated sarcoma, angiosar-coma, leiomyosarcoma, and lymphoma.

Malignant hepatic tumors of childhood have been associated with a number of genetic syndromes and environmental risk factors. Hepatoblastoma has been reported in children with Beckwith–Wiedemann syn-drome, familial adenomatous polyposis (which includes Gardner syndrome), and isolated hemihypertrophy. The strongest association has been reported in infants born at less than 1500 g. Additional associa-tions may include maternal smoking (inde-pendent of birth weight), use of infertility treatment, fetal alcohol syndrome, use of oral contraceptives during pregnancy, and occupational exposure to metals, petro-leum, paints, and pigments. HCC is seen in association with hereditary tyrosinemia, biliary cirrhosis, glycogen storage diseases, hemochromatosis, ataxia telangiectasia, and α_1-antitrypsin deficiency. Infection with hepatitis B or C has been identified as a risk factor for HCC as have exposure to alcohol, anabolic steroids, aflatoxin, and certain carcinogens such as pesticides and vinyl chloride.

Clinical presentation

The most common presenting signs of a malignant hepatic tumor in childhood are generalized abdominal enlargement or an asymptomatic abdominal mass palpated by the family or physician. Patients with HCC may present with constitutional symptoms including weight loss, anorexia, emesis, and abdominal pain. Rarely, children may present with jaundice in HCC or in cases with biliary tree involvement. Occasionally, males with hepatoblastoma present with signs of isosexual precocious puberty due to excessive production of the beta subunit of human chorionic gonadotropin (β-HCG) that is converted to testosterone. Lung metastases (typically asymptomatic) may occur at presentation in up to 20% to 30% of children with hepatoblastoma and HCC. Extrahepatic extension may include peritoneal implants as well as spread to regional and distant lymph nodes, bone, bone marrow, and rarely the central nervous system. Liver tumors may also invade into adjacent intra-abdominal structures.

Diagnosis and staging

Work up of a suspected hepatic mass should include laboratory measurement of liver function with coagulation studies in addition to transaminases, total bilirubin, and alkaline phosphatase. Patients should have a baseline complete blood count (CBC) in addition to metabolic studies as patients may present with thrombocytosis and/or leukocytosis. Patients with suspected hepatoblastoma should have elevation of α-fetoprotein (AFP) and, less commonly, of β-HCG. In certain cases with an extremely high AFP, the value reported out may be falsely low due to overwhelming of the assay (hook effect). When the index of suspicion is high, serial dilution of serum can allow for more accurate reporting. Those with HCC may also have elevation in AFP but not to the same magnitude as hepatoblastoma. β-HCG may be elevated in patients with carcinoma of the biliary tract. Of note, carcinoembryonic antigen (CEA) and vitamin B_{12} binding capacity may be elevated in some cases of HCC. Imaging studies should begin with abdominal and specifically liver ultrasound with Doppler flow to characterize the tumor as well as the relationship between tumor and hepatic vessels. CT or MRI should also be obtained prior to surgical intervention. Angiography may be required to help with surgical planning, but is rarely needed now due to the excellent resolution of current generation CT and MRI. Evaluation for metastatic disease should include chest CT.

AFP is the most sensitive marker for disease, especially in hepatoblastoma. Patients with small-cell undifferentiated histology have a poorer prognosis and tend to have low serum AFP, which is a poor prognostic marker. Decline in AFP levels with courses of treatment is prognostic and AFP should be followed for normalization after surgical resection and as a marker for potential disease recurrence. Of note, serum AFP levels vary with age in infancy, declining to adult levels by around 6 to 8 months of age. In addition, AFP has a long serum half-life of 5 to 6 days and therefore may take several weeks to normalize in cases with an extremely high level at presentation.

In cases where clinical presentation, imaging, and tumor markers are highly suggestive of hepatoblastoma, patients should undergo a primary resection if it is deemed safe and feasible. In cases where a complete resection is not feasible or the diagnosis is uncertain, the patient should first undergo biopsy. A current Children's Oncology Group clinical trial hopes to determine whether patients who undergo a complete resection with a favorable histology (i.e., pure fetal histology) can be safely observed without adjuvant chemotherapy. Patients who cannot obtain a complete resection or have a less favorable histology will receive chemotherapy. In the past, chemotherapy for hepatoblastoma has consisted of cisplatin, 5-FU (fluorouracil), and vincristine (C5V). For patients with higher risk disease (i.e., small-cell undifferentiated histology or higher stage), the addition of other chemotherapeutic agents such as doxorubicin and irinotecan is being explored. Patients should receive chemotherapy in order to facilitate total resection when feasible, and if not feasible, prior to orthotopic liver transplantation. Consolidative chemotherapy is given after resection to treat any residual microscopic metastatic disease. Patients with gross metastatic disease at presentation have a poor prognosis, as do patients with recurrent disease.

In general, HCC has a poor prognosis and often presents with multifocal liver and metastatic disease. Previous studies treated pediatric patients with a similar chemotherapeutic regimen as hepatoblastoma (i.e., C5V) with disappointing results. Gross total surgical resection remains the mainstay of cure for HCC. In cases where resection is not safe or feasible at presentation, neoadjuvant chemotherapy may be of benefit and allow for a later total resection or for orthotopic liver transplantation.

A distinct pathologic variant, fibrolamellar HCC, has been associated with a higher resection rate and improved survival compared to other forms of HCC. Novel targeted agents have shown a modest benefit at best, but may have promise when used as part of multimodal therapy.

Radiation therapy has not been proven to be effective in the treatment of hepatoblastoma and HCC, but it may have a role in palliation of lung metastases. Similarly, high-dose chemotherapy with autologous stem cell rescue has not as yet been found beneficial. Local therapies including hepatic artery chemoembolization, percutaneous radiofrequency ablation, and percutaneous ethanol injection may be beneficial in patients with localized yet unresectable HCC.

Adrenocortical carcinoma

Adrenocortical carcinoma (ACC) is a rare malignancy in childhood and adolescence with peaks in both the first and fourth decades of life. The incidence varies worldwide with an interestingly high incidence in southern Brazil. ACC has been reported in association with specific genetic syndromes such as Beckwith–Wiedemann syndrome, isolated hemihypertrophy, Li-Fraumeni syndrome, and in association with congenital adrenal hyperplasia and multiple endocrine neoplasia type 1 (MEN-1 syndrome). Germline mutations in the p53 tumor suppressor gene have been implicated in the majority of pediatric cases in the United States and Brazil.

ACC may be functionally inactive or secrete hormones such as glucocorticoids, sex steroids and their precursors, and mineralocorticoids. Benign adrenocortical tumors are more common and must be carefully differentiated from ACC. Patients frequently present with clinical signs and symptoms of excessive cortisol production (Cushing's syndrome) or excessive androgen production (virilization). Other less common symptoms include abdominal pain and weight loss. The diagnosis is made based on the presence of elevated concentrations of adrenocortical hormones and their intermediates in the serum or urine. Baseline studies should include a 24-hour free cortisol, dexamethasone suppression test, basal cortisol, and adrenocorticotropic hormone (ACTH) to measure glucocorticoid secretion; testosterone, estradiol, androstenedione, dehydroepiandrosterone sulfate (DHEA-S), and 17-OH-progesterone to measure sex steroids and their precursors; and aldosterone and renin in patients with hypertension or hypokalemia to rule out mineralocorticoid excess. Pheochromocytoma can be ruled out by checking catecholamines and metanephrines. Imaging with CT or MRI of the abdomen confirms the presence of a suprarenal mass. FDG-PET may be utilized in equivocal cases or if CT/MRI are negative with positive hormone markers. FDG-PET is negative in benign adrenocortical tumors. Many patients present with large primary tumors and evidence of metastatic disease involving the lungs, liver, or bones. CT of the chest, abdomen, and pelvis in addition to bone scan should be done for staging purposes prior to surgical resection. ACC are locally aggressive tumors with a thin pseudocapsule; an open adrenalectomy should be performed to prevent extensive hemorrhage or tumor rupture. Surgical resection is the only known curative therapy for ACC, both for primary and metastatic sites. Surgery is also indicated in recurrent disease to prolong survival.

Due to the poor response to chemotherapy, patients with advanced disease have a very poor prognosis. A tumor weight < 200 g (<5 cm in diameter in adults) is a good prognostic factor. Patients with localized disease should undergo aggressive gross total surgical resection. Patients with large tumors (>200 g) without metastatic disease may also benefit from radical retroperitoneal lymph node dissection (RPLND). Patients with advanced disease (invasive or metastatic) should be treated with aggressive surgical resection of the primary tumor, RPLND, and resection of metastatic lesions in addition to chemotherapy. If resection of metastases is not feasible, resection of the primary tumor may not be of benefit. Mitotane, a synthetic derivative of the insecticide dichlorodiphenyltrichloroethane (DDT), has a specific cytotoxic effect on adrenocortical cells. It has shown benefit in a subset of patients with invasive, metastatic, or recurrent disease. Mitotane may have benefit in patients with localized, fully resected disease, although this question has not been clearly answered. Mitotane levels greater than 14 mg/L seem to be most beneficial. As mitotane is an adrenocorticolytic agent, replacement with hydrocortisone and fludrocortisone is necessary to prevent adrenal insufficiency. For patients that progress on mitotane or have side effects that limit its usage, chemotherapy with cisplatin, etoposide, and doxorubicin may be beneficial. ACC is considered radioresistant, so this is not a therapeutic option.

Thyroid tumors

The incidence of malignant thyroid carcinoma in children is very low, comprising less than 2% of pediatric cancers. The peak incidence is in the older adolescent age group, 15 to 19 years of age, with a preponderance in females. Childhood thyroid carcinomas are clinically and biologically distinct from those seen in adults. The majority of thyroid carcinomas are papillary or follicular variants of papillary carcinoma. Exposure to head and neck irradiation is associated with an increased risk of thyroid carcinoma, particularly the papillary variant. An increased incidence has been seen in children receiving therapeutic radiation with a median latency of 13 years and has also been observed in survivors following the Chernobyl nuclear accident. Genetics plays a major role in patients with medullary carcinoma with many children having a positive family history. Inherited medullary carcinoma is also seen in association with MEN types 2A and 2B or as part of familal medullary carcinoma. MEN types 2A and 2B are caused by germline mutations in the RET (rearranged during transfection) protooncogene. Patients with MEN type 2A develop medullary thyroid carcinoma, pheochromocytoma, and parathyroid tumors. Patients with MEN type 2B may develop medullary carcinoma or pheochromocytoma and are associated with a marfanoid body habitus, mucosal neuromas, and ganglioneuromatosis. A high incidence of papillary carcinoma of the thyroid is seen in familial adenomatous polyposis coli and Cowden disease.

Patients typically present with a painless solitary thyroid nodule (approximately 70% to 75%) and up to 35% to 40% present with palpable cervical adenopathy. If the tumor has invaded locally, patients may present with dysphagia or dysphonia. Children are more likely than adults to present with advanced or metastatic disease (primarily lungs). Pulmonary metastases classically appear as miliary lesions. Staging in children is based on the presence or absence of metastases. Younger children may have an increased risk of recurrence. Presence of metastatic disease, age, size of tumor, and degree of extrathyroid invasion are predictive of outcome.

The initial evaluation of the child with a thyroid nodule should include thyroid ultrasound as well as measurement of free thyroxine (FT4) and thyroid-stimulating hormone (TSH). Up to 20% of thyroid nodules in children will be malignant, and younger age, past history of irradiation, and family history are all highly predictive of malignant disease. Ultrasound characteristics may guide the clinician in the diagnosis as malignant tumors are more likely to have indistinct margins, vascularity, an absence of an echogenic halo around the nodule, and presence of calcifications. Nuclear medicine thyroid scintigraphy (usually with I^{123}) can be utilized but is not diagnostic and delivers quite a bit of radiation. The majority of thyroid nodules are cold on thyroid scan but most of these are benign follicular adenomas. Image-guided fine needle aspiration is recommended to obtain tissue diagnosis. Surgical removal may be considered in higher risk patients with suspicious features on imaging, positive family history, or past history of irradiation. When a thyroid carcinoma is diagnosed, staging is completed with a neck ultrasound, CT, or MRI to evaluate lymph nodes, chest CT to evaluate for metastasis, and possibly a neck MRI to assess for degree of local invasion.

Surgical resection is key to curative therapy in thyroid carcinoma. Patients should undergo a total or subtotal thyroidectomy. No specific recommendations are currently available in children with regard to lymph node dissection. When lymph node involvement is confirmed on imaging or by biopsy, a modified lateral neck dissection is recommended. Following surgery, a diagnostic whole body scan with I^{123} or I^{131} is recommended to define areas of residual disease. Radioiodine ablation is then recommended and has been shown to reduce the incidence of locoregional recurrence. Lifetime thyroid replacement is required after surgery and radioablation.

Suggested Reading

Khara L, Silverman A, Bethel C, et al. Thyroid papillary carcinoma in a 3-year-old American boy with a family history of thyroid cancer: a case report and literature review. J Pediatr Hematol Oncol 23:e118–e121, 2010.

Litten JB, Tomlinson GE. Liver tumors in children. Oncologist 13:812–820, 2008.

Lohmann D. Retinoblastoma. Adv Exp Med Biol 685:220–227, 2010.

Ribeiro RC, Pinto EM, Zambetti GP. Familial predisposition to adrenocortical tumors: clinical and biologic features and management strategies. Best Pract Res Clin Endocrinol Metab 24:477–490, 2010.

Sinnott B, Ron E, Schneider AB. Exposing the thyroid to radiation: a review of its current extent, risks, and implications. Endocr Rev 31:756–773, 2010.

23 Histiocytic Disorders

Histiocytes (composed of dendritic cells and monocytes/macrophages; also called tissue macrophages) are cells of the mononuclear phagocytic system that fight infection and clear debris. Histiocytic disorders occur due to abnormal proliferation or activity of these cells and have a wide variety of clinical presentations, from the localized and mild to the generalized and severe.

The classification of these conditions can be as confusing as the conditions themselves. The most recent World Health Organization (WHO) classification was developed in 1997 and is presented in Table 23.1. While most of the histiocytic disorders are considered nonmalignant conditions, many are treated similarly to malignant disease, and the mortality of several conditions is quite high. The etiology of most types is unknown, but appears secondary to poorly understood pathophysiological mechanisms. This chapter focuses on the more common presentations of disease, specifically Langerhans cell histiocytosis (LCH) and hemophagocytic lymphohistiocytosis (HLH). Less common disorders include juvenile xanthogranuloma (including Erdheim–Chester disease) and sinus histiocytosis with massive lymphadenopathy (Rosai–Dorfman disease).

Langerhans cell histiocytosis

LCH is now the accepted umbrella term for a wide variety of other conditions previously described, including histiocytosis X, eosinophilic granuloma, Hand-Schüller–Christian syndrome, Letterer–Siwe disease, Hashimoto–Pritzker syndrome, self-healing histiocytosis, pure cutaneous histiocytosis, Langerhans cell granulomatosis, Langerhans cell (eosinophilic) granulomatosis, type II histiocytosis, and nonlipid reticuloendotheliosis. The pathogenesis of LCH is poorly understood. Immune dysregulation likely plays a role and may be reactive, occurring secondary to trauma and infection, especially in those patients with remitting disease. A neoplastic process may also be possible in cases that are systemic and widely disseminated. LCH is a misnomer as the Langerhans cell, an epidermal dendritic cell, is not the sole culprit; rather, like other histiocytic disorders, LCH is due to abnormalities in the mononuclear phagocytic system. Diagnosis is based on histologic features of these Langerhans cells (characterized by Birbeck granules on electron microscopy) in addition to specific immunophenotypic markers (CD1a and CD207).

Handbook of Pediatric Hematology and Oncology: Children's Hospital & Research Center Oakland, Second Edition. Caroline A. Hastings, Joseph C. Torkildson, and Anurag K. Agrawal.
© 2012 John Wiley & Sons, Ltd. Published 2012 by John Wiley & Sons, Ltd.

Table 23.1 Classification of histiocytic disorders.

Group	Cell of origin	Condition
Disorders of varied biological behavior "Excludes disorders that are considered to be malignant while recognizing a wide scope of severity ranging from self-limited to lethal disease"	Dendritic cell	Langerhans cell histiocytosis Secondary dendritic cell processes Juvenile xanthogranuloma and related disorders Solitary histiocytomas of various dendritic cell phenotypes
	Macrophage	Hemophagocytic lymphohistiocytosis (familial and sporadic; commonly elicited by viral infections) Secondary hemophagocytic syndromes Infection-associated Malignancy-associated Other Rosai-Dorfman disease (sinus histiocytosis with massive lymphadenopathy) Solitary histiocytoma with macrophage phenotype
Malignant disorders	Monocyte	Leukemias (FAB and revised FAB classifications) Monocytic leukemia (M5A and B) Acute myelomonocytic leukemia (M4) Chronic myelomonocytic leukemia Extramedullary monocytic tumor or sarcoma (monocytic counterpart of granulocytic sarcoma)
	Dendritic cell	Dendritic cell-related histiocytic sarcoma (localized or disseminated) Specify phenotype; follicular dendritic cell, interdigitating dendritic cell, etc.
	Macrophage	Macrophage-related histiocytic sarcoma (localized or disseminated)

Abbreviations: FAB, French-American-British.

LCH most often presents in the bone as a solitary or as multifocal lesions and may also be localized to the skin or lymph nodes. Bone lesions may be painful or painless. On plain film, lesions appear lytic, often with a "punched out," beveled appearance and may have an associated periosteal reaction with soft tissue swelling. Skin lesions are scaly, erythematous papules often involving the scalp. Localized disease in these areas portends a good prognosis with chance for spontaneous remission due to "burning out" of the underlying immune reaction. Observation is generally favored in this situation, with certain caveats:

1. Vertebral lesions have an inherent risk of causing vertebral compression (vertebra plana) or spinal cord compression if significant soft tissue swelling exists, therefore radiation therapy should be considered.

2. Large or symptomatic solitary lesions may benefit from surgical curettage or resection, intralesional steroid injection, or radiation therapy.

3. For solitary bone lesions, the recommendation for observation excludes sites that put the patient at increased risk for the development of diabetes insipidus (facial bones and anterior/middle cranial fossa). For these "special sites," and for multifocal bone, skin, or lymph node involvement, chemotherapy with 12 months of prednisone and vinblastine is recommended.

Systemic disease, which involves multiple organs including the bone marrow, liver, spleen, or lungs, has a much worse prognosis, especially in those patients without an early response to therapy. Poor responders likely will require more intensive therapy including, potentially, hematopoietic stem cell transplantation.

Hemophagocytic lymphohistiocytosis

Like other histiocytic disorders, immune dysregulation is the key feature in HLH. This condition presents with prolonged and excessive activation of macrophages, histiocytes, and cytotoxic T-lymphocytes (CTL). Natural killer (NK) cells, vital to antigen recognition and killing as well as contraction of the immune response from T-cells and histiocytes, often have decreased activity, in part allowing for this hyperproliferative immune response. Viral infection by Epstein–Barr virus is the most common known acquired cause, although multiple other viruses have been implicated, and often the pathogen is not identified. Familial HLH can occur secondary to multiple known genetic causes that lead to NK and CTL dysfunction. The familial causes are outlined in Table 23.2. An underlying genetic predisposition may still require a "second hit," such as a viral infection, to develop HLH.

Clinical findings are secondary to the chronic inflammatory state and most notably include fever, splenomegaly, cytopenias, and hepatitis. Diagnostic criteria for HLH are summarized in Table 23.3. For the patient with high

Table 23.2 Genetic mutations associated with HLH.

Gene	Pathophysiology
Perforin 1 (PRF1)	Synthesized in natural killer and cytotoxic T-cells, permeabilizes target membrane allowing granzyme B to initiate apoptotic pathways
MUNC 13–4 (UNC13D)	Important for cytolytic granule fusion to target membrane
RAB27A (Griscelli syndrome)	Docking of secretory granules
Syntaxin (STX11/STXBP2)	Failure of degranulation when encountering susceptible targets
LYST (Chédiak-Higashi syndrome)	Involved in maturation of cytolytic enzyme granules
AP3B1 (Hermansky–Pudlak syndrome type II)	Polarization/intracellular movement of cytolytic granules
SH2D1A (X-linked lymphoproliferative syndrome)	Polarization/intracellular movement of cytolytic granules

Table 23.3 Diagnostic criteria for hemophagocytic lymphohistiocytosis.

Diagnosis by molecular criteria (summarized in Table 23.2)
OR
Five of the following eight criteria:
Fever
Splenomegaly
Bicytopenia (i.e., hemoglobin <9 g/dL, platelets $< 100 \times 10^9$/L, neutrophils $< 1 \times 10^9$/L)
Hemophagocytosis in bone marrow, spleen, lymph nodes, or central nervous system
Fasting hypertriglyceridemia (≥ 265 mg/dL) and/or hypofibrinogenemia (≤ 150 mg/dL)
Low or absent natural killer activity
Ferritin ≥ 500 mcg/L
CD25 (soluble IL-2 receptor) >2400 U/mL (based on reference level)

clinical suspicion for HLH, treatment should be initiated promptly even while pending pertinent laboratory evaluation. Current therapy includes dexamethasone, etoposide, and cyclosporine. For patients that have a complete response after 8 weeks, treatment can be stopped. For those that have not responded completely or relapse after stopping therapy, hematopoietic stem cell transplantation is the treatment of choice.

Excessive activation of macrophages and T-lymphocytes may also lead to a secondary or reactive HLH known as macrophage activation syndrome (MAS). Clinical criteria for MAS are similar to HLH and the underlying pathogenesis is due to an autoimmune condition, most commonly systemic onset juvenile idiopathic arthritis (adult Still's disease). Multiple other autoimmune diseases have been reported to cause MAS. NK cells are vital in the prevention of autoimmunity; decreased NK activity could result in both the development of an autoimmune disease and secondary HLH. Often it is difficult to separate the symptoms of MAS from the underlying autoimmune disease or primary HLH. Patients may have leukocytosis, thrombocytosis, and hyperfibrinogenemia secondary to the underlying inflammatory state, but these levels will trend down with the development of MAS. Fevers may become nonremitting, and due to worsening liver dysfunction, there may be a paradoxical improvement in inflammatory markers such as the erythrocyte sedimentation rate (ESR) and fibrinogen with a resultant improvement in inflammatory symptoms such as arthritis. Treatment for MAS includes pulse steroids and cyclosporine. Duration of therapy is dependent on clinical response; patients that do not respond or relapse may benefit from primary HLH therapy although outcomes are poor.

Case study for review

You are seeing a 6-year-old child that presents to the emergency department with 3 weeks of an erythematous and painful diffuse and spreading rash. Fever began soon after the rash with associated weakness, malaise, and anorexia. Initial laboratory tests include the following:

Complete blood count:

$$\begin{array}{ccc} & 12.5 & \\ 19.8 & \diagup\!\!\!\!\diagdown & 150 \end{array}$$

Differential: 35% segs, 44% bands, 6% lymphs, and 12% monos

ESR: 47 mm/h   CRP: 6.3 mg/dL
Complete metabolic panel:

$$\frac{131 \mid 103 \mid 12}{3.7 \mid 28 \mid 0.7} < 222$$

Total protein 5.2 g/dL
Albumin 2.1 g/dL
AST 146 U/L
ALT 44 U/L
Total bili 0.3 mg/dL

On examination, the patient is alert and interactive, but seems somewhat uncomfortable from the rash. There is mild splenomegaly and no hepatomegaly. The patient is started on antibiotics for presumed sepsis/toxic shock with initial resolution of fever. Cultures are all normal. Due to worsening labs and rash, as well as no source of infection, the differential diagnosis is revisited. The patient again becomes febrile.

1. What findings in the initial laboratory tests suggest sepsis as well as HLH and MAS?

The patient has elevated inflammatory markers (CRP and ESR). Hyponatremia and hypoalbuminemia are often seen with an underlying inflammatory condition. There are no significant cytopenias, making HLH less likely. In addition, the high CRP makes HLH less likely.
    You review the lab trends:

Hemoglobin: 12.5 → 10.3 → 8.9
Platelets: 150 → 98 → 67
White blood cell count: 18.4 → 28.7 → 39.7
    (continued left shift)
ESR: 50 → 47
CRP 6.3 → 12.9 → 18.1
Fibrinogen: 441 → 387 mg/dL

A ferritin is sent and is very elevated at 68,300 mcg/L. Fasting triglycerides are 253 mg/dL.

2. How do these lab values help with the differential?

The patient continues to have signs of an underlying inflammatory picture and hypercytokinemia. Sepsis should still be considered on the differential with the continued elevated ESR, CRP, and fibrinogen. The worsening bicytopenia though should make HLH and MAS higher on the differential. The extremely elevated ferritin is relatively specific for HLH and MAS, and a level this high is concerning for MAS. The decreasing ESR and fibrinogen also raise the concern that the patient is moving for symptoms of an underlying autoimmune disorder to frank MAS. Finally, the elevated white blood cell count with neutrophilia makes MAS much more likely than HLH.

Suggested Reading

Arceci RJ. When T cell and macrophages do not talk: the hemophagocytic syndromes. Curr Opin Hematol 15:359–367, 2008.

Filipovich AH. Hemophagocytic lymphohistiocytosis (HLH) and related disorders. Hematol Am Soc Hematol Educ Prog 127–131, 2009.

Filipovich A, McClain K, Grom A. Histiocytic disorders: recent insights into pathophysiology and practical guidelines. Biol Blood Marrow Transplant 16:S82–S89, 2010.

24 Hematopoietic Stem Cell Transplantation

Hematopoietic stem cell transplantation (HSCT) has become increasingly accepted as a therapeutic modality for a variety of malignant and nonmalignant conditions. HSCT involves the ablation of the recipient's bone marrow with high doses of chemotherapy as well as, in some cases, radiation therapy in order to allow engraftment of the donor's stem cells. Collected stem cells can either be allogeneic (from a separate donor) or autologous (from the patient). The rationale for HSCT is based on the logarithmic dose–response curve for many chemotherapeutic agents: a much higher dose effectively increases tumor killing at the cost of profound myelosuppression. Secondarily, multidrug therapy is required to overcome resistance and heterogeneity within the malignant cell population.

allogeneic transplantation is generally recommended for hematologic malignancies due to the underlying bone marrow involvement (Table 24.1). In addition to the effectiveness of high-dose chemotherapy in tumor killing, there is benefit of a "graft-versus-leukemia" (or lymphoma) effect in allogeneic transplant in which the immunosensitized donor T-cells can theoretically kill residual malignant cells. In contrast, autologous transplant is generally reserved for patients with solid tumors and no evidence of bone marrow involvement after failure of standard chemotherapeutic regimens (Table 24.2). Recommendations for allogeneic HSCT in nonmalignant conditions are summarized in Table 24.3.

Types of transplantation

Stem cells for allogeneic transplantation are collected from bone marrow, peripheral blood, or umbilical cord blood (UCB), whereas stem cells for autologous transplantation are collected most commonly from peripheral blood. Collection of stem cells from peripheral blood occurs after mobilization with granulocyte colony-stimulating factor (G-CSF). The usual volume of bone marrow required to ensure successful

Transplantable conditions

Diseases treated using HSCT can be divided into malignant and nonmalignant conditions. Recommendations for malignant conditions are continually being updated due to changes in the effectiveness of standard chemotherapy and the risks and benefits of HSCT. In pediatric patients,

Handbook of Pediatric Hematology and Oncology: Children's Hospital & Research Center Oakland,
Second Edition. Caroline A. Hastings, Joseph C. Torkildson, and Anurag K. Agrawal.
© 2012 John Wiley & Sons, Ltd. Published 2012 by John Wiley & Sons, Ltd.

Table 24.1 Malignant conditions potentially benefiting from allogeneic transplant.

Acute lymphoblastic leukemia (ALL) in first remission and high risk for relapse
Relapsed ALL in second remission
Acute myelogenous leukemia (AML)
Juvenile myelomonocytic leukemia (JMML)
Hodgkin or non-Hodgkin lymphoma in second or subsequent partial or complete remission
Myelodysplastic syndromes (MDS)
Relapsed, refractory, or familial hemophagocytic lymphohistiocytosis

engraftment of donor cells is 10 to 20 mL/kg of recipient body weight. Younger donors have a higher proportion of marrow repopulating cells. Peripheral blood stem cells are collected via apheresis and identified by the presence of a cell surface marker, CD34 (cluster of differentiation). In general, 5×10^6 CD34$^+$ cells/kg are required to ensure engraftment. For allogeneic transplant, the physician must balance the risks, benefits, and availability of cells derived from bone marrow, peripheral blood, and UCB. Peripheral blood has the highest yield of CD34$^+$ cells (with G-CSF mobilization), whereas UCB has the lowest (due to the volume of UCB). The risk of graft-versus-host disease (GVHD) is lowest after UCB

Table 24.2 Malignant conditions potentially benefiting from autologous transplant.

High risk neuroblastoma
High risk brain tumors (medulloblastoma/ PNET)
Metastatic retinoblastoma
Recurrent high risk germ cell tumors
Relapsed Hodgkin or non-Hodgkin lymphoma
Relapsed Wilms tumor

Abbreviation: PNET, primitive neuroectodermal tumor.

transplantation and highest after peripheral blood stem cell transplant (PBSCT). Engraftment of donor cells occurs earliest after PBSCT. Availability of allogeneic stem cells is often limited by the lack of an eligible donor.

Donor matching in allogeneic transplantation

The major histocompatibility complex (MHC) is a large genomic region on chromosome 6 that encodes the human leukocyte antigen (HLA) system. MHC is vital for the immune system to recognize self versus nonself and varies greatly between individuals. MHC is divided into two major classes, class I and class II. MHC class I molecules are found on nucleated cells and present the MHC to cytotoxic T-cells and natural killer cells. MHC class I includes HLA-A, HLA-B, and HLA-C. MHC class II molecules are located on antigen-presenting cells (B-cells and macrophages) and present the MHC to T helper cells. MHC class II includes HLA-DP, HLA-DQ, and HLA-DR. Many other minor histocompatibility complexes are important in the immune response; however, current donor matching for HSCT is limited to class I and II molecules.

Identification of a suitable donor requires matching the recipient's MHC class I and II antigens with those of the donor. Greater disparity between donor and recipient leads to increasing risk of rejection of the donor cells and, if engraftment occurs, GVHD. Matched family member donor grafts have been found to be the least immunogenic. Unfortunately, 60% to 70% of patients will not have a matched family donor. In these cases, unrelated volunteer donors can be found through bone marrow donor registries, such as the National Marrow Donor Program in the United States

Table 24.3 Nonmalignant conditions benefiting from allogeneic transplant.

Congenital syndromes

Immunodeficiency syndromes	SCID, congenital agammaglobulinemia (Bruton's), DiGeorge syndrome, Wiskott–Aldrich syndrome, chronic mucocutaneous candidiasis, lymphoproliferative syndromes
Hematologic disorders	Sickle cell disease, β-thalassemia, Fanconi anemia, Shwachman–Diamond syndrome, Diamond–Blackfan anemia, dyskeratosis congenita, chronic granulomatous disease, Chédiak–Higashi syndrome, leukocyte adhesion deficiency
Metabolic disorders	Storage diseases, lysosomal diseases, mucolipidosis, mucopolysaccharidoses

Acquired syndromes

Severe aplastic anemia

Paroxysmal nocturnal hemoglobinuria

Abbreviation: SCID, severe combined immunodeficiency syndrome.

and Bone Marrow Donors Worldwide that coordinates multiple worldwide registries. Due to the unavailability of a matched donor in many cases, partially matched donors must be used with increasing risk of immune reactions.

Currently, HLA matching is limited to HLA-A, HLA-B, HLA-C, HLA-DR, and HLA-DQ. National Marrow Donor Program retrospective reviews on HLA matching in unrelated donor bone marrow transplantation have shown that mismatches at MHC class I (HLA-A, HLA -B, and HLA -C) and MHC class II DR (specifically HLA-DRB1) each had a separate, significant effect on survival and risk of GVHD. Additionally, an increasing number of mismatches led to decreasing survival. HLA-DQB1 was also found to have an additive negative effect in patients with other mismatches. UCB transplantation has been shown to not require the same level of HLA matching, and matching is limited to HLA-A, HLA-B, and HLA-DR. UCB transplantation is thought to be less immunogenic secondary to the decreased

alloreactivity of these immature cells. Ultimately, the physician must balance the availability of a matched donor with other factors such as the patient's disease stage, remission status, and general condition. In most cases, disease stage has a greater impact on survival than the level of HLA mismatch.

Pretransplant preparative regimens

High-dose chemotherapy, with or without radiation, is administered in order to maximize tumor killing and, in patients undergoing allogeneic transplant, to affect a sufficient amount of immunosuppression to overcome recipient rejection of the HSCT. Commonly used conditioning agents, their mode of action, and potential side effects are summarized in Table 24.4.

Engraftment and graft failure

Evidence of donor replacement of the recipient's bone marrow begins with increasing

Table 24.4 Common agents used in pretransplant preparative regimens.

Agent	Mode of action	Common potential risks
Antithymocyte globulin	Alteration of function and elimination of T-cells	Fever and chills, pruritus, anaphylaxis, serum sickness
BCNU (Carmustine)	Alkylation leading to DNA damage	Nausea and vomiting, pulmonary infiltrates and fibrosis, transaminitis, nephrotoxicity
Busulfan	Alkylating agent	Nausea and vomiting, electrolyte abnormalities, seizures, mucositis, alopecia, hyperpigmentation, sterility
Carboplatin	Inhibits DNA synthesis by forming DNA cross-links	Nausea and vomiting, type I hypersensitivity, renal impairment and electrolyte wasting, ototoxicity
Cyclophosphamide	Alkylating agent, elimination of T regulatory cells, immunosuppressant	Fluid retention (SIADH), hemorrhagic cystitis, nausea, vomiting, and anorexia, cardiomyopathy, sterility
Etoposide	Inhibits topoisomerase II causing DNA strand breakage	Hypotension, nausea, skin blisters or erythema, nephropathy, hemorrhagic cystitis, alopecia, stomatitis, transaminitis
Fludarabine	Purine analog inhibiting DNA synthesis, immunosuppressant	Nausea, vomiting, and anorexia, mucositis, hemolytic anemia
Melphalan	Alkylating agent	Nausea and vomiting, mucositis
Thiotepa	Alkylating agent	Nausea, vomiting, and anorexia, sterility, excretion through the skin
Topotecan	Inhibits topoisomerase I causing DNA strand breakage	Nausea, vomiting, and anorexia, diarrhea, mucositis, peripheral neuropathy
Total body irradiation	Antitumor activity, immunosuppressant	Fever, myelosuppression, mucositis, alopecia, diarrhea, skin reactions and hyperpigmentation, parotitis, pancreatitis, multiple late effects including risk of secondary malignancy

Abbreviation: SIADH, syndrome of inappropriate antidiuretic hormone. See Chapter 30 and Formulary for more information.

white blood cell counts and decreasing transfusion dependency. Engraftment is defined to occur when the transplant recipient achieves three consecutive days of an absolute neutrophil count (ANC) $> 0.5 \times 10^9$/L. Due to the volume of CD34$^+$ stem cells, engraftment of donor cells occurs earliest after PBSCT and latest after UCB transplantation.

Engraftment syndrome, characterized by fever, rash, as well as pulmonary symptoms and weight gain (secondary to capillary leak), may take place during the initial rapid rise in the white blood cell count. After infection has been ruled out, a short course of intravenous steroid therapy can alleviate symptoms.

Primary graft failure is defined as a lack of engraftment within 6 weeks after transplant. Chimerism studies, either of the peripheral blood or bone marrow, measure percentage of donor and recipient cells and thus also help determine marrow engraftment or primary graft failure. Factors in graft failure include: a nonmyeloablative preparative regimen, insufficient volume of stem cells (i.e., UCB transplant), increased immunogenicity due to mismatched HSCT, and the use of myelosuppressive agents (i.e., medications for GVHD). Secondary graft failure (graft rejection) occurs after the initial wave of engraftment secondary to the continued presence of recipient cytotoxic T-cells. Chimerism studies must again be utilized to show that the majority of cells are of host origin. Other causes of graft failure including infection and recurrence of an underlying hematological malignancy should be ruled out.

Complications of hematopoietic stem cell transplantation

HSCT recipients have a unique set of potential complications that must be well understood when caring for these patients. The pretransplant preparative regimen can lead to a number of posttransplant complications as outlined in Table 24.4. A common complication is veno-occlusive disease (VOD) of the liver, also known as sinusoidal obstructive syndrome (SOS). The profound immunosuppression that occurs both before and after engraftment puts HSCT

patients at high risk for infection with a variety of organisms. Finally, immunogenic donor T-cells can lead to GVHD due to the recognition of host alloantigens as foreign. Multiple late sequelae of HSCT must also be considered.

Infections

Practitioners must be cognizant of the many potential infectious complications in the HSCT patient. Infection prophylaxis is an important aspect of supportive care and is outlined in more detail below (text and Table 24.12). The duration of severe neutropenia (ANC $< 0.5 \times 10^9$/L) and time to engraftment are significant risk factors, as the large majority of patients will have a documented infection after 4 to 5 weeks of neutropenia. Even though the white blood cell count recovers in weeks after transplant, immune reconstitution takes months to years depending on the type of transplant (autologous vs. allogeneic) as well as the continued use of immunosuppressive agents to prevent or treat GVHD. The presence of a central venous catheter is a secondary risk factor. Infections tend to occur at different times after transplant as outlined in Table 24.5. Work up of fever in the posttransplant period is outlined in Table 24.6. Engraftment syndrome, GVHD, and medications such as G-CSF can all be causes of fever in the posttransplant period but are diagnoses of exclusion. *Clostridium difficile* should be considered in the patient with associated symptoms such as fever, abdominal pain, and diarrhea.

Veno-occlusive disease/sinusoidal obstructive syndrome

Veno-occlusive disease (VOD), also called sinusoidal obstructive syndrome (SOS), results from hepatic injury caused by high-dose chemotherapy or total body irradiation leading to fibrosis of small hepatic

Table 24.5 Common infections seen at different time points following hematopoietic stem cell transplantation.

First 30 days	Bacterial	Gram-negative aerobes and anaerobes
		Staphylococcus epidermidis
	Fungal	*Aspergillus* species
		Candida
	Viral	Herpes simplex type I reactivation
30–120 days	Fungal	*Candida albicans* and *C. tropicalis*
		Aspergillus
		Other *Candida* sp., *Trichosporon* sp., *Fusarium* sp.
		Pneumocystis jiroveci[*]
	Viral	Cytomegalovirus (CMV)
		Adenovirus
		Epstein-Barr virus (EBV)
		Human herpesvirus 6 (HHV-6)
	Protozoal	*Toxoplasma* sp.

[*]Formerly *Pneumocystis carinii*, generally considered to be a fungal organism.

vessels. VOD/SOS typically occurs in the first 30 days after allogeneic transplant and presents with worsening weight gain, jaundice, and hepatomegaly. Treatment of VOD/SOS is supportive; general guidelines are outlined in Table 24.7.

Graft-versus-host disease

GVHD occurs due to the proliferation of donor T-cells that recognize host antigen as foreign. Direct effects of the T-lymphocytes and cytokine response lead to the signs and symptoms of GVHD. Acute GVHD can begin within weeks of transplantation; chronic GVHD is defined as GVHD lasting beyond 100 days after transplant. Signs and symptoms of acute and chronic GVHD are summarized in Table 24.8, grading of GVHD is outlined in Table 24.9, and prophylaxis and treatment are described in Table 24.10. Patients should be checked daily for signs and symptoms of acute GVHD while hospitalized following HSCT.

Late sequelae

Multiple late effects must be considered and are summarized in Table 24.11.

Supportive care in transplant patients

Routine care for the HSCT patient is a unique and vital aspect of preventing infections and a multitude of other potential complications including bleeding, transfusion-associated GVHD, and CMV reactivation, as well as ABO incompatibility between recipient and donor.

Infection prophylaxis

Due to profound immunosuppression, HSCT patients are at risk for reactivation of latent viral infections in addition to fungal and bacterial infection. Guidelines for infection prophylaxis and surveillance are outlined in Table 24.12.

Diet

Due to the pretransplant preparative regimen, patients will have an extended period of anorexia requiring total parenteral nutrition (TPN). Triglycerides should be followed weekly while on TPN in addition to routine monitoring of electrolytes. Trace elements should be included in the TPN.

Table 24.6 Evaluation and empiric treatment of fever in the posttransplant period.

Rule out bacterial infection	Daily blood cultures from central catheter (aerobic and anaerobic) while febrile
	Consider noncatheterized urinalysis and culture
Rule out pneumonia	Chest radiography at first fever and then as clinically indicated
Rule out fungal infection	Daily fungal cultures from central catheter while febrile
	Careful skin exam; if concern for infection perform skin biopsy
	CT of the chest and/or sinuses if with localizing signs or symptoms
Rule out occult infection	Consider CT of the chest ($\pm$ sinuses, abdomen, pelvis) if asymptomatic with prolonged fevers (i.e., $\geq$5–7 days) without a source
	Consider galactomannan antigen testing if with persistent fever
Rule out viral infection	CMV serology; consider studies for adenovirus, HHV-6, EBV, BK virus (urine) if prolonged fever (i.e., $\geq$5–7 days) and consistent clinical symptoms
Rule out pneumonia or interstitial pneumonitis	CT of the chest if with consistent symptoms or CXR equivocal
Treatment	If not on empiric antibiotic therapy (see Table 24.12), begin antipseudomonal cephalosporin (i.e., ceftazidime or cefepime) $\pm$ aminoglycoside (i.e., tobramycin) or carbapenem (i.e., meropenem)*
	If with prolonged fevers (i.e., $\geq$5–7 days), consider switching empiric cephalosporin to carbapenem for broader (anaerobic) coverage. Addition of an echinocandin (i.e., micafungin) for broader fungal coverage with prolonged fevers (i.e., $\geq$3–7 days)
	Consider vancomycin for staphylococcal and streptococcal coverage if patient worsening clinically
	Directed antimicrobial coverage or further studies based on positive work-up

*Based on institutional preference.
Abbreviations: CT, computed tomography; CMV, cytomegalovirus; HHV-6, human herpesvirus 6; EBV, Epstein–Barr virus; CXR, chest radiography.

Once the patient is eating, it is vital that the patient's family be aware of the bone marrow transplant low microbial diet of acceptable foods and appropriate methods of handling, preparation, and storage in order to prevent infection from food-borne pathogens.

Transfusion guidelines

Due to immunosuppression, all HSCT patients should receive irradiated blood products in order to eliminate the risk of transfusion-associated GVHD. In addition, packed red blood cell (PRBC) transfusions should be CMV negative for HSCT recipients who are identified as CMV seronegative during the pretransplant period. CMV seronegative platelets are not routinely required as leukofiltered platelets are considered sufficiently leukoreduced to prevent transmission of CMV. In order to diminish the risk of spontaneous bleeding, platelet level is kept above 20×10^9/L after HSCT. This threshold is increased to above 50×10^9/L in certain cases, including patients with sickle cell disease, brain tumor

Table 24.7 Treatments for veno-occlusive disease/sinusoidal obstructive syndrome.

Supportive care	Fluid and sodium restriction
	Spironolactone therapy (in lieu of loop diuretics) for sodium and water diuresis (e.g., aldactone 1–3 mg/kg/day div BID PO)
Antioxidant therapy	N-acetylcysteine. Loading dose of 150 mg/kg IV over 15 min, followed by 50 mg/kg over 4 hours. Maintenance dose of 100–150 mg/kg/day
	Vitamin C, vitamin E, selenium (can be added to parenteral nutrition)
Thrombolytic therapy	TPA. 0.1 mg/kg/h IV for 4 hours over 4 consecutive days; maximum dose 5.0 mg/h
	Heparin. Initial bolus of 20 units/kg IV (max 1000 units), concomitantly with TPA infusion, then 150 units/kg/day. Dose adjusted to keep PTT just at or slightly above ULN
	Antithrombin III. Loading dose of 50 U/kg IV every 8 h for the initial 24 h followed by 50 U/kg daily
	Defibrotide is an experimental agent with fibrinolytic and antithrombotic properties that has shown potential benefit for prophylaxis of VOD/SOS and possible therapeutic benefit in severe disease. Patients must be off all other thrombolytic therapies. In experimental study given at 25 mg/kg/day div Q6 h IV for at least 21 days

Abbreviations: TPA, tissue plasminogen activator; PTT, partial thromboplastin time; ULN, upper limit of normal; VOD/SOS, veno-occlusive disease/sinusoidal obstructive syndrome.

Table 24.8 Signs and symptoms of acute and chronic graft-versus-host disease.

Acute GVHD	Skin	Mild maculopapular rash to generalized erythroderma; can be nonspecific
	GI	Secretory diarrhea, nausea, vomiting, anorexia, stomatitis, hepatic dysfunction
	Hematologic	Anemia, thrombocytopenia
	Ocular	Photophobia, hemorrhagic conjunctivitis
	Pulmonary	Interstitial pneumonitis, alveolar hemorrhage
Chronic GVHD	Skin	Sclerodermatous changes, contractures, alopecia
	GI	Xerostomia, oral atrophy with depapillation of tongue, oral erythema and/or lichenoid lesions, esophagitis, cholestasis, malabsorption, hepatic dysfunction
	Hematologic	Thrombocytopenia
	Ocular	Dry eyes, keratoconjunctivitis sicca (conjunctival and/or corneal inflammation caused by dryness)
	Pulmonary	Interstitial pneumonitis, bronchiolitis obliterans
	Other	Arthritis, immunologic abnormalities

Abbreviations: GVHD, graft-versus-host disease; GI, gastrointestinal.

Table 24.9 Grading of graft-versus-host disease.

Clinical grade	Skin	Liver (TB, mg/dL)	Diarrhea (children; <70 kg) (mL/kg/day)	Diarrhea (adults; ≥ 70 kg) (mL/day)
I	<25% involvement, maculopapular	1.5–3.0	10–15	500–1000, nausea/vomiting
II	25–50% involvement, maculopapular	3.0–6.0	16–20	1000–1500, nausea/vomiting
III	>50% involvement, maculopapular or generalized erythroderma	6.0–15.0	21–25	>1500, nausea/vomiting
IV	Desquamation/bullae	>15	>25, pain/ileus	>2500, pain/ileus

Abbreviation: TB, total bilirubin; adapted from Lanzkowsky P. Hematopoietic stem cell transplantation. In: Manual of Pediatric Hematology and Oncology, 5th ed. New York: Elsevier, 2011.

Table 24.10 Agents used for prophylaxis and treatment of graft-versus-host disease.

Agent	Mode of action	Common potential risks
Cyclosporine	Inhibits T-cell activation	Hypomagnesemia, bicarbonate wasting, renal insufficiency, nausea, vomiting, hyperglycemia, gingival hypertrophy, hirsutism, hypertension, seizures, paresthesias, tremors
Methotrexate	Cell cycle specific; inhibits T-cells as they divide	Transaminitis, mucositis, renal insufficiency, effusions, nausea, vomiting, anorexia, bone marrow suppression
Tacrolimus	Inhibits T-cell activation	Hypomagnesemia, hyperkalemia, renal insufficiency, hypertension, seizures, paresthesias, nausea, vomiting, hyperglycemia
Methylprednisolone	Immunosuppressant; mechanism not well understood	Hypertension, increased blood sugars, increased appetite, insomnia, mood swings, acne, truncal obesity
Mycophenolate mofetil (MMF)	Inhibits T-cell proliferative response	Nausea, vomiting, anorexia, bone marrow suppression, multiple others
Antithymocyte globulin (ATG)	Alteration of function and elimination of T-cells	Fever and chills, pruritus, anaphylaxis, serum sickness
Etanercept/infliximab	TNF-α inhibitors; consideration in refractory GVHD	Severe immunosuppression

Abbreviations: TNF, tumor necrosis factor; GVHD, graft-versus-host disease.

Table 24.11 Late effects of hematopoietic stem cell transplantion.

Late effect	Underlying cause
Endocrine disorders (gonadal failure, delayed pubescence, growth hormone deficiency, hypothyroidism)	TBI
Sterility	TBI, busulfan, cyclophosphamide, thiotepa
Secondary malignancy	TBI, busulfan, ATG, cyclophosphamide, etoposide, genetic factors
Cataracts	TBI
Renal insufficiency	Cyclosporine, other nephrotoxic drugs
Pulmonary disease	Chronic GVHD, BCNU
Cardiomyopathy	Anthracycline therapy, TBI, chronic GVHD
Avascular necrosis	Steroid therapy
Leukoencephalopathy	IT methotrexate
Immunological dysfunction	Chronic GVHD, immunosuppressive therapy
Posttransplant lymphoproliferative disorder	Immunosuppressive therapy
Poor dentogenesis (in young children)	TBI
Decreased bone mineral density	Multiple factors

Abbreviations: GVHD, graft-versus-host disease; TBI, total body irradiation; ATG, antithymocyte globulin; IT, intrathecal; adapted from Lanzkowsky P. Hematopoietic stem cell transplantation. In: Manual of Pediatric Hematology and Oncology, 5th ed. New York: Elsevier, 2011.

patients, and patients with severe mucositis, VOD/SOS, or problems with hemostasis (e.g., epistaxis and GI bleeding). A lower threshold of 10×10^9/L can be utilized in stable patients who are out of the immediate posttransplant period. Hemoglobin levels are usually kept above 8 to 9 mg/dL depending on institutional practice. Platelet transfusions should be limited to 1 pheresed unit (see Chapter 5). ABO blood types of both the donor and recipient must be considered when transfusing platelets and PRBCs. Appropriate transfusion in ABO-incompatible donor and recipient is summarized in Table 24.13.

Immune reconstitution

Even with the recovery of white blood cell counts and specifically lymphocyte counts, HSCT patients take months to years to recover immune function. Loss of memory B-lymphocytes due to the pretransplant preparative regimen leads to loss of antibody secondary to vaccination and lifetime environmental exposures. Immune recovery is variable but generally occurs once the patient is off immunosuppressant therapy, and therefore is often earlier in patients undergoing autologous transplantation. Once there is sufficient evidence of immune reconstitution, HSCT patients will proceed with revaccination. Studies of immune reconstitution, which begin once the absolute lymphocyte count is $>1 \times 10^9$/L and the patient is off immunosuppressive therapy, are summarized in Table 24.14.

Case study for review

A 14-year-old boy is on the bone marrow transplant unit after receiving an HSCT for

Table 24.12 Routine infection prophylaxis and surveillance in transplant patients.

Prophylaxis for	
PCP	TMP-SMX until 2 days prior to transplant, then restarted once ANC $>0.75 \times 10^9$/L for 2–3 consecutive days; for at least six months (until PRP >1 mcg/mL or per institutional guidelines, see Table 24.14)
HSV	If seropositive, at least 30 days of acyclovir (until off immunosuppressive therapy; until HSV blastogenesis present if with recurrent infection)
VZV	If seropositive, at least 180 days of acyclovir (until VZV blastogenesis present)
Candida albicans	Fluconazole until immune reconstitution to *Candida*; hold if transaminases increased to >2–3× ULN
Bacterial infection	Anti-pseudomonal cephalosporin (i.e., ceftazidime or cefepime) ± aminoglycoside (i.e., tobramycin) or carbapenem (i.e., meropenem)*; start with first fever or once ANC drops to $<0.5 \times 10^9$/L if afebrile, continue until afebrile and ANC $> 0.5 \times 10^9$/L for 2 days
Routine surveillance	
CMV	Weekly serology
Occult bacterial infection	Weekly to three times weekly blood culture if on steroids and afebrile (controversial)
Pneumonia	Weekly chest radiograph (controversial)
Deficient IgG	Monthly quantitative IgG; replace with IVIG if IgG < 400 mg/dL

*Based on institutional preference.

Abbreviations: PCP, *Pneumocystis jiroveci* pneumonia; TMP-SMX, trimethoprim-sulfamethoxazole; PRP, polyribose phosphate; ANC, absolute neutrophil count; HSV, herpes simplex virus; VZV, varicella zoster virus; ULN, upper limit of normal; CMV, cytomegalovirus; IgG, immunoglobulin G; IVIG, intravenous immune globulin.

acute myelogenous leukemia (AML) in remission. His stem cell reinfusion took place 14 days ago. He has been having daily fevers up to 39.5 °C for 3 days with negative blood cultures to date. He is not in any respiratory distress and his physical exam is unremarkable except for a mild rash. His laboratory tests are remarkable for a WBC count that has been increasing, most recently 0.2×10^9/L. He has a double lumen central catheter and is on total parenteral nutrition. He has moderate-to-severe mucositis that is improving. His weight has been stable and his tests are otherwise unremarkable. His medications include ceftazidime, tobramycin, fluconazole, and acyclovir.

1. What is the differential for fever at this point after HSCT?

Differential diagnosis:

Bacterial infection (Gram-negative rods, *Staphylococcus epidermidis*, *Streptococcus viridans* species)
Viral infection (CMV, herpes simplex I)
Fungal infection (*Candida*, *Aspergillus*)
Engraftment syndrome

Table 24.13 Transfusion in ABO-incompatible transplantation.

Recipient type	Donor type	Transplant incompatibility	Choice for PRBC transfusion	Choice for plasma	First-choice platelets	Second-choice platelets
A	O	Minor	O	A, AB	A	AB, B, O
A	B	Major	O	AB	AB	A, B, O
A	AB	Major	A, O	A, AB	AB	A, B, O
B	O	Minor	O	B, AB	B	AB, A, O
B	A	Major	O	AB	AB	B, A, O
B	AB	Major	B, O	B, AB	AB	B, A, O
O	A	Major	O	A, AB	A	AB, B, O
O	B	Major	O	AB	B	AB, A, O
O	AB	Major	O	AB	AB	A, B, O
AB	O	Minor	O	AB	AB	A, B, O
AB	A	Minor	A, O	AB	AB	A, B, O
AB	B	Minor	B, O	AB	AB	B, A, O

Abbreviation: PRBC, packed red blood cell.

Table 24.14 Immune reconstitution studies following bone marrow transplantation.

Test		Interpretation
Blastogenesis	Viral panel (CMV, HSV, VZV)	Measures response to CMV, HSV, and VZV and defines length of acyclovir prophylaxis
	Mitogens (Concanavalin A, pokeweed, phytohemagglutinin)	Concanavalin A measures T- and B-cell function Pokeweed measures B-cell function Phytohemagglutinin measures T-cell function, must be reactive before PCP prophylaxis is discontinued
	Antigens (tetanus toxoid, *Candida albicans*)	Lack of response to tetanus toxoid indicates need for revaccination Response to *Candida* defines length of fluconazole prophylaxis
PRP	(If done by institution)	Measurement of T- and B-cell function; indicates need for PCP prophylaxis as well as ability to respond to conjugated vaccines

Abbreviations: CMV, cytomegalovirus; HSV, herpes simplex virus; VZV, varicella zoster virus; PCP, *Pneumocystis jiroveci* pneumonia; PRP, polyribose phosphate.

2. What medications would you consider adding based on the above differential?

The patient is well covered for Gram-negative infections with ceftazidime and tobramycin. Gram-positive infections usually have a positive blood culture, although vancomycin should be considered if the patient is clinically worsening (i.e., respiratory distress or hypotension). The patient is at risk for *S. epidermidis* secondary to the central catheter and *S. viridans* secondary to mucositis, neither of which is covered with ceftazidime and tobramycin. Fungal infection must be seriously considered. Fluconazole will cover *Candida albicans* but not other candidal species or *Aspergillus*. You should consider discontinuing fluconazole and starting an antifungal agent with a broader spectrum of activity such as an echinocandin (i.e., micafungin). Micafungin has a broader spectrum of activity than fluconazole, but only has moderate coverage against *Aspergillus* and does not cover most mold species. Finally, the addition of steroids for engraftment syndrome with fever and rash should be a consideration if infection is relatively well ruled out after negative blood cultures and chest radiography.

After a few days the patient defervesces but has developed an increase in his bilirubin. The infectious work up has been negative to date. On looking at his fluid status for the last 48 hours, you note that he is 2 L positive and his weight has increased by 2 kg from the time of his transplant.

3. What is the differential diagnosis for hyperbilirubinemia and weight gain at this point after transplant?

Differential diagnosis:

    Veno-occlusive disease/sinusoidal obstructive syndrome

Viral infection

Engraftment syndrome

Heart failure (secondary to infection, fluid overload, and previous anthracycline therapy)

Graft-versus-host disease

At this time point after transplant, with a negative infectious work up, VOD/SOS is the most likely diagnosis. If the patient is having increasing WBC counts with rash and diarrhea, engraftment syndrome is possible but should be a diagnosis of exclusion. Although GVHD is a possible cause of hyperbilirubinemia and weight gain, it is less likely this soon after HSCT. Heart failure is a possibility secondary to toxicity from therapy or an underlying infection and should be ruled out with echocardiogram.

4. What would be changes in therapy that you should institute?

Most patients with VOD/SOS ultimately recover with supportive care alone. Fluid and sodium restriction should be initiated in addition to starting spironolactone therapy. An abdominal ultrasound with Doppler flow should be undertaken to look for hepatic fibrosis and changes in portal venous flow. Antioxidants including vitamin C, E, and selenium should be added to the TPN. If the patient develops increasing weight gain and liver dysfunction, more aggressive interventions such as antithrombin III therapy or defibrotide should be instituted.

Suggested Reading

Copelan EA. Hematopoietic stem-cell transplantation. N Engl J Med 354:1813–1826, 2006.

Coppell JA, Richardson PG, Soiffer R, et al. Hepatic veno-occlusive disease following stem cell transplantation: incidence, clinical course, and outcome. Biol Blood Marrow Transplant 16:157–168, 2010.

Ferrara JL, Levine JE, Reddy P, Holler E. Graft-versus-host disease. Lancet 373:1550–1561, 2009.

Lanzkowsky P. Hematopoietic stem cell transplantation. In: Manual of Pediatric Hematology and Oncology, 5th ed. New York: Elsevier, 2011.

Wayne AS, Baird K, Egeler RM. Hematopoietic stem cell transplantation for leukemia. Pediatr Clin N Am 57:1–25, 2010.

25 Supportive Care of the Child with Cancer

Much of the dramatic improvement in outcomes in pediatric oncology over the last 50 years can be attributed to the development of novel chemotherapeutic agents and an increase in therapeutic intensity. With this increased intensity, supportive care has become a vital component in preventing, recognizing, and treating the potential side effects of this therapy. The practitioner should be familiar with the potential risks of chemotherapy as outlined in Chapter 30, guidelines for transfusional supportive care as described in Chapter 5, and treatment for febrile neutropenia as discussed in Chapter 27. Here we discuss infection prophylaxis, antiemetic therapy, and the use of hematopoietic growth factors. Specific supportive care information for patients after hematopoietic stem cell transplantation (HSCT) is discussed in Chapter 24.

Infection prophylaxis

Children receiving chemotherapy for treatment of their malignancies are susceptible to acquiring infection from bacterial, viral, fungal, and protozoal organisms. They are chronically immunosuppressed as a direct result of chemotherapy, and at times severely myelosuppressed. While inpatient they have an increased exposure to nosocomial organisms as well. Many of these children have central venous catheters and may intermittently have mucosal breakdown secondary to chemotherapy, both factors disrupting the integrity of the body's physical defense barriers. Poor nutrition also plays a significant role in host susceptibility. Certain standards of care are indicated to minimize the risk of acquiring infection in these children. Infection prophylaxis remains the cornerstone of supportive care in children with malignancies, decreasing morbidity and mortality.

General measures for the prevention of infection include avoidance of crowded environments, wearing a mask in public when severely neutropenic (i.e., absolute neutrophil count [ANC] $<0.5 \times 10^9$/L), and careful hand washing (by the patient and all those who have direct contact). Good nutrition and proper dental hygiene cannot be overemphasized. Oral hygiene should include daily brushing (with a soft brush) and oral rinsing with tap water or saline solution. Cleanliness of the perianal area is important, especially in the neutropenic state. Constipation should be avoided with an age-appropriate diet, and, if necessary, a stool softener (e.g., docusate sodium) or laxative (e.g., MiraLax). Rectal suppositories and rectal temperatures should be avoided to decrease the possibility of a

Handbook of Pediatric Hematology and Oncology: Children's Hospital & Research Center Oakland, Second Edition. Caroline A. Hastings, Joseph C. Torkildson, and Anurag K. Agrawal.
© 2012 John Wiley & Sons, Ltd. Published 2012 by John Wiley & Sons, Ltd.

mucosal tear and infection with enteric organisms.

Trimethoprim/sulfamethoxazole (TMP/ SMX) prophylaxis is indicated in immunosuppressed children to reduce the risk of acquiring *Pneumocystis jiroveci* pneumonia (PCP) due to T-lymphocyte dysfunction secondary to chemotherapy. Current prophylactic dosing is 5 mg/kg/day of the TMP component in two divided doses on two to three successive days per week. Evidence indicates that this regimen also provides good general antibacterial prophylaxis, although probably more effectively in patients given daily prophylaxis, which must be balanced with potential allergy or intolerance to TMP/SMX and especially secondary to myelosuppression from the therapy. For patients unable to take TMP/ SMX, inhaled pentamidine or oral dapsone may be given. Pentamidine is preferred but due to the need for a cooperative patient who can appropriately inhale the medication, is usually limited to children above the age of 7 years. The dose is 300 mg inhaled on a monthly basis. Dapsone is given once weekly at 4 mg/kg, with a maximum dose of 200 mg. It is dispensed as 25 and 100 mg tablets. Patients should commence prophylaxis at the time of diagnosis and continue until 3 months after completion of therapy to ensure T-lymphocyte immune reconstitution. Prophylaxis with TMP/SMX should be discontinued one day prior to the administration of high-dose IV methotrexate (doses >1 g/m^2) and restarted after the serum methotrexate level has fallen to below 1×10^{-7} M due to competitive excretion between TMP/SMX and methotrexate and the risk for delayed methotrexate clearance. Temporary interruption of TMP/SMX or a change to an alternative therapy may be necessary for prolonged marrow suppression or transaminitis rather than decreasing the dose of maintenance chemotherapy for children with acute lymphoblastic leukemia (ALL).

Fungal prophylaxis is indicated in severely myelosuppressed patients. Mouth care with brushing and oral rinsing is routinely recommended for the prevention or treatment of mouth sores and yeast. Fluconazole (3 mg/kg/day PO or IV) is indicated in patients that are at very high risk of developing infection (i.e., acute myelogenous leukemia [AML], relapsed acute lymphoblastic leukemia [ALL] patients). The most common fungal infections in patients receiving intensive chemotherapy include candidiasis and aspergillosis. Efforts to prevent invasive fungal disease (especially *Aspergillus* sp., an airborne organism) include respiratory isolation, laminar air flow rooms, and high-efficiency particulate air filters. Patients should not have live plants in the room, play in dirt or gardens, or be in proximity to construction work. Some patients may benefit from the addition of an echinocandin (e. g., micafungin 1.5–2 mg/kg IV daily) for broader prophylactic fungal coverage while inpatient with prolonged fevers and severe neutropenia (see Chapter 27).

Prophylaxis for subacute bacterial endocarditis is recommended for patients with central venous catheters undergoing invasive procedures that could cause transient bacteremia and seeding of the catheter or heart valves. Such interventions include dental cleaning or procedures and potentially surgery involving the gastrointestinal or genitourinary tract (controversial). The standard regimen is the same as recommended by the American Heart Association for children with congenital heart disease: amoxicillin 50 mg/kg (maximum 2 g) orally 1 hour prior to the procedure. Azithromycin may be given to penicillin-allergic patients (15 mg/kg, max 500 mg, 1 hour prior to the procedure).

Viral prophylaxis and treatment

Common viral infections may be particularly virulent in immunocompromised children. These viruses include varicella zoster

(VZV), herpes simplex (HSV), cytomegalovirus (CMV), Epstein–Barr virus, hepatitis types A and B, respiratory syncytial virus, and rubeola (measles). Infection with these viruses may result in prolonged viral excretion, increased morbidity, or death. At the time of diagnosis, an immunization and infection history should be determined. In addition, serologies for VZV, HSV, and CMV should be obtained as potential future exposure to and infection with these agents will result in different treatment recommendations depending on the potential for primary infection versus reactivation. CMV serology should also be known in determining whether a potential HSCT patient needs CMV-negative blood (see Chapter 5).

The child exposed to **varicella or zoster** with known negative varicella immune status (negative titers [IgG] and no history of varicella infection) should receive Varicella Zoster Immune Globulin (VariZIG) within 96 hours of exposure (of note, VariZIG remains an investigational agent in the United States and requires institutional review board approval and completion of an investigational new drug form). Parents should be counseled on the risk of exposure for the child with negative immune status and the need for immediate evaluation and treatment if exposed. The dosage is one vial (125 units) per 10 kg, with a minimum dose of 125 units and a maximum of 625 units (5 vials), intramuscularly. Administration of VariZIG extends the incubation period from 14 to 28 days and decreases, but does not eliminate, the possibility of clinical infection with VZV (the incubation period generally is shortened in the immunocompromised patient who does not receive VariZIG). If VariZIG is not available then intravenous immune globulin can be given at 400 mg/kg. Myelosuppressive chemotherapy may need to be stopped 7 days after the exposure and held until the end of the incubation period. The decision to hold chemotherapy during the incubation period should be based on the intensity of exposure, condition of the patient, and intensity of the chemotherapy. If >96 hours have passed since exposure, the patient should be given acyclovir at 80 mg/kg/day (max dose 800 mg/dose) divided QID PO for 7 days. In the event of varicella or zoster infection, chemotherapy should be stopped and IV acyclovir should be given, 30 mg/kg/day divided TID for 7 to 10 days, until all lesions are crusted and no new lesions have appeared for 24 to 48 hours. Monitor renal function and fluid status daily due to potential nephrotoxicity from acyclovir. Of note, it is safe for household contacts to receive varicella vaccination as transmission from healthy recipients rarely occurs. If skin lesions occur after vaccination, exposure should be avoided until all lesions have crusted over.

Children with a history of recurrent **herpes simplex** infections are at an increased risk of reactivation with subsequent courses of chemotherapy or during and after HSCT. Acyclovir administered prophylactically can prevent or decrease the severity of recurrent herpes infection; the recommended oral dose is 200 mg TID-QID for children above 2 years of age. Immunocompromised patients with active HSV infection should receive IV acyclovir (30 mg/kg/day or 1500 mg/m^2/day divided q8h). HSCT guidelines for HSV and VZV prophylaxis are summarized in Chapter 24.

Immunization during chemotherapy

Patients receiving chemotherapy, or who are otherwise immunocompromised, should not receive live virus vaccines (MMR, live attenuated influenza vaccine [LAIV; FluMist®], varicella, rotavirus, and oral polio). Siblings or household contacts should not receive oral polio although MMR, varicella, and rotavirus are safe as transmission is rare. Limited information is available regarding risk of transmission with LAIV; since an inactivated form of influenza vaccination is available, this should be the preferred immunization in family members as well as health care providers. Although varicella vaccination has been shown to be safe in patients with ALL in maintenance, the benefits and risks of this immunization should be weighed carefully. Consideration should be given to the likelihood of developing a protective response while still on chemotherapy and the potential to develop active infection with administration of a live attenuated vaccine. This must be weighed with the significant risks from natural varicella infection in the immunocompromised, although the chance of infection has decreased significantly with herd immunity.

Inactivated vaccines (e.g., DTaP, Tdap, Hepatitis A, Hepatitis B, pneumococcal, Hib, IPV, meningococcal, and influenza) can be safely given during therapy, although response will be significantly attenuated based on the level of immunosuppression. Yearly influenza vaccination is reasonable during therapy as the potential benefit of immunization outweighs the risks, especially for children with ALL in maintenance. In order to increase the chance of an appropriate antibody response, vaccination should be spaced out from chemotherapy as much as feasible. Due to potential risks of pneumococcal and Hib infection in patients with Hodgkin lymphoma (HL) some experts recommend vaccination against these pathogens prior to starting therapy. Although not immunocompromised, untreated patients with HL have an underlying B-lymphocyte dysfunction and the benefits of immunization prior to therapy are often significantly diminished. Evidence is lacking to make firm recommendations.

Catch-up immunizations should occur after the completion of therapy. Most sources feel that waiting 3 to 6 months after therapy completion will produce sufficient immune reconstitution to allow an appropriate response to inactivated vaccines. Patients who had not previously completed their primary vaccination series should restart from the beginning. Patients who previously completed the primary series can have antibody titers drawn to determine what protection they have lost, if any. Children above 5 years of age (not including patients with HL) have a small risk of developing significant disease from pneumococcus or *Hemophilus influenza*, but revaccination against these pathogens should be considered in all patients after therapy. Postvaccination titers can be considered although the likelihood of an insufficient response is minimal in patients who are vaccinated ≥ 6 months after chemotherapy has been completed. Little evidence exists as to the appropriate and safe timeframe to receive live vaccinations after chemotherapy. In general, we recommend waiting 12 months after therapy completion before reimmunizing with MMR and varicella. HSCT guidelines are briefly described in Chapter 24.

Prevention of chemotherapy-induced nausea and vomiting

Antiemetics are a vital component of the supportive care regimen for patients receiving chemotherapy or radiation. There are three types of chemotherapy-induced nausea and vomiting (CINV): (1) anticipatory, (2) acute, and (3) delayed. Anticipatory emesis occurs before chemotherapy is administered and may be a result of nausea and vomiting experienced during previous cycles of therapy. Acute emesis occurs within the first 24 hours of therapy; delayed emesis occurs at least 24 hours after therapy has been completed. Poor control of nausea and vomiting may prolong, or result in, hospitalization and lead to dehydration and electrolyte abnormalities. The single most important factor in CINV is the emetogenic potential of a particular chemotherapeutic agent, which, in pediatric patients, is also dose dependent for some drugs (Table 25.1).

Multiple agents are useful for the prevention and treatment of CINV. Recognition of the chemoreceptor trigger zone and the importance of the $5-HT_3$ receptor have been instrumental in better controlling CINV. Cytotoxic chemotherapy appears to be associated with release of local mediators such as 5-HT and substance P from the enterochromaffin cells of the small intestine. The release of these local mediators subsequently stimulates vagal afferents that initiate vomiting. $5-HT_3$ receptors and substance P receptors (called neurokinin-1) are located both peripherally (vagal nerve terminals) and centrally in the chemoreceptor trigger zone; thus, $5-HT_3$ and substance P antagonists may have both peripheral and central effects in inhibiting vomiting.

The major pediatric antiemetics, and their specific mechanisms of action and dose, are summarized in Table 25.2.

Hematopoietic growth factors in children with cancer

Several hematopoietic growth factors have been approved for clinical use in children including granulocyte colony-stimulating factor (G-CSF, filgrastim) granulocyte–macrophage colony-stimulating factor (GM-CSF, sargramostim), and erythropoietin (EPO, epoetin alfa). The indications for each of these growth factors are based on limited evidence in pediatric patients and are generally derived from adult data. Here we summarize general recommendations for the use of these agents in pediatric oncology.

Granulocyte colony-stimulating factor

G-CSF is a lineage specific cytokine that stimulates the proliferation of neutrophils (granulocytes). As patients may have prolonged periods of myelosuppression after chemotherapy, G-CSF is recommended for adult patients with: (1) the expectation for prolonged myelosuppression to prevent episodes of febrile neutropenia and infection, (2) a history of febrile neutropenia, (3) the history of a delay between chemotherapy cycles, and (4) a diagnosis of febrile neutropenia. Pediatric evidence is minimal compared to adult studies but supports the use of G-CSF for patients with two of these four scenarios: (1) prevention of febrile neutropenia and infection (primary prophylaxis), and (2) treatment of febrile neutropenia. Although infection-related morbidity has not been shown to decrease with G-CSF usage in these scenarios, risk of infection and length of hospitalization have been shown to be significantly reduced in meta-analyses, with potential benefits for quality of life and decreased cost from shorter hospitalization. GM-CSF has shown similar results to G-CSF but has not been shown to be superior in clinical studies. In general, G-CSF is the colony-stimulating factor of choice in pediatric patients. Clinical studies have also established that the appropriate dose of G-CSF and GM-CSF are 5 mcg/kg/day and $250 \, mcg/m^2$/day respectively, given SC or IV. It should be noted that the IV dose may be less effective than the SC dose. A longer lasting pegylated form of G-CSF (pegfilgrastim) has been shown to be equally efficacious in adult studies with

Table 25.1 Emetogenic potential of common pediatric chemotherapeutic agents.

High (>90%)	Moderate–high (60–90%)	Moderate (30–60%)	Moderate–low (10–30%)	Minimal (<10%)
Cytarabine (>1000 mg/m^2)	Cytarabine (250–1000 mg/m^2)	Carboplatin	Cytarabine (<250 mg/m^2)	Bleomycin
Cisplatin (>50 mg/m^2)	Cisplatin (<50 mg/m^2)	Cyclophosphamide	Etoposide	Decadron
Cyclophosphamide	Cyclophosphamide	(<750 mg/m^2)	Mercaptopurine	Prednisone
(>1500 mg/m^2)	(750–1500 mg/m^2)	Daunomycin	Methotrexate	Fludarabine
	Dactinomycin	Doxorubicin (<60 mg/m^2)	(50–250 mg/m^2)	Methotrexate
	Doxorubicin (>60 mg/m^2)	Idarubicin	Topotecan	(<50 mg/m^2)
	Methotrexate (>250 mg/m^2)	Ifosfamide	Vinblastine	Thioguanine
		Irinotecan	Radiation therapy	Vincristine

Table 25.2 Common pediatric antiemetic agents.

Agent	Mechanism of action	Dose	Comments
Ondansetron	5-HT$_3$ receptor antagonist	0.15 mg/kg q8h IV/PO (max 32 mg/day)	Well tolerated; common side effects include headache, fatigue, constipation, diarrhea. Also available as orally disintegrating tablet
Lorazepam	Interaction with GABA receptor; poorly understood antiemetic effects	0.25–0.5 mg q4–6 h IV/PO, max dose 2 mg	Used as adjunctive; can be utilized for anticipatory nausea. At higher doses has more sedation/anxiolytic effect than antiemetic effect
Diphenhydramine	H1 histamine receptor antagonist	0.5–1 mg/kg q6 h IV/PO, max dose 50 mg	Used as adjunctive; can be utilized for anticipatory nausea. Higher dose used for prevention of dystonic reaction with metoclopramide
Metoclopramide	Dopamine antagonist	1 mg/kg q4–6 h IV/PO, max dose 50 mg	Used as adjunctive; higher dose required for antiemetic effect as compared to prokinetic. Must be given with diphenhydramine at higher dose
Decadron	Poorly understood	5 mg/m^2 q6 h IV/PO	Used as adjunctive; cannot be used in malignancies where steroids are part of the treatment regimen
Scopolamine	Anticholinergic	Transdermal patch for adolescents/adults	Must be changed q72 h; patient must be advised to not touch patch and then rub eyes as this will lead to mydriasis
Dronabinol	Cannabinoid; agonist antiemetic effect	5 mg/m^2 q2–4 h, max dose 15 mg/m^2 in adults	No established pediatric dosing. Teens and young adults should be advised to not smoke cannabinoids that can contain impurities or increase the risk of fungal infection
Aprepitant	Neurokinin-1 receptor antagonist	80–125 mg daily PO in adults	Pediatric dosing not established; insufficient studies in pediatric patients to date

less frequent dosing; pediatric randomized controlled studies are lacking.

Primary prophylaxis

G-CSF should be given to patients receiving multiagent chemotherapy who are expected to experience a high incidence of febrile neutropenia or severe, prolonged neutropenia (i.e., ANC $<0.5 \times 10^9$/L for 7 or more days). G-CSF should not be given on the same days patients are given myelosuppressive chemotherapy or radiation therapy. G-CSF is generally not administered to patients with myeloid leukemia due to the theoretical risk of stimulating proliferation of the leukemic clone.

Treatment of febrile neutropenia

Pediatric guidelines are not clear but treatment should be considered in patients with profound neutropenia (ANC $<0.1 \times 10^9$/L), uncontrolled primary disease, pneumonia, hypotension, multiorgan failure, and invasive fungal infection.

Duration

G-CSF should be started between 1 to 5 days after the last dose of myelosuppressive chemotherapy or radiation. G-CSF should be continued until the ANC is greater than 1.5×10^9/L for 1 to 2 days following the expected neutrophil nadir from chemotherapy. Specific protocols may call for different ANC thresholds.

Monitoring

Once G-CSF is initiated, a complete blood count (CBC) and differential should be monitored at least weekly.

Adverse effects

The most common side effects of G-CSF are bone pain and elevation of uric acid, LDH, or alkaline phosphatase. Occasionally G-CSF has been reported to cause fever, nausea and vomiting, diarrhea, splenomegaly, and erythema at the injection site.

Recombinant human erythropoietin

Erythropoietin induces proliferation and differentiation of red blood cell progenitors. The recombinant product erythropoietin alfa (rHuEPO) has been approved in pediatric patients although administration of rHuEPO to oncology patients with chemotherapy-induced anemia remains controversial. A second recombinant, darbopoietin alfa, which has a two- to threefold longer half-life, has been approved in adult patients only.

Meta-analysis of adult data has shown that although rHuEPO decreases transfusion requirements in cancer patients, there is a significant increase in venous thromboembolism and, potentially, mortality. Pediatric data are limited but have not to date shown a significant difference in survival with the use of rHuEPO, although quality of life may be improved. In addition, venous thromboembolism has not been seen in pediatric patients. Concern remains that the decrease in adult survival rates with rHuEPO may be secondary to the ubiquitous expression of the EPO-receptor on tumor cells and therefore tumor upregulation with rHuEPO usage. Conclusive *in vivo* data are lacking.

Pediatric guidelines for rHuEPO therefore include the following: (1) use of rHuEPO is not recommended in pediatric oncology patients, and (2) rHuEPO should be considered on a case-by-case basis in special populations where blood product usage is relatively contraindicated. Specifically, Jehovah's Witnesses forbid blood product transfusion and therefore the potential risks and benefits of rHuEPO should be discussed with the practicing patient and their family. A candid discussion should occur between the provider, patient, family, and potentially patient advocate, to discuss this complex situation. Although rHuEPO may ameliorate some transfusion need, it may not be able to eliminate this need completely. Additionally, the patient and family should be made aware of the theoretical risks regarding survival with rHuEPO usage.

Suggested Reading

Feusner J. Guidelines for Epo use in children with cancer. Pediatr Blood Cancer 53:7–12, 2009.

Hesketh PJ. Chemotherapy-induced nausea and vomiting. N Engl J Med 358:2482–2494, 2008.

26 Central Venous Catheters

Indwelling central venous catheters (CVCs) have revolutionized the care of children with cancer by simplifying the administration of therapy, increasing safety, decreasing pain, and improving quality of life by reducing physical and psychological stress. Peripheral venous access can become increasingly difficult in young children. Additionally, peripheral administration of certain antineoplastic drugs may cause injury due to extravasation. CVCs provide a safe, accessible route for infusion of chemotherapy, total parenteral nutrition, blood products, antibiotics, pain medications, hematopoietic stem cells, and other medications and infusions. These devices also allow for frequent and convenient blood sampling, which can be taught to home care providers. CVCs are now an integral aspect of management of cancer or chronic illness in children.

The optimal type and timing of placement of a CVC are not standardized. Many types of CVCs are available and are divided between temporary (peripherally inserted central catheters) and more permanent, tunneled catheters. Tunneled catheters can either be entirely under the skin or have an external portion that allows access. This chapter focuses on the permanent catheters, placed to provide access for months to years.

These catheters are typically made of plastics with flexible silicone rubber tubing. They are surgically placed (and removed) by experienced practitioners via a percutaneous or cut down technique. The patient should be assessed for bleeding risk by having a platelet count and coagulation studies checked preoperatively. External right atrial catheters are typically inserted into the subclavian, internal jugular, or external jugular vein and are tunneled to an exit site on the anterior or lateral chest. Placement in other locations may be necessary for patients with a history of thrombosis, multiple previous CVCs, or in the patient with compression of the upper venous system due to tumor. The location of the catheter tip should be confirmed by fluoroscopy or chest radiography to be at the junction of the superior or inferior vena cava and the right atrium prior to the catheter being used. Ultrasonography or angiography may assist the surgeon in determining the most accessible vein for CVC placement. External CVCs have a Dacron cuff attached to the catheter wall that is positioned 1–2 cm from the skin exit site. This allows for the growth of fibrous tissue (scar) into the cuff, preventing migration and loss of the line. Surgeons will typically place sutures externally as well that

Handbook of Pediatric Hematology and Oncology: Children's Hospital & Research Center Oakland,
Second Edition. Caroline A. Hastings, Joseph C. Torkildson, and Anurag K. Agrawal.
© 2012 John Wiley & Sons, Ltd. Published 2012 by John Wiley & Sons, Ltd.

may be removed after healing. Totally implanted catheters (ports) are secured to the deep fascia on the anterior chest wall with sutures. Ports are made of nonimmunogenic materials and some now allow for high-pressure infusion of contrast for radiographic imaging. The silicone membrane of the reservoir is accessed by a special non-coring needle (Huber) and is self-sealing with needle removal. Topical anesthesia is typically applied over the reservoir prior to internal catheter access.

The most frequently used tunneled external catheters are Broviac, Hickman, and Leonard. Totally implantable catheters include Medi-Port, Port-a-Cath, BardPort, and PowerPort. Single lumen external catheters and ports are used most commonly in children, but double and triple lumen catheters and ports are available. Patients that require pheresis for stem cell collection early in their course of therapy may benefit from the placement of a pheresible catheter, such as a Medcomp. These lines require meticulous maintenance and are not repairable, unlike the standard external tunneled catheters. Due to the larger lumen size required for a pheresible catheter and associated risk of thrombosis, these lines are not always feasible for long-term access in smaller children. The Bard PowerLine is becoming a popular double lumen pheresible catheter due to the higher flow rates that are possible through them. In addition, they can frequently be placed in children who are too small to safely receive a conventional double lumen catheter (see Table 26.1).

The decision about the type of CVC to be placed is based on multiple factors including length and intensity of therapy; frequency of lab draws; the need for multiple lumens to

Table 26.1 Common tunneled central venous catheters and related care.

Catheter type	Saline flush	Heparin	Site care
Hickman Broviac	≤10 kg: 5 mL/lumen >10 kg: 10 mL/lumen after access	10 units/mL 2 mL q24 hours PRN after catheter access or blood draw	Dressing change weekly or per institution policy (or when wet, dirty) Type of dressing per institution (tegaderm, Mepore, etc.)
Pheresible catheter	10 mL each lumen q24 hours	100 units/mL >30 kg: 2 mL/lumen 15–30 kg: 1.5 mL/lumen <15 kg: 1 mL/lumen q24 hours and after access	Dressing change weekly or per institution policy (or when wet, dirty) Do not use iodine or iodine-based disinfectants
Mediport	10 mL q24 hours and PRN when accessed Flush 20 mL after blood draw	10 units/mL 2 mL q24 hours and PRN while accessed 100 units/mL 2 mL with deaccess and monthly*	Huber needle changed weekly if continuously accessed; dress securely when accessed; apply topical anesthetic prior to port access

*<10 kg, give 2 mL of 10 units/mL.

Table 26.2 Type of central venous catheter to be placed by diagnosis.

CVC type	Number of lumens	Diagnosis
External	Single	ALL, high risk
		Solid tumors, not metastatic
		Neuroblastoma, low and intermediate risk
		Non-Hodgkin lymphoma
External	Double	AML
		Neuroblastoma, advanced stage
		Brain tumors requiring Head Start/HSCT
		Solid tumors, advanced stage
Internal	Single	ALL, standard and high risk
		Wilms tumor
		Hodgkin and non-Hodgkin lymphoma
		Malignant glioma

Abbreviations: ALL, acute lymphoblastic leukemia; AML, acute myelogenous leukemia; CVC, central venous catheter; HSCT, hematopoietic stem cell transplantation.

support simultaneous administration of chemotherapy, hydration, pain medication, parenteral nutrition, antibiotics, and other agents; age; and lifestyle. In general, external and multilumen devices are associated with greater risk, primarily due to an increased incidence of infection and thrombosis. Ports are becoming increasingly more popular, especially with lower intensity therapies and in older children and adolescents. Ports are cosmetically more satisfactory, do not require routine care, and allow for easy bathing and swimming. However, ports may be difficult to place and access in obese or very thin patients. Additionally, the use of ports for routine blood draws is limited due to their need to be accessed prior to use. An external CVC should be used in patients requiring frequent laboratory monitoring. External CVCs and ports may be used immediately after placement. In the case of a port, the surgeon should be asked to access the device when it is placed, prior to development of postoperative edema. This allows immediate use, decreasing patient discomfort and reducing the

potential for introduction of infection. Ultimately, in cases where an external catheter is not essential, the decision on the type of catheter to utilize must include a discussion with the patient and the family reviewing the pros and cons of each type of device. Table 26.2 summarizes the type of CVC to consider based on diagnosis and subsequent therapy intensity.

Maintenance

External catheters require daily heparin flushes and periodic dressing changes (see Table 26.1). Families require detailed education on the care and potential complications of CVCs. They should be taught sterile technique to access the CVC for blood draws or flushes and to provide external care. Frequency of dressing changes may be dependent on institution policy, type of CVC, and local factors such as a wet, dirty, or loose dressing. At all times, the CVC exit site should be kept dry and clean. Patients are instructed to protect it during bathing and not immerse the dressing or exit site in a bath, hot tub, or pool. Should this occur, the dressing should be changed immediately with careful cleansing of the exit site. Ports require less care, and heparin flushes, which are required only monthly, are typically performed by the health care team. No dressing is needed for implantable devices when they are not accessed. Each institution has a standardized approach to the care and maintenance of CVCs that is followed by staff, family members, and home health care agencies.

Complications: mechanical

The use of CVCs can result in a number of short- and long-term complications. Immediate complications related to CVC placement include malposition, hemorrhage, pneumothorax, chylothorax, arterial cannulation, cardiac dysrhythmia, and failure to place the line. Rarely, complications may occur due to the anesthetic required for surgical placement. Long-term complications include mechanical failure, catheter breakage, leakage, and port extrusion. Mechanical failures have been reported in up to 10% of patients and may result in removal of the CVC. Some types of external CVCs may be repaired if the break is distal to the catheter exit site. Children with implanted ports are at risk for the Huber needle becoming dislodged during infusion, leading to extravasation with resultant skin irritation or breakdown. These require careful periodic assessment.

Complications: infectious

Infection is the most common complication of CVCs. Most catheter-related infections arise by one of two mechanisms: (1) infection at the exit site with migration of the pathogen along the external catheter surface, and (2) contamination of the hub, leading to intraluminal colonization and consequent seeding of the pathogen into the circulation (see Chapter 27 for common pathogens and management of fever in patients with CVCs). Patients with CVCs require constant attention for prevention and early recognition of infection. Despite the meticulous techniques used by health care providers and caregivers to maintain sterility, many children with CVCs will develop a line infection or bacteremia. Infection is often related to organisms that are ubiquitous but can lead to true infection in the immunosuppressed patient (such as gut and skin flora), or be due to organisms introduced with venous access or with blood product or medication/fluid administration. Coagulase-negative staphylococci, *Staphylococcus aureus*, aerobic Gram-negative bacilli, and *Candida albicans* most commonly cause catheter-related bloodstream infection. Additionally, development of a thrombus in the catheter may serve as a nidus for infection. Occasionally, despite best efforts and appropriate antibiotic therapy, the line may be colonized and need to be removed. Recent techniques for catheter sterilization include antibiotic and ethanol locks. Additionally, many manufacturers have created antibacterial substances bonded to the catheters.

Risk factors for CVC infection include the placement of an external catheter, young patient age, multilumen catheter, early placement (i.e., within 2 weeks of diagnosis of acute lymphoblastic leukemia [ALL]), stem cell transplant, solid tumor, lack of perioperative prophylactic antibiotics, high-intensity protocol, and placement during periods of neutropenia. These factors must be weighed against the benefits of early line placement, type of line placed, and number of catheter lumens. The relatively higher infection rate seen with external catheters favors the use of implanted catheters when possible.

Approximately 50% of catheter-related infections occur locally at the exit site, along the tunneled catheter or as a "pocket" infection around the implanted reservoir. Skin irritation may occur with external CVCs and requires alteration of the prescribed exit site care and dressing to avoid repeated irritation, skin breakdown, infection, and pain. Patients with local catheter infections typically have local signs and symptoms with tenderness on palpation, erythema, purulent drainage, lack of healing, swelling, and pain. Severely neutropenic patients may only have pain and tenderness as these symptoms do not require the presence of neutrophils. If drainage is present, the site should be cultured. Tunnel infections are characterized by a spreading cellulitis along the subcutaneous tract of long-term catheters. The catheter should be removed if the administration of appropriate parenteral antibiotics does not result in resolution of the signs and symptoms within 24 to 48 hours. When evaluating a child with fever and a CVC, palpate along the tunnel to assess for tenderness or to express drainage. Pocket abscesses may need to be surgically drained and packed and almost always will require removal of the reservoir and catheter. Site infections with minor exit site erythema and tenderness are treated with topical antibiotics and monitored with careful, daily assessment; systemic antibiotics should be added for clinical worsening, lack of improvement, or a positive blood culture from the line. Tunnel and pocket infections should be treated with both topical and systemic antibiotics, as well as a daily sterile dressing change. The patient should be treated systemically with broad-spectrum antibiotics providing good Gram-positive coverage and be monitored for the development of an abscess requiring surgical drainage. The antibiotic regimen may be altered with culture results, but if the patient is neutropenic it should include both broad-spectrum and directed antibiotic therapy. Site infections provide an opportunity to review meticulous local CVC management with the caregivers.

In addition to site infections, colonization of the catheter may occur. In this case, the patient will have repeatedly positive cultures with the same organism, often without systemic symptoms of infection. In cases of colonization, cultures may become quickly positive and may persist through appropriate antibiotic therapy. At times, catheters may be reseeded from distant sites of occult infection (e.g., cardiac vegetations, osteomyelitis, deep abscesses).

The CVC should always be considered the source of infection in a patient who presents with fever until proven otherwise. Fever, chills, or hypotension temporally related to line flushing increase the likelihood of a line infection. Broad-spectrum empiric antibiotics should be administered after drawing cultures from each lumen of the CVC. Persistent bacteremia despite appropriate antibiotic coverage (>72 hours), signs of sepsis (hypotension, chills, persistent fever, cool extremities, delayed capillary refill), or infection with fungus or water-borne bacteria (e.g., pseudomonas, stenotrophomonas) warrant CVC removal. If placement of a new CVC is deemed necessary, the patient should first complete an appropriate course of antibiotic therapy allowing for sufficient healing time and decreasing the risk of subsequent reinfection of the new CVC.

CVC infection may be overdiagnosed, resulting in either prolonged antibiotic administration or unnecessary removal of the catheter. Differential time to positivity is a reliable diagnostic technique to differentiate a true line infection from bacteremia. Paired blood samples (aerobic and anaerobic) from a peripheral vein and the central catheter are obtained and compared with respect to time to positivity. If the culture from the catheter turns positive 2 or more hours before the peripheral culture, this is diagnostic of a catheter-related infection. A positive differential time to positivity may not change management, although consideration should be given to the type and duration of systemic antibiotic therapy, utility of an antimicrobial or ethanol lock, and the need for catheter removal. Additional factors include the type of catheter, prior history of infection, current neutrophil count, likelihood of short term recovery, and current chemotherapeutic regimen. When a specific pathogen has been identified, antibiotic therapy should be targeted, with additional broad empiric coverage in the neutropenic patient (see Chapter 27). The possibility of an infected catheter-related thrombus should be considered, and treatment may also involve thrombolytic agents or anticoagulation.

Assessment and management of catheter-related thrombosis

Venous thromboembolism is another common complication of long-term CVCs. The extent of thrombosis may include the catheter tip (ball-valve clot), the length of the catheter (fibrin sheath), or the catheterized vessel (e.g., the upper limb with or without the central vasculature of the neck or mediastinum). Catheter-related venous thromboembolism can result in significant morbidity, and subclinical thrombosis may occur in up to 50% of patients with CVCs. The risk of thrombosis is influenced by catheter location, insertion technique, catheter kinking or compression by a mass or other structure, ratio of the catheter size to the intraluminal vessel diameter, blood flow rheology, genetic predisposition, and administration of prothrombotic medications or infusions (e.g., asparaginase and total parenteral nutrition). Primary thromboprophylaxis

is not currently recommended as standard practice; however, it may be warranted in certain situations with documented increased risk.

Thrombosis should be suspected in patients whose catheter does not flush or draw easily or in the event of suggestive clinical findings (pain or swelling in extremity, prominent vasculature or swelling on side of neck/chest with CVC, inability to successfully access an implanted port). It should be noted that a line that does not draw or flush might be occluded by the vessel wall or a valve. Patients suspected of having a thrombosis should undergo imaging to confirm this and determine the extent (see Figure 26.1). Based on the timing of line dysfunction or symptom development, the age of the clot can be approximated. Additionally, pertinent family history of thrombosis should be sought out to help guide the necessity of genetic evaluation for thrombophilia (see Chapter 10). Finally, environmental and medication prothrombotic factors should be considered (e.g., immobilization, steroids, and other medications).

Treatment of thrombosis may require thrombolytic therapy, anticoagulation, or catheter removal. Below are guidelines for the assessment and treatment of a suspected CVC-associated thrombus:

• Examine the catheter for any kinks in the tubing.
• Reposition the patient; flush the CVC with normal saline (if possible) and again attempt to withdraw blood. Have the patient hold their hands above their head, turn, cough, or hold their breath.
• Attempt a tissue plasminogen activator (TPA) dwell if the catheter can be flushed:
  ○ Infants <3 months receive 0.25 mg (0.5 mL) per lumen; older children receive 0.5 mg (1 mL) per lumen. Dwell should be administered for 30 minutes.
  ○ After the first dwell, attach an empty 3 mL syringe and attempt to withdraw blood. If

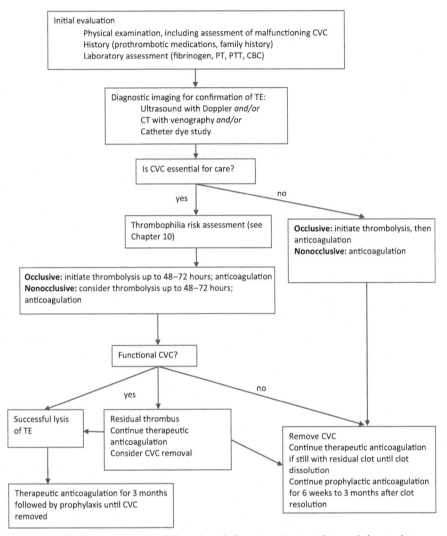

Figure 26.1 Evaluation of suspected thromboembolism in patients with tunneled central venous catheters. Abbreviations: CVC, central venous catheter; PT, prothrombin time; PTT, partial thromboplastin time; CBC, complete blood count; TE, thromboembolism; CT, computed tomography.

successful, obtain blood work and flush line per protocol. If unsuccessful, instill a second TPA dwell for an additional 30 minutes.
- If the TPA dwell is unsuccessful, further workup is required to determine the extent of thrombus.
  - Obtain a chest radiograph to confirm appropriate line position.
  - Obtain further imaging studies such as a dye study of the line, ultrasound with Doppler flow, or CT with venography to evaluate for thrombosis location and extent. Assess for sleeve thrombus, mechanical failure of the CVC, or migration of the catheter outside the vessel.

- If a thrombus is identified and the time from symptom onset is <14 days, thrombolytic therapy with low-dose systemic TPA should be attempted if the catheter can be flushed
  - Infants < 3 months receive 0.06 mg/kg/h for 6 to 24 hours; older children receive 0.03 mg/kg/h. If no clinical improvement in 24 hours, double the dose to 0.06–0.12 mg/kg/h (max dose 2 mg/h).
  - Systemic TPA can be given for up to 96 hours.
  - Monitor the fibrinogen level and maintain above 100 mg/dL with cryoprecipitate.
- Monitor the patient for signs of sepsis as bacteria can be released into the bloodstream with dissolution of the thrombus.
- If the catheter becomes functional after administration of systemic TPA, obtain a follow-up radiographic study to assess for clot resolution.
- Remove the catheter if the thrombus cannot be cleared after 24 to 48 hours.

If the thrombus dissolves, or is stabilized with normal CVC function, determination should be made as to the current necessity of the line and risk for recurrent thrombosis. If the CVC can be safely removed, some practitioners recommend short-term prophylactic anticoagulation to mitigate the risk for rethrombosis (usually 6 weeks to 3 months of low-molecular-weight heparin [LMWH]). If the line needs to be maintained and the clot has resolved, the patient should continue on therapeutic LMWH for 3 months and then switch over to prophylactic LMWH until the line is removed. For the patient with a stable clot and a functional CVC, therapeutic anticoagulation with LMWH should be continued until approximately 3 months after clot dissolution and then switched to prophylactic anticoagulation until line removal (see Chapter 10 and Formulary for dosing guidelines). Additionally, if the patient is determined to have a genetic predisposition to thrombosis based on family history or a personal history of previous thromboembolism, a thrombophilia trait workup should be sent (see Chapter 10 for details). If the patient has multitrait thrombophilia and therefore a higher risk of rethrombosis, every effort should be made to remove the CVC once the risk of having an indwelling line outweighs the benefit (i.e., maintenance therapy in the ALL patient).

If the patient on prophylactic anticoagulation develops rethrombosis, management should be the same as with the initial clot with systemic low-dose TPA followed by therapeutic anticoagulation with LMWH until clot dissolution. If the patient is on therapeutic anticoagulation with clot extension, the CVC will need to be removed. In cases where the clot cannot be dissolved or stabilized and the line needs to be removed, 3 to 5 days of anticoagulation is recommended for clot stabilization prior to catheter removal. Special circumstances will warrant disruption in anticoagulation, such as lumbar punctures to administer intrathecal chemotherapy or other surgical procedures. In general, LMWH should be held for 24 hours in advance of these procedures and resumed 12 to 24 hours after procedure completion, depending on the nature of the procedure and risk of postoperative bleeding. Additionally, LMWH should be held during periods of moderate thrombocytopenia (i.e., $<50 \times 10^9$/L) to minimize additional risk of bleeding. If the CVC is removed and it is necessary to place a new catheter, consideration should be given to anticoagulation prophylaxis to prevent recurrence of thrombosis.

Suggested Reading

Gallieni M, Pittiruti M, Biffi R. Vascular access in oncology patients. CA Cancer J Clin 58:323–346, 2008.

Hirsh J, Guyatt G, Albers GW, et al. Antithrombotic and thrombolytic therapy: American College of Chest Physicians evidence-based clinical practice guidelines (8th edition). Chest 133:71S–109S, 2008.

McLean TW, Fisher CJ, Snively BM, Chauvenet AR. Central venous catheters in children with lesser risk acute lymphoblastic leukemia: optimal type and timing of placement. J Clin Oncol 23:3024–3029, 2005.

Shivakumar SP, Anderson DR, Couban S. Catheter-related thrombosis in patients with malignancy. J Clin Oncol 27:4858–4864, 2009.

27 Management of Fever in the Child with Cancer

Children with cancer are at an increased risk for serious bacterial, viral, and fungal infections. Many factors contribute to this susceptibility in immunocompromised children. The two most important determinants of susceptibility to bacterial and fungal infection are the number of circulating neutrophils (absolute neutrophil count; ANC) and the duration of severe neutropenia. Other factors include:

- Underlying disease: leukemia, especially acute myelogenous leukemia (AML), advanced stage lymphoma, or other metastatic solid tumors are at higher risk due to increased therapy intensity.
- Remission status: patients not in remission are at higher risk.
- Type of therapy with dose- or time-intensive therapies: administration of high-dose cytarabine and stem cell transplant confer the highest risk.
- Nutritional status: malnutrition adversely affects immune function.
- Disruption of protective barriers such as skin, mucocutaneous tissues, gastrointestinal tract, and exit sites of catheters.
- Defects in humoral immunity related to therapy, impaired splenic function, or B-cell malignancies.

- Defects in cellular immunity such as seen in patients with T-cell malignancies or those receiving steroids or radiation; persistence of lymphopenia due to chemotherapy.
- Colonization from endogenous microflora.
- Presence of indwelling catheters or shunts.

The **ANC** is calculated by multiplying the percentage of neutrophils (segmented neutrophils + bands) by the total white blood cell (WBC) count.

Example: WBC $= 1.0 \times 10^9$/L, segmented neutrophils $= 10\%$, bands $= 10\%$
ANC $= 20\% \times 1.0 \times 10^9$/L $= 0.2 \times 10^9$/L

ANC $< 1.5 \times 10^9$/L is defined as neutropenia
ANC $< 1.0 \times 10^9$/L is defined as moderate neutropenia
ANC $< 0.5 \times 10^9$/L represents severe neutropenia
ANC < 0.1 to 0.2×10^9/L represents profound neutropenia

In general, patients with an ANC of less than 0.5×10^9/L or those with dropping counts after chemotherapy are considered severely neutropenic. The ANC at time of presentation with respect to the most recent chemotherapy gives important information. For

Handbook of Pediatric Hematology and Oncology: Children's Hospital & Research Center Oakland, Second Edition. Caroline A. Hastings, Joseph C. Torkildson, and Anurag K. Agrawal.
© 2012 John Wiley & Sons, Ltd. Published 2012 by John Wiley & Sons, Ltd.

instance, if a child is neutropenic without recent myelosuppressive therapy, infection (and less likely relapse of a hematologic malignancy) should be considered as the most likely etiology due to marrow suppression. In general, the expected nadir in ANC occurs 7 to 14 days from the start of myelosuppressive chemotherapy. This timing should be considered when assessing the patient and determining the management plan. Practitioners may also utilize the absolute phagocyte count (APC), which is the summation of the ANC and absolute monocyte count, in determining the risk of bacterial infection as monocytes also possess bacteria-fighting ability. An increasing monocyte count is often seen prior to and often heralds neutrophil recovery.

Fever is defined as a single temperature of 38.3°C (101.0°F) or greater, two temperatures of 38.0 to 38.2°C (100.4 to 100.9°F) within a 24-hour period, or a temperature of 38.0 to 38.2°C (100.4 to 100.9°F) persistently for 1 hour, taken in the axilla, orally, or by tympanic probe. Generally, oral and tympanic temperatures are preferred since the axillary temperature can be affected by outside temperature. Oral temperatures preferably are taken without any recent hot or cold oral intake. **Once a fever is documented, it should be considered as real no matter what the underlying circumstances are**, even if the patient defervesces without any intervention. Patients who develop a low-grade fever (38.0°C to 38.2°C) should be monitored without antipyretics to determine if a fever spike will occur. Rectal temperatures should never be taken in potentially neutropenic children.

Fever and neutropenia

Every oncology patient who presents with febrile neutropenia (FN) is considered septic until proven otherwise. These children may have fever as their only symptom of infection. It should be noted that neutropenia will not prevent the patient from having a temperature spike with infection; one exception is the patient on steroids (such as in acute lymphoblastic leukemia [ALL] induction) who may not mount a fever with an underlying infection. A careful clinical examination is critical as the patient's status may change quickly and dramatically.

Septic shock results from overwhelming infection with microorganisms in the blood leading to central vascular dilation with resultant circulatory failure and inadequate tissue perfusion. Symptoms of septic shock include hypotension, tachycardia, tachypnea, clammy extremities (although can be warm with initial sepsis), decreased urine output, and deterioration of mental status. Although septic shock can be seen with any organism, the usual culprits with acute and overwhelming sepsis are Gram-negative rods.

The most common organisms causing bacteremia and sepsis are:
- Gram-positive: Staphylococci (coagulase-negative, *Staphylococcus aureus* including methicillin-resistant [MRSA]), streptococci (α-hemolytic) including *Streptococcus viridans* and *S. mitis*
- Gram-negative: Enterobacteriaceae (*E. coli, Enterobacter, Klebsiella, Serratia*), *Pseudomonas aeruginosa, Stenotrophomonas maltophilia, Acinetobacter* sp.
- Anaerobic: *Clostridium difficile, Bacteroides* sp., *Proprionobacterium acnes*
Other pathogens infecting cancer patients include:
- Fungi: *Candida* sp., *Aspergillus* sp., zygomycetes, cryptococci
- Viruses: Herpes simplex virus (HSV), varicella zoster virus (VZV), cytomegalovirus (CMV), Epstein–Barr virus, respiratory syncytial virus, adenovirus, influenza, parainfluenza, human herpesvirus 6

• Other: *Pneumocystis jiroveci, Toxoplasma gondii, Strongyloides stercoralis,* cryptosporidium, *Bacillus* sp., atypical mycobacterium

Initial evaluation of febrile neutropenia

See Figure 27.1.

1. History and physical examination

a. Determination of vitals and evaluation for shock.

b. Meticulous physical examination with particular attention to sites of occult infection such as the skin, exit sites of catheters, sites of recent bone marrow aspiration, oral cavity, and perianal areas. Even subtle evidence of inflammation (faint erythema, tenderness, or minimal

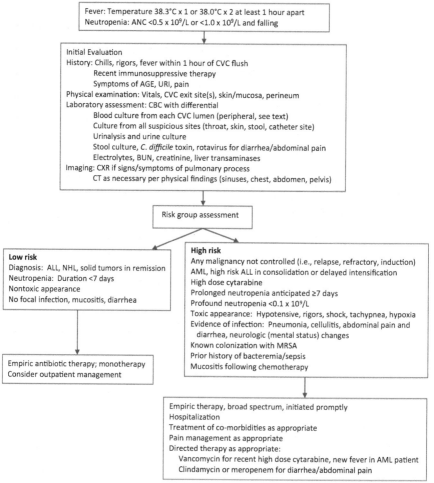

Figure 27.1 Evaluation and initial management of febrile neutropenia in the child with cancer. (Abbreviations: CVC, central venous catheter; AGE, acute gastroenteritis; URI, upper respiratory infection; CBC, complete blood count; BUN, blood urea nitrogen; CXR, chest radiography; CT, computed tomography; ALL, acute lymphoblastic leukemia; NHL, non-Hodgkin lymphoma; AML, acute myelogenous leukemia; MRSA, methicillin-resistant *Staphylococcus aureus*).

discharge) may represent a source of infection as neutropenia diminishes classic inflammatory changes. **Pain**, however, is always a concerning finding and should be considered a potential clue to site and source of infection.

2. **Laboratory evaluation**

   a. Complete blood count (CBC) with manual differential to determine ANC.

   b. Blood cultures from each lumen of the central venous catheter (CVC); peripheral culture is necessary if the child does not have a central line or it is unobtainable from the central line. Controversy still exists as to utility of a peripheral blood culture when cultures are taken from the line as delayed time to positivity between these two sources can help determine the existence of a line infection versus bacteremia (see Chapter 26). Do not flush the catheter after labs are obtained in the patient with a recent history of high fever, hypotension, chills, or rigors within 1 hour of flushing the catheter, suggestive of a line infection. See below under *Initial management*.

   c. Serum chemistries to include electrolytes, liver, and renal function studies.

   d. Urinalysis and urine culture (no catheter sample for neutropenic patients).

   e. Chest radiograph only if the patient has ausculatory signs or symptoms of infection or respiratory compromise.

   f. If the child has tenderness over the sinuses, perform diagnostic imaging to evaluate for sinusitis (plain radiographs and/or CT).

   g. Patients with symptoms of esophagitis should be evaluated for viral or fungal causes with serologies and culture, if possible.

   h. Cultures and bacterial Gram stain or fungal stains from suspicious sites such as the oropharynx, skin breakdown sites, and catheter sites.

   i. If diarrhea is present, send a stool sample for stool culture, rotavirus, and *C. difficile* antigen.

   j. In contrast to nononcology patients, a lumbar puncture (LP) is not routinely done as part of a serious bacterial infection evaluation in patients with FN and an oncologic diagnosis. If an LP appears clinically indicated, evaluation for increased intracranial pressure with appropriate imaging (i.e., head CT) should be done and the pediatric oncology attending notified *prior* to the procedure. An adequate platelet count and at least near-normal coagulation studies are also required in advance of the LP.

   k. If another implanted device is present (e.g., ventriculoperitoneal shunt or Ommaya reservoir), do not attempt to obtain a culture without speaking to the appropriate attending physicians. Intervention by a neurosurgeon may be required. It is uncommon for these devices to be the source of infection if it has been more than 2 to 4 weeks since they were inserted.

Initial management

Risk stratification models for pediatric oncology patients with FN to determine which patients are low risk and could potentially be managed as outpatients and which are higher risk and should be monitored as inpatients have yet to be validated and widely accepted. Adult studies suggest that patients with predicted time of severe neutropenia of ≤7 days and no concerning clinical signs including focal infection such as pneumonia, new abdominal pain, or hypotension can be safely managed as outpatients. With the lack of data in pediatric patients, we continue to recommend that parenteral broad-spectrum antibiotics be started immediately and the patient admitted to the hospital. FN is considered an oncologic emergency and all measures should be taken to ensure prompt evaluation and treatment, with a *goal of ≤60 minutes between presentation and the initiation of antibiotics*. Antibiotics should be chosen based on microbial prevalence and antibiotic sensitivity patterns at each institution. In general, due to the more acute risk from Gram-negative organisms, broad coverage for these organisms (including *Pseudomonas*) should be initiated. Many combinations of antibiotics are effective and acceptable regimens include:

1. Monotherapy:

    Fourth generation cephalosporin (antipseudomonal β-lactam)

    Cefepime 150 mg/kg/day intravenous (IV) divided q8h

    Carbapenem

    Imipenem 50 mg/kg/day IV divided q6–8h

    Meropenem 60 to 120 mg/kg/day IV divided q8h

    Piperacillin/Tazobactam

    Zosyn 240 to 300 mg/kg/day IV divided q8h

2. Dual therapy (antipseudomonal β-lactam plus an aminoglycoside):

    Ceftazidime 100 to 150 mg/kg/day IV divided q8h *and*

    Tobramycin 7.5 mg/kg/day IV divided q8h or 7–9 mg/kg/dose IV daily

Other antibiotics used in specific circumstances (see below) are:

1. Anaerobic drugs:

    Clindamycin 40 mg/kg/day IV divided q6–8h

    Metronidazole 30 mg/kg/day (loading dose 15 mg/kg) IV divided q6h

2. Vancomycin 60 mg/kg/day IV divided q8h

Patients with AML receiving high-dose cytarabine (Ara-C) should have vancomycin as part of their empiric regimen in combination with broad-spectrum coverage due to the high risk of *S. viridans* infection with its accompanying septic shock and acute respiratory distress syndrome. Cytarabine is known to alter mucosal integrity and allow entry of this organism. Patients with *S. viridans* sepsis have a high rate of morbidity and mortality. They typically require prolonged hospitalization following chemotherapy until neutrophil recovery occurs to allow emergent initiation of treatment in the event of fever or other signs of impending shock or sepsis. Other indications for vancomycin in the empiric regimen include:

- Presentation with hypotension or other evidence of shock
- Mucositis due to chemotherapy
- Patients with prior history of α-hemolytic streptococcus bacteremia
- Catheter site infection or other skin breakdown
- Patients colonized with resistant organisms treatable only with vancomycin
- Vegetations on echocardiogram

Anaerobic therapy should be considered in patients who have significant mucosal breakdown, perianal skin breakdown, peritoneal signs, or in cases of typhlitis with presumed or proven *C. difficile* infection. For patients on dual therapy with an aminoglycoside, trough levels should be monitored weekly due to the risks of nephro- and ototoxicity, especially in those receiving other nephro- or ototoxic drugs (e.g., vancomycin, furosemide). For patients on therapy with vancomycin, trough levels should be monitored for toxicity as well as medication effectiveness, with goal trough levels of 10 to 15 mcg/mL. Dose increases are often required in pediatric patients to reach these levels. Monitor daily electrolytes, fluid balance, renal function studies, and ensure adequate hydration. Patients with renal dysfunction should receive renal dosing with more frequent trough levels to prevent toxicity.

Any patient that presents with hypotension, chills, rigors, or fever immediately following, or within 1 hour, of central venous catheter flushing should be seen emergently due to the risk of bacteremia and septic shock. In our practice, we elect not to use the central venous line for IV fluids or medication administration initially in this situation due to the risk of infusing a large amount of bacteria into the bloodstream and worsening the signs of clinical sepsis. Patients should have central catheter cultures, placement of a peripheral IV with peripheral cultures, administration of broad-spectrum antibiotics, and a fluid bolus (e.g., NS/LR 20 mL/kg), if necessary. The central catheter should not be flushed or utilized until the patient improves clinically with defervescence, resolution of hypotension, and negative follow-up blood cultures. If the line cannot be flushed, a TPA dwell can be attempted; if unsuccessful, the line will need to be removed (see Chapter 26). It is advisable to give an IV fluid bolus prior to reusing the catheter in the event the patient again develops symptoms of bacteremia with hypotension following the flush. In the event the initial blood culture from the catheter is positive, the clinician will need to decide whether to remove the catheter or attempt to reuse it depending on the patient's clinical condition and the type of organism that is growing. Patients that have persistent fever and Gram-negative organisms may do best with removal of the line; patients that have defervesced and are looking clinically well can generally have their line reused and ultimately salvaged.

Modification of initial antibiotic treatment

Patients should be assessed daily for changes in vital signs, persistence of fever or change in the fever curve, presence of new symptoms or signs of infection with a meticulous physical examination, and results of prior cultures and diagnostic imaging performed (see Figure 27.2). The status of catheters should be assessed (site, function, and concern for thrombosis). Daily blood cultures and a CBC with differential should be done on persistently febrile patients. Determination of the ANC is also important for patients who have defervesced and have negative cultures to determine the length of appropriate therapy. When the neutropenic child becomes afebrile (no fever for 24 hours) and cultures are negative (obtained daily while febrile), broad-spectrum coverage should be continued until there is evidence of adequate marrow recovery and an appropriate period of therapy for any initially positive cultures has been provided. Resolution of neutropenia is defined as an ANC of $>0.5 \times 10^9$/L and evidence of bone marrow recovery is an ANC of $>0.2 \times 10^9$/L and rising on 2 consecutive days. Some practitioners also use an APC of $>0.5 \times 10^9$/L as sufficient evidence of recovery from neutropenia. When the patient no longer has fever, has negative blood cultures, and has signs of neutrophil recovery, the antibiotics may be safely discontinued and the child discharged, assuming an appropriate treatment length for any positive cultures has been provided. Should the child have any local evidence of infection such as diarrhea or skin breakdown, appropriate therapy should continue, but in the outpatient setting.

Modification should be made to the initial broad-spectrum antibiotic regimen if a source of infection is found to explain the initial fever, or the fever persists for more than 3 to 7 days. If the source of the infection is a catheter site with accompanying signs or symptoms of inflammation (discharge, palpable tenderness, local abscess), vancomycin should be added for Gram-positive coverage. If the source is perianal, gingival, or intra-abdominal,

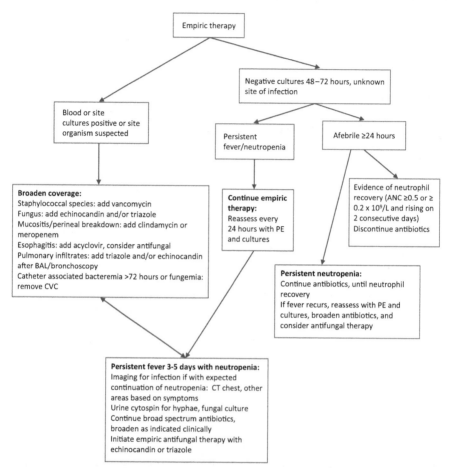

Figure 27.2 Ongoing management of fever and neutropenia. (Abbreviations: ANC, absolute neutrophil count; PE, physical examination; BAL, bronchoalveolar lavage; CVC, central venous catheter; CT, computed tomography).

anaerobic coverage should be added to the regimen (clindamycin, metronidazole, or meropenem).

Vancomycin is the most effective antibiotic against skin flora such as coagulase negative staphylococci (i.e., *S. epidermidis*) as well as mouth flora, most commonly streptococcal species (*S. viridans, Peptostreptococcus*). Vancomycin is also effective against bacillus nonanthracis species that can be true pathogens in the immunocompromised patient. Finally, though rarely seen, MRSA should be a consideration in the very sick patient. Vancomycin should be used judiciously due to emerging resistance patterns such as vancomycin-resistant enterococcus (VRE). Vancomycin should *not* be part of the empiric antibiotic regimen unless the institutional experience and susceptibility patterns require it or there are special circumstances (see above).

Protracted fever may signify the presence of a second or previously untreated infection. Patients should be reassessed daily for new signs or symptoms of infection and appropriate interventions and studies performed. Antibiotic-induced colitis may occur after any antibiotic. *C. difficile* overgrowth may be asymptomatic, lead to mild diarrhea, or may have moderate-to-severe diarrhea and abdominal pain. The patient may also develop pseudomembranous colitis with peritoneal signs, mucosal erosions, and bloody diarrhea. Since *C. difficile* is a normal bowel inhabitant, the toxin must be documented to diagnose this condition. If oral therapy is possible, vancomycin (40 mg/kg divided q8h) or metronidazole (30 mg/kg divided q6h) may be given; in the patient unable to tolerate oral medications, IV metronidazole (same as PO dose) should be given. Abdominal pain may also be due to infection with aerobic Gram-negative bacteria, enterococcus (which no cephalosporin covers *in vivo*), or anaerobes.

If the patient is determined to have a **catheter-associated bacteremia** with a specific organism, broad-spectrum antibiotics should be continued with addition of antibiotics as needed to ensure adequate coverage of the identified organism until sensitivity patterns are reported. If daily cultures are persistently positive with the same organism for 72 hours after initiation of appropriate antibiotics, it will be necessary to remove the catheter. In addition, several organisms including *S. aureus*, *Pseudomonas*, *B. cereus*, *Corynebacterium*, *Mycobacterium* sp., *Stenotrophomonas*, and fungi usually require line removal. General care measures are as follows:

- Hand washing with clean or sterile gloves prior to manipulation of CVC.
- Monitor CVC site on a daily basis; change CVC dressing weekly.
- Assess site for skin infection (including tunnel infection) with any fever.

- In multilumen devices, the antibiotic infusion should be rotated among the lumens as infection may not be limited to one lumen. If one particular lumen has the positive blood culture, it is reasonable to run the majority of the antibiotic through this lumen.
- Daily blood cultures while febrile or if growth is present (from each lumen of CVC), until afebrile and negative cultures for 3 days.
- Assess cardiac valves for vegetations with an echocardiogram for repeatedly positive cultures with Gram-positive organisms.
- If bacteremia persists for more than 3 days of appropriate therapy, the catheter should be removed.

For patients with a history of multiple positive cultures or a difficult to eradicate organism, consideration should be made for the use of ethanol or vancomycin lock therapy to possibly prevent the need for line removal. Ethanol locks should not be used with polyurethane catheters (PowerLine, MedComp) as ethanol will damage the catheter material.

Duration of therapy

When a pathogen has been identified, its antibiotic susceptibility pattern must be determined and appropriate antibiotic coverage provided along with broad-spectrum coverage until the patient is afebrile and has evidence of bone marrow recovery. Once the child is afebrile and the ANC recovers, antibiotics can be tailored to the specific organism for a 10- to 14-day course, with day 1 being the day of the first negative culture.

Patients that defervesce but do not have recovery of the ANC should continue on broad-spectrum antibiotics to prevent secondary infection. Some practitioners may discontinue antibiotics after 14 days if the patient continues to be neutropenic but afebrile, although our general practice is to continue until count recovery.

Empiric antifungal therapy

When FN persists for 4 to 7 days, empiric treatment should be broadened to include fungal prophylaxis. The risk of fungal infection is directly related to the duration of neutropenia, which is secondary to the severity of chemotherapy or radiation cytotoxicity. Thus, patients undergoing more intensive therapy such as for AML, relapsed ALL, and hematopoietic stem cell transplantation are at highest risk of an invasive fungal infection. The major causative fungi are *Aspergillus* and *Candida*, with mortality as high as 30% to 60% with documented invasive disease. Fungal infections can be difficult to detect due to the frequent absence of localizing signs or symptoms and lack of means of detection by culture. *Prompt diagnostic assessment and initiation of antifungal empiric therapy* are paramount for improving outcomes in these patients.

Empiric antifungal therapy prevents fungal overgrowth in patients with prolonged neutropenia. It also provides early treatment of clinically occult infection. Clinical trials have found that antifungal treatment of children with persistent or recurring fever reduced morbidity and mortality from invasive fungal disease. This is especially true in patients with profound neutropenia not receiving antifungal prophylaxis. The current recommendation is that high risk groups (i.e., those expected to have neutropenia >7 days) should receive antifungal prophylaxis during episodes of prolonged FN.

A meticulous physical examination, laboratory assessments, and radiographic studies in search of deep-seated infections are also warranted after this 4 to 7 day time frame. Particular attention should be paid to the skin examination as it can reveal

fungal nodules. Fungal cultures should be sent from the blood and urine as well as any suspicious skin site. In addition, the patient should have a serum galactomannan performed to screen for *Aspergillus* infection. CT imaging of the chest, as well as imaging of other symptomatic areas, should be performed. It should be noted that in the severely neutropenic patient, areas of infection may not be appreciated on imaging until neutrophil recovery has occurred. In these cases, the patient will generally have continued or new fevers with count recovery that should alert the clinician to the need for repeat CT imaging which should include the sinuses, chest, and abdomen.

Commonly used antifungal agents for empiric therapy in prolonged FN include:
1. Echinocandins

   Micafungin

   Prophylaxis 1 to 2 mg/kg IV daily
   Treatment 3 to 4 mg/kg IV daily
   Caspofungin
   Anidulafungin
2. Triazoles

   Voriconazole
   Posaconazole
3. Amphotericin B
4. Lipid formulations of amphotericin B

The echinocandins have replaced amphotericin B as the empiric antifungal agent of choice due to their once daily dosing, significantly decreased side effect profile, and broad coverage. Echinocandins are fungicidal to most *Candida* species and at least fungistatic against *Aspergillus* species. They also have limited activity against *Fusarium* species and *Zygomycetes*. The triazoles are derivatives of fluconazole with broad-spectrum antifungal activity and limited side effects. Of note, the triazoles are fungicidal against *Aspergillus* species. In general, we utilize the echinocandins as first-line empiric therapy and consider adjustment in patients that are worsening clinically or have signs consistent with *Aspergillus* infection. Patients on either an echinocandin or triazole should be monitored closely for hepatic toxicity; voriconazole may also cause visual disturbance that is more common in adult patients. Posaconazole may provide better coverage against *Aspergillus* species but is only available as an oral medication and clinical trial data are limited in pediatric patients.

Amphotericin B remains the most widely active antifungal agent but has generally been replaced due to its significant toxicity profile, most notably nephrotoxicity and infusional toxicity. Fever, chills, nausea, metabolic abnormalities, hypokalemia and other electrolyte disturbances, and hepatic toxicity can all occur. In order to treat, and possibly prevent, some of these complications, several measures are taken. Patients with a history of nephrotoxicity may benefit from receiving pre- and postinfusion NS boluses and diuretics. Premedications including acetaminophen, diphenhydramine, and meperidine may be given to treat or prevent acute symptoms related to the infusion (fever, chills, rigors, nausea). Hydrocortisone can also be added to address infusion-related toxicity. Use of liposomal formulations of amphotericin B (Ambisome and Abelcet) results in significantly fewer adverse events, but they are much more expensive than amphotericin B.

Viral infection

Immunosuppressed children are able to tolerate many viral infections without difficulty. However, defects in cellular immunity predispose them to unusually severe infections with certain viruses, particularly the herpes family of viruses. Primary varicella infection is associated with high morbidity and mortality. In transplant patients, primary infection or reactivation with cytomegalovirus (CMV) is an important cause of interstitial pneumonitis, marrow aplasia, and other infections. Antiviral drugs are available for a limited number of infections including herpes simplex virus (HSV), varicella zoster virus (VZV), CMV, and influenza and should be utilized in the treatment of immunocompromised patients. Other patients may also be candidates for prophylaxis (e.g., solid organ transplant patients and patients with a prior history of infection on therapy).

Patients with documented infection with HSV should be treated with IV acyclovir (30 mg/kg/day if <12 years; 15 mg/kg/day for ≥12 years divided TID for 7 to 14 days). Infection with VZV is potentially life threatening and therefore chemotherapy should be stopped while treating with IV acyclovir (30 mg/kg/day divided TID for 7 to 10 days or until all lesions are crusted and no new lesions have appeared for 24 to 48 hours). It is important to monitor renal function and ensure adequate fluid intake due to potential nephrotoxicity from acyclovir.

Patients with symptomatic primary CMV infection or reactivation can be treated with ganciclovir (10 mg/kg/day IV divided q12h for 2 to 4 weeks until resolution of viremia by polymerase chain reaction). Patients with persistent infection may require longer therapy or may have resistant disease and require alternate therapy with foscarnet or cidofovir. Of note, ganciclovir can be myelosuppressive, whereas foscarnet and cidofovir are quite nephrotoxic. Concomitant therapy with intravenous immune globulin (IVIG) may be beneficial especially in the setting of CMV pneumonitis. Data regarding prophylactic therapy in this setting is lacking, although once daily dosing can be considered in patients that complete a course of antiviral therapy and remain neutropenic or severely immunocompromised.

Patients who develop influenza while on therapy should be treated with neuraminidase inhibitors (i.e., oseltamivir for children ≥ 1 year of age, twice daily for 5 days) to reduce symptom duration and severity of disease. Oseltamivir may also be given as daily prophylaxis for 5 days to patients that have been exposed to the virus. If given as treatment, it is most effective when given within 48 hours of symptom onset.

Pneumocystis jiroveci pneumonia

Pneumocystis jiroveci is now considered an atypical fungus and is a ubiquitous organism that may cause severe or fatal pneumonitis in immunocompromised patients (most notably patients with HIV and those being treated for cancer). Patients typically develop a rapid onset of fever in association with tachypnea and other symptoms of respiratory compromise such as nasal flaring and intercostal retractions. Lung sounds may be clear and typically patients do not have rales. Hypoxemia is evident by pulse oximetry and arterial blood gas. Chest radiography or CT shows an interstitial pattern. Without appropriate therapy, patients rapidly progress to respiratory failure.

Diagnosis is made by demonstrating the organism by Gomori methanamine silver stain on a sample obtained by induced sputum, bronchoalveolar lavage, percutaneous needle biopsy, or open lung biopsy. Patients who are at risk and present with the classic signs and symptoms should be treated while awaiting definitive diagnosis, given the rapidity of clinical deterioration.

For documented or highly suspected infection with *P. jiroveci*, trimethoprim/sulfamethoxazole (TMP/SMX) is the treatment of choice, at a dose based on the TMP component of 15 mg/kg/day IV divided q8h for 14 to 21 days. If the patient fails to respond to TMP/SMX within 72 hours, or develops this infection while on prior TMP/SMX prophylaxis with good compliance, initiate therapy with pentamidine, 4 mg/kg IV daily. In patients with moderate or severe proven infection, concomitant administration of corticosteroids may be beneficial with IV methylprednisolone or prednisone given 2 to 4 times per day for 5 to 7 days, followed by a taper over 1 to 2 weeks.

New sites of infection

New or persistent fever and neutropenia may be associated with the development of new sites of infection due to continued severe immunosuppression. Particular symptoms may provide clues to site and potential pathogen.

1. Burning retrosternal pain may be esophagitis from *Candida* sp. or HSV. Cytotoxic treatment may also cause severe pain due to mucosal erosions. Empiric micafungin or acyclovir, or both, may be needed. Esophagitis may also be bacterial, especially as a result of Gram-positive aerobes.

2. Pulmonary infiltrates may be due to resistant bacteria, *Pneumocystis*, fungi, or viruses. Neutropenic patients may not show evidence of pulmonary infiltrates due to lack of an appropriate local inflammatory response. However, with the recovery of the ANC, these sites of infection may become evident. If FN has been less than 7 days, pulmonary infiltrates are very likely to be of bacterial origin. If the neutropenia persists for greater than 7 days, the patient is at particularly high risk for fungal infection. Bronchoalveolar lavage or induced sputum may identify *Pneumocystis*, viruses, or fungi. The risks and benefits of open lung biopsy and pursuing an aggressive diagnostic

evaluation must be considered. It is important to remember that the child may rapidly become very ill and this decision must be made expeditiously after discussion between the oncologist, surgeon, radiologist, pulmonologist, as well as the patient and family.

Other supportive measures

Granulocyte colony-stimulating factor (G-CSF) may be indicated in the setting of FN; however, there are no specific standards for its use. Therapy with 5 mcg/kg/day subcutaneously is recommended under certain conditions in which the clinical course is likely to worsen before the anticipated marrow recovery (see Chapter 25). Patients who remain severely neutropenic with life-threatening infections should receive G-CSF. Granulocyte transfusions may be considered in the setting of profound neutropenia and sepsis, especially an invasive bacterial or fungal infection that is not improving on appropriate therapy with expected continuation of profound neutropenia (see Chapter 5). However, such transfusions are becoming increasingly more difficult to obtain.

Fever in the nonneutropenic oncology patient

The febrile, nonneutropenic patient remains susceptible to infection secondary to immune dysfunction and often secondary to the presence of a CVC. These patients should have a careful assessment with history, physical examination, and pertinent laboratory studies as in the febrile neutropenic patient. Patients with localizing findings should have appropriate diagnostic procedures. Clinical judgment must be utilized to determine the risk for the patient without an obvious source of infection. Issues in the social history such as family reliability, compliance, and ability to travel to the outpatient center must be factored into a decision plan. If the patient has recently received chemotherapy and is expected to reach a nadir in the next few days, consideration should be given to more frequent assessment or hospital admission.

As with the neutropenic patient, blood cultures should be drawn and empiric antibiotics initiated. The risk for *Pseudomonas* is significantly decreased in the patient without severe neutropenia and therefore ceftriaxone IV/IM at 50 mg/kg (maximum 2 g) can be given daily while febrile in the outpatient setting in the otherwise well-appearing child for at least the first 48 hours, while awaiting results of the blood culture. Hospitalization may be required in patients who are persistently febrile with a dropping ANC and in those with a positive blood culture or the development of localizing signs.

Suggested Reading

Donowitz GR, Maki DG, Crnich CJ, et al. Infections in the neutropenic patient—new views of an old problems. Hematol Am Soc Hematol Educ Prog 113–139, 2001.

Freifeld AG, Bow EJ, Sepkowitz KA, et al. Clinical practice guideline for the use of antimicrobial agents in neutropenic patients with cancer: 2010 update by the Infectious Disease Society of America. Clin Infect Dis 52:e56–e93, 2011.

Pizzo PA. Fever in immunocompromised patients. N Engl J Med 341:893–900, 1999.

28 Acute Pain Management in the Inpatient Setting

Pain is a common problem for children with hematologic or oncologic conditions, as it can result both from the condition itself and from its management. A number of studies have demonstrated that effective pain management not only increases a patient's comfort level but can also effect long-term changes in a patient's pain threshold, and, in critically ill patients, it has been demonstrated to improve morbidity and mortality. Despite this, other studies have demonstrated that pediatric pain management is often suboptimal. This results from perceptions on the parts of both parents and care providers that pain is less frequent or less severe than is the case, or from concerns of causing dependence or addiction.

The management of chronic pain is a frequent challenge for pediatric hematologists and oncologists, but is outside the scope of this chapter. For pain management at the end of life, see Chapter 29. For pain management in patients with sickle cell disease, see Chapter 3.

The World Health Organization analgesic ladder

In 1986 the World Health Organization presented the analgesic ladder as a framework that physicians could use when developing treatment plans for cancer pain, paving the way for significant improvements in its management. Over the subsequent 25 years, it has undergone much scrutiny and several modifications have been proposed. A recent adaptation is presented in Figure 28.1.

The cornerstone of the ladder rests on five simple recommendations that remain valid today:

1. The oral form of medication should be chosen whenever possible.

2. Analgesics should be given at regular intervals. It is necessary to respect the duration of the medication's efficacy and to prescribe doses at specific intervals in accordance with the patient's level of pain. The dose should be adjusted until the patient is comfortable.

3. Analgesics should be prescribed according to pain intensity as evaluated by a scale of intensity of pain. The prescription must be given according to the level of the patient's pain and not according to the medical staff's perception of the pain.

4. Dosing of pain medication should be adapted to the individual. The correct dosage is one that will allow adequate relief of

Handbook of Pediatric Hematology and Oncology: Children's Hospital & Research Center Oakland, Second Edition. Caroline A. Hastings, Joseph C. Torkildson, and Anurag K. Agrawal.
© 2012 John Wiley & Sons, Ltd. Published 2012 by John Wiley & Sons, Ltd.

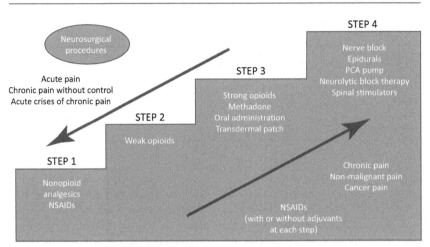

Figure 28.1 Adaptation of the World Health Organization analgesic ladder. Abbreviations: NSAID, non-steroidal anti-inflammatory drug; PCA, patient-controlled analgesia.

pain. The dosing should be adapted to achieve the best balance between the analgesic effect and the side effects.

5. Analgesics should be prescribed with a constant concern for detail. The regularity of analgesic administration is crucial for the adequate treatment of pain.

It is important to remember that these are guidelines and that there are situations where a stepwise approach to pain is not the best choice for management. For example, management of sickle cell vaso-occlusive crises typically involves early introduction of step 3 medications without waiting for the patient to fail step 1 and 2 therapies.

Assessment of pain

The accurate and reproducible assessment of pain is essential to effective management, allowing the provider to determine when intervention is necessary and to more objectively measure the response to intervention. However, the subjective nature of pain and the impact of developmental stage

on the best method of assessment have made its measurement a challenge. As a result, a variety of pediatric pain assessment scales have been developed to assist in this process.

Neonates and infants

The Neonatal Infant Pain Scale (NIPS), developed at the Children's Hospital of Eastern Ontario, is a widely used method of assessing pain in this patient population. It evaluates a series of six parameters, with a range of scores between 0 and 7. Scores above 3 are considered indicative of a pain level sufficient to require intervention. The scale is presented in Table 28.1. Its major limitation is that it may underestimate the level of pain in infants who are too ill to respond appropriately or are receiving a paralyzing agent.

Preverbal/Nonverbal children

Pain assessment for children who are unable to describe their pain or use an interactive pain assessment scale due to young age, cognitive dysfunction, injury, or medical interventions such as intubation requires

Table 28.1 The Neonatal Infant Pain Scale (NIPS).

Parameter	0 points	1 point	2 points
Facial expression	Relaxed	Contracted/grimacing	–
Cry	Absent	Mumbling	Vigorous
Breathing patterns	Relaxed	Different than basal	–
Arms	Relaxed	Flexed/stretched	–
Legs	Relaxed	Flexed/stretched	–
State of arousal	Sleeping/calm	Uncomfortable	–

an alternative similar to the NIPS that allows the subjective evaluation of pain-related behaviors by another individual. One of the more commonly used assessment tools is the Face, Legs, Activity, Cry, Consolability (FLACC) Behavior Scale. Developed at the University of Michigan as a tool to assess postoperative pain, it has been shown to reliably measure pain in a variety of clinical situations. It is presented in Table 28.2. The range of possible scores is from 0 to 10, consistent with other commonly used numerical rating scales used for older children.

School aged and older children

Children 5 years of age and older have been shown to have the ability to accurately rate their level of pain using a numerical rating scale. A commonly used tool is the Wong–Baker FACES scale, presented in Figure 28.2. Developed in the early 1980s, it remains one of the most widely used tools for assessing pain in both children and adults.

When pain assessment scales are used appropriately they can be very valuable in helping the care team know whether their pain management interventions are

Table 28.2 The Face, Legs, Activity, Cry, Consolability (FLACC) Scale.

Parameter	0 Points	1 Point	2 Points
Face	No particular expression or smile	Occasional grimace, or frown, withdrawn or disinterested	Frequent to constant frown, clenched jaw, quivering chin
Legs	Normal position or relaxed	Uneasy, restless, or tense	Kicking or legs drawn up
Activity	Lying quietly, normal position, moves easily	Squirming, shifting back and forth, or tense	Arched, rigid, or jerking
Cry	No cry	Moans, whimpers, or occasional complaint	Crying steadily, screams or sobs, frequent complaints
Consolability	Content, relaxed	Reassured by occasional touching, hugging, or being talked to; distractible	Difficult to console or comfort

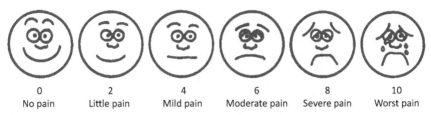

0	2	4	6	8	10
No pain	Little pain	Mild pain	Moderate pain	Severe pain	Worst pain

Figure 28.2 The Wong–Baker FACES Pain Rating Scale.

appropriate or need to be adjusted. However, there is no "magic number" that indicates when interventions need to be initiated. Studies consistently show that there is little correlation between a child's pain score and their perception as to whether or not they need pain medication. Therefore, in situations where patients are likely to have pain, it is essential to question them regularly regarding their need for medication.

Pain pharmacology

Pain can be subdivided into two categories, nociceptive and neuropathic. Acute pain in children is most often nociceptive, and a variety of drugs can be used to treat this pain. Much of the information regarding this therapy is empiric, as there are few formal drug studies for many of these agents, especially in children less than 12. Nonsteroidal anti-inflammatory drugs (NSAIDs), opiates, muscle relaxants, local anesthetics, and tramadol can be used. Some other adjuvant therapies can also be utilized, such as psychological intervention, distraction, and biofeedback.

When treating pain in neonates it is important to remember that several factors can modify their response and clearance of drugs. They have increased body water content and decreased fat, which can alter drug distribution. A relative increase in blood flow to the brain and a somewhat "leaky" blood–brain barrier can cause a prolongation of drug effect. Renal clearance of drugs can be relatively decreased up to 1 year of age. Hepatic enzymes are initially immature, but these mature quickly. Children 2 to 6 years of age develop a larger relative hepatic size for weight and often metabolize drugs more quickly than younger or older children; this can translate to a need for larger doses of drug given more frequently to achieve adequate analgesia. Variations in age, weight, blood flow, and organ function can all affect effective drug dosing.

Step 1 therapy: nonopioid analgesics

Drugs that are commonly used for step 1 therapy of pain in children are presented in Table 28.3. These should be first-line therapy for pain unless the clinical situation dictates that therapy should begin at a higher step.

The use of NSAIDs in children with cancer is generally discouraged due to the common occurrence of thrombocytopenia in this population and concern for an increased risk of bleeding due to an inhibition of platelet function. However, there have been no large, controlled trials demonstrating the validity of this concern. Several clinical trials have demonstrated that ibuprofen can safely be used following dental surgery, tonsillectomy, and neurosurgery in healthy children and *in vitro* data suggest that ibuprofen causes no significant prolongation of the platelet function assay PFA-100.

Step 2 therapy: weak opioids

Patients whose pain is inadequately controlled with step 1 therapy or who are being weaned from step 3 therapy require

Table 28.3 Step 1 pain therapy medications.

Drug	Dose	Comments

Ibuprofen	1–3 months: 5 mg/kg 3–4 times daily
	3 months–1 year: 50 mg 3 times daily
	1–4 years: 100 mg 3 times daily
	4–7 years: 150 mg 3 times daily
	7–10 years: 200 mg 3 times daily
	10–12 years: 300 mg 3 times daily
	12–18 years 300–400 mg 3 times daily
	Maximum dose 30 mg/kg/day; 2.4 g/day
		• Block conversion of arachi-
		   donic acid into prostaglan-
		   dins and thromboxanes
		• Nonselective; variably impair
		   platelet function
		• Ketorolac can affect renal
		   function or bone growth with
		   prolonged use

Naproxen	5 mg/kg/dose 2 times daily Maximum dose 15 mg/kg/day	
Ketorolac	0.5 mg/kg/dose IV/IM every 6 hours Maximum dose 30 mg Maximum 20 doses	

Acetaminophen	15 mg/kg/dose every 4–6 hours
	Maximum 5 doses/day; maximum 4 g/day
		• Has no antiplatelet effect
		• Can be hepatotoxic
		• Avoid rectal dosing in neu-
		   tropenic patients
		• Parenteral form recently
		   licensed in United States

Abbreviations: IV, intravenous, IM, intramuscular.

treatment with step 2 agents. In the United States, the most common agents used are those that combine acetaminophen with a weak opioid. These include codeine or hydrocodone, although there is some disagreement about the inclusion of hydrocodone in the weak opioid category. Commonly used agents in this category are presented in Table 28.4.

It is important to remember that the designation "weak opioid" does not translate to "without side effects." The use of codeine and hydrocodone can cause the same side effects seen with stronger opioids: respiratory depression, hypoxia, nausea, vomiting, pruritus, constipation, physical tolerance, and dependence. Although the Food and Drug Administration (FDA) classifies them as Schedule III medications, the risks of abuse and diversion still exist.

Step 3 therapy: strong opioids

Patients not responding to step 2 therapy or whose condition indicates the need for stronger pain therapy at the outset are candidates for step 3 therapy. All of the medications in this category are strong opioids. They act by binding to μ-receptors in the spinal cord and central nervous system (CNS). These receptors are also found throughout the body, and binding to peripheral sites accounts for many of the side effects seen with opiate therapy. Opioids vary both by their duration of action and by the emotional effect they produce. Meperidine and oxycodone typically cause euphoria; conversely, morphine more commonly causes dysphoria. Equivalent doses of the strong opioids and the pharmacokinetics of their oral formulations are presented in Table 28.5.

Table 28.4 Step 2 pain therapy medications.

Drug	Dose	Comments
Codeine	0.5–1 mg/kg q4–6 hour Max: 60 mg/dose	• Comes as 30 and 60 mg tablets • Up to 35% of children are inefficient metabolizers of codeine to morphine; they will achieve minimal benefit from this product
Acetaminophen with codeine	0.5–1.0 mg/kg/dose of codeine q4–6 hour Max: 2 tablets/dose; 15 mL/dose	• Tablet: 300 mg/15 mg, 300 mg/30 mg • Liquid: 120 mg/12 mg per 5 mL • Up to 35% of children are inefficient metabolizers of codeine to morphine; they will achieve minimal benefit from this product
Acetaminophen with hydrocodone	>2 years: 0.135 mg/kg/dose hydrocodone <40 kg: do not exceed 5 mg hydrocodone per dose >40 kg: do not exceed 7.5 mg hydrocodone per dose	• Tablet: 5 mg/500 mg • Liquid: 7.5 mg/500 mg per 15 mL • Elixir contains 7% alcohol

Oral starting doses of step 3 medications are presented in Table 28.6. It is important to remember that patients with severe chronic pain will often be on doses much larger than this due to tolerance. Tactics such as narcotic substitution can be used to deal with tolerance or with side effects resulting from large doses. However, these steps should be performed under the guidance of individuals who are well versed in such measures. Transdermal fentanyl has not been included; practitioners familiar with its usage should transition patients to this agent when deemed necessary.

Step 4 therapy

As can be seen in Figure 28.1, step 4 therapy does not introduce new medications. Patient-controlled analgesia (PCA) pumps are listed; this does not refer to short-term PCA pump use such as following surgery or to deal with postchemotherapy mucositis or sickle cell vaso-occlusive crisis. Rather, it refers to long-term, ambulatory PCA pump use for severe chronic pain. With the increased availability of highly concentrated oral narcotics and novel delivery systems, the use of home PCA therapy has declined significantly. Additional step 4 therapies include nerve blocks, epidural injections, and other alternative interventions routinely provided by a specialized pain service.

Nonpharmacologic approaches to pain

The effectiveness of psychological interventions to decrease the perception of pain and the anxiety associated with it, and to improve the quality of life in patients

Table 28.5 Strong opioid characteristics.

Medication	Equianalgesic doses (mg)		Pharmacokinetic profile (oral formulations unless specified)	
	IV	PO	Onset	Duration
Morphine sulfate	10	30		
IR			IV: 2–4 minutes	IV: 2–4 hours
CR (MS Contin/Oromorph)			20–30 minutes	3–6 hours
ER (Kadian)			2–4 hours	8–12 hours
			1–2 hours	12–24 hours
Hydromorphone	1.5	4.5	20–30 minutes	2–4 hours
Oxycodone		20		
IR			20–30 minutes	4–6 hours
CR (for regular, not prn use)			2–4 hours	8–12 hours
Fentanyl	180 mg oral morphine/24 hour = 100 mcg transdermal fentanyl/hour		TD: 12–16 hours	TD: 48–72 hours
	1 mg IV morphine = 10 mcg IV fentanyl		IV: 1–5 minutes	IV: 0.5–2 hours
Methadone	Conversion ratios: - Oral: IV = 2:1 - Oral morphine: methadone based on 24-hour morphine total	Oral morphine: methadone ratio	• Interindividual variability exists; methadone should be used by experienced clinicians only • Doses may need to be decreased after several days of administration; monitor vital signs daily and consult a specialist • May cause QT interval prolongation at higher doses	
	24 hour oral morphine total (mg)			
	<30	2:1		
	31–99	4:1		
	100–299	8:1		
	300–499	12:1		
	500–999	15:1		
	>1000	20:1		

Abbreviations: IV, intravenous; IR, immediate release; CR, controlled release; ER, extended release; TD, transdermal.

Table 28.6 Step 3 oral pain therapy medications.

Drug	Oral dose	Comments
Oxycodone	• Instant release: 0.05–0.15 mg/kg/ dose up to 5 mg/dose q4–6 hour • Sustained release: for patient taking >20 mg/day of oxycodone can administer 10 mg q12 hour	
Morphine	• 0.3–0.6 mg/kg/dose every 12 hours for sustained release • 0.2–0.5 mg/kg/dose q4–6 hour prn for immediate release tablets or solution	• Injection (mg/mL): 1, 2, 4, 5, 10 • Injection, preservative free (mg/mL): 1, 5 • Oral solution (mg/mL): 2, 4, 20 • Tablet (IR) (mg): 10, 15, 30 • Tablet (ER) (mg): 15, 30, 60, 100, 200
Hydromorphone	0.03–0.08 mg/kg/dose PO q4–6 hour; max: 5 mg/dose	
Methadone	0.03–0.08 mg/kg/dose PO q4–6 hour; max: 5 mg/dose	

Abbreviations: IR, immediate release; ER, extended release.

with chronic pain, has been clearly demonstrated in a number of clinical settings. These include:

• Minimizing postoperative pain and anxiety through the use of preoperative interventions before painful procedures. These include the explanation of the event in developmentally appropriate terms, minimizing wait times once the patient arrives in the operating room, child-friendly waiting spaces, and cognitive-behavioral therapies (CBT) such as directed imagery, deep breathing, and role playing. These interventions are typically provided and coordinated by the child-life program.

• The use of CBT, relaxation therapy, and biofeedback to decrease the perception of pain among children suffering from chronic pain caused by cancer, headache, and abdominal pain.

• The use of CBT, relaxation, self-hypnosis, biofeedback, and social support groups to decrease painful episodes and improve quality of life in patients with sickle cell disease.

It is vital that child-life workers become involved with children admitted with a possible diagnosis of cancer very shortly after admission. Data indicate that psychological interventions are most effective in decreasing anxiety related to painful procedures when initiated before the first painful experience. It is also important to obtain input from a psychologist early on for children with conditions causing chronic pain so that appropriate interventions can be started.

Suggested Reading

Friedrichsdorf SJ, Kang TI. The management of pain in children with life-limited illnesses. Pediatr Clin N Am 54:645–672, 2007.

Verghese ST, Hannallah RS. Acute pain management in children. J Pain Res 3:105–123, 2010.

29 Palliative Care

The World Health Organization defines pediatric palliative care as care that "aims to improve the quality of life of patients facing life-threatening illnesses, and their families, through the prevention and relief of suffering by early identification and treatment of pain and other problems, whether physical, psychosocial, or spiritual." It is the active total care of the child's body, mind, and spirit, and also involves giving support to the family. It begins when illness is diagnosed, and continues irrespective of whether or not a child receives disease-directed treatment. It requires that health providers evaluate and alleviate a child's physical, psychological, and social distress at all times during their treatment. To be effective, it requires a broad multidisciplinary approach that includes the family and makes use of available community resources. However, it can be successfully implemented even if community resources are limited. Palliative care can and should be provided in tertiary-care facilities, community health centers, and at home.

This definition contains several concepts that deserve consideration. It contains the broadly defined term "life-threatening" that includes situations in which a cure is possible, instead of the more limited "life-limiting" that includes only those conditions for which there is no realistic hope of cure.

There is a role for palliative care for all children diagnosed with cancer, even those whose cancers have an excellent prognosis with appropriate therapy. It also applies to the large number of children with life-threatening nononcologic conditions. The definition stresses the importance of "early identification and treatment of pain and other problems." Palliative care is not synonymous with "end-of-life" care; palliative care must begin at the time of diagnosis and continue on throughout the period of disease-directed therapy. It also must include many resources from throughout the patient's and family's range of experience: physicians, nurses, social workers, psychologists, spiritual counselors, and a variety of other support personnel chosen because of each child's unique situation. During any hospitalization, an important responsibility of the medical team is to ensure that each child has access to all needed services and is being supported to the greatest extent possible.

Individualized care planning and coordination

At the time of diagnosis, parents and caregivers of children with life-threatening illness have two goals: a care-directed goal of

Handbook of Pediatric Hematology and Oncology: Children's Hospital & Research Center Oakland, Second Edition. Caroline A. Hastings, Joseph C. Torkildson, and Anurag K. Agrawal.
© 2012 John Wiley & Sons, Ltd. Published 2012 by John Wiley & Sons, Ltd.

cure and a comfort-directed goal of decreasing suffering. Introducing palliative care principles early on in the care process is respectful and supportive of these goals. A model developed by the Palliative and End-of-Life Care Task Force at St. Jude Children's Hospital, the Individualized Care Planning and Coordination model is designed to facilitate this introduction (Figure 29.1). Although developed to assist in making care decisions for children undergoing bone marrow transplantation, the model is useful in helping to define what care options are acceptable to the patient and family given the prognosis and goals of treatment. Key concepts in this model include the establishment of a close and caring relationship with the patient and family, clarifying patient and family values and priorities, determining the goals of care based on the patient's and family's understanding of prognosis, and allowing them to choose from

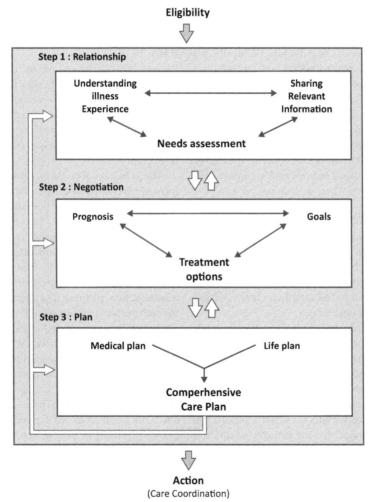

Figure 29.1 The Individualized Care Planning and Coordination Model.

available goal-directed treatment options. From this foundation, the members of the care team can coordinate the provision of care to ensure the social, psychological, and emotional needs of the patient and family are addressed at the same time that appropriate medical care is provided.

End of life care

Despite the tremendous advances made in the care of children with cancer over the past 50 years, at the present time one in five children diagnosed with cancer will ultimately die of their disease. The death of a child affects the physical and psychological well-being of family members for the rest of their lives. Events occurring around the time of death, both positive and negative, play a critical role in defining how family members grieve and ultimately come to terms with the event. Families who have lost a child have identified several needs regarding end-of-life care. These include the need to have complete information honestly communicated, to have easy access to essential staff members who will be supportive, to have assistance in coordinating necessary services, to have their relationship with their child maintained as much as possible, and to be allowed to feel that their child's life and death has meaning.

Research studies involving pediatric palliative care are limited, but they have identified several important shortcomings in the level of palliative care provided to children. Several studies have demonstrated a lack of successful management of pain and other distressing symptoms. Other studies have demonstrated that the majority of children dying of life-threatening diseases die in the hospital, often in the intensive care unit. The impact of this outcome on the appropriateness of care provided and its effect on the family's bereavement process are not totally clear. Studies have also demonstrated that significant levels of parental dissatisfaction with hospital staff can arise from confusing, inadequate, or uncaring communication regarding treatment and prognosis as well as discrepancies between parents and care providers in understanding the terminal condition. When a language barrier exists between family and staff, these problems are often exacerbated.

Common symptoms at the end of life

Pain

Parents and caregivers report that their child's pain is the symptom they fear most. A large survey of parents whose children died of cancer revealed that 75% of them felt their child suffered pain at the end of life, but only 37% felt the pain was successfully managed.

The principles of pediatric pain management are presented in Chapter 28 and pain management at the end of life follows these same principles. However, it becomes particularly important to clarify and understand the goals of treatment as elucidated by the patient and parents. The desire to maintain alertness and interaction early in treatment may give way to a desire to keep the patient comfortable, even if it means the patient will be more sedated and less aware. Acceding to the family's wishes that the patient not be hooked up to monitors might outweigh concern that the doses of pain medications being used could result in respiratory depression. These decisions often run counter to what physicians see as their primary goal of care, to prolong life as long as possible. Working through some of these difficult philosophical issues with the help of a mentor can be essential to working comfortably and effectively in this type of setting.

Nausea and vomiting

Nausea and vomiting at the end of life can be triggered by many different stimuli. A variety of toxins such as medications and their metabolites, urea resulting from renal failure, or metabolic byproducts of hepatic failure can all stimulate the chemoreceptor trigger zone and cause nausea. Increased intracranial pressure and a variety of emotional and sensory stimuli can mediate nausea and vomiting through cortical pathways. The gastrointestinal (GI) tract can stimulate the vomiting center in response to local receptor stimulation caused by obstruction, stasis, toxins, or drugs. In addition, pharyngeal stimulation by mucous or mucosal breakdown can also trigger the vomiting center.

A stepwise approach to the management of nausea and vomiting in the palliative care setting is outlined in Table 29.1. A key feature of this approach is to ensure that the interventions selected are in keeping with the patient's and family's goals of care.

A number of medications can be tried to control nausea and vomiting. The ideal agent is one that targets the specific cause of the patient's distress if such an agent can be identified. A list of useful medications is outlined in Table 29.2.

Opioids frequently cause nausea and vomiting due to a direct effect on the chemotherapy trigger zone or secondarily to their effect on GI motility leading to gastroparesis and constipation.

Table 29.1 Management of nausea and vomiting.

Step	Objective	Intervention
1	Attempt to identify causes	History (timing, quality, severity of nausea; description of vomiting)
		Physical exam focused on neurological, abdominal symptoms
		Medication history (opioids, chemotherapy, antibiotics, NSAIDs, other drugs)
2	Initiate environmental changes	Small meals
		Minimize strong smells
		Create a comfortable environment
		Provide support for emotional distress
3	Clarify scope of interventions that will be acceptable to patient and family	Discuss goals of care with patient and family
4	Choose treatment based on etiology and goals of care	Chemically induced: stop medications if possible, opioid rotation if felt to be cause; antiemetics
		Increased ICP: surgical treatment if possible (shunt insertion, shunt revision), medical therapy (steroids, antiemetics)
		Obstruction/ileus: surgical management if consistent with goals of care; medical management (steroids, octreotide, opioids with scopolamine, haloperidol)
		Other/unknown cause: trial of antiemetics

Abbreviations: NSAIDs, nonsteroidal anti-inflammatory drugs; ICP, intracranial pressure.

Table 29.2 Medications for treatment of nausea and vomiting.

Drug	Dose
Metoclopramide (prokinetic/ dopamine antagonist)	Prokinetic dose: 0.1 mg/kg/dose IV or orally every 6 hours Dopamine antagonist (antiemetic) dose: 0.5–1 mg/kg/dose IV or orally every 6 hours; use with diphenhydramine to prevent extrapyramidal symptoms
Ondansetron (serotonin receptor antagonist)	0.45 mg/kg/day IV or orally; may be dosed once daily or divided every 8 hours
Scopolamine (anticholinergic)	For children >40 kg: 1.5 mg patch behind ear every 72 hours
Meclizine (antivertigo agent)	For children >12 years of age: 25–75 mg/day orally in up to 3 divided doses
Dexamethasone (anti- inflammatory)	Antiemetic: 10 mg/m^2 IV or orally daily; maximum dose 20 mg daily Increased ICP: increase dosing frequency to 2–4 times daily, with a maximum dose of 40 mg/day
Octreotide (somatostatin analogue)	5–10 mg/kg/day (continuous 24-hour IV infusion or divided twice daily subcutaneously)
Dronabinol (cannabinoid)	For children aged 6 years and older; 2.5–5 mg/m^2/dose every 4–6 hours. Not recommended for children who have clinical depression
Lorazepam (benzodiazepine)	0.025 mg/kg/dose IV or orally every 6 hours

Abbreviations: IV, intravenous; ICP, intracranial pressure.

Constipation

Constipation often causes pain and distress for children at the end of life, both physically and psychologically. Prevention of constipation should therefore be a primary goal of end-of-life care.

One of the most common causes of constipation are opioids, which decrease GI motility and fluid secretion, leading to hard, dry stools. Unlike other narcotic side effects, constipation does not seem to decrease with ongoing use. Patients and families should be informed ahead of time about this side effect, as children in severe pain may not consider regular bowel movements a priority. Once well established, constipation may require quite aggressive and unpleasant therapies to correct it.

Other factors that contribute to constipation in terminal patients include poor oral intake of fluids and food, decreased physical activity, neurological dysfunction, and intestinal obstruction due to presence of tumor.

Assessment
History

- Stool frequency, consistency, and associated discomfort
- Abdominal pain, nausea, vomiting, and anorexia
- Neurological symptoms: urinary problems, lower extremity numbness, weakness, and paresthesias
- Diarrhea (sign of encopresis or obstipation?)
- Prior episodes, previously effective therapies

Physical Examination

- Abdominal palpation

- External rectal exam (digital exam rarely needed and may be dangerous)
- Neurologic exam

Medications

- Stool softeners (docusate): rarely effective alone
- Osmotic agents (Miralax™, magnesium sulfate, and lactulose): effective for long-term use; Miralax requires 4 to 8 oz. of fluid which can be a limitation
- Stimulants (senna, bisacodyl): often useful and necessary in the end-of-life setting when less concern exists regarding development of dependence

Anorexia and weight loss

Anorexia or loss of appetite is a familiar symptom in children with cancer. It can occur at any point in treatment; institutional studies indicate that it affects as many as 40% of children with cancer at diagnosis and the prevalence increases to as high as 70% in children with advanced stage disease. Early in treatment it is most often a side effect of chemotherapy or radiation, or a result of stomatitis, dysphagia, constipation, pain, or depression. As the child's cancer becomes progressive, it is often a component of the anorexia/cachexia syndrome, a complex set of central nervous system (CNS) and metabolic abnormalities caused by a combination of tumor byproducts and host cytokine release.

Step 1: assessment

State of primary disease
Diet and fluid history
Nausea/vomiting/constipation
Oral lesions (including candidiasis)
Medication history
History of prior eating disorder
Sense of smell

Step 2: environmental changes

Small meals
Regular mouth care
Comfortable environment

Table 29.3 Appetite stimulants for cancer-associated anorexia.

Drug	Dose
Cyproheptadine (Periactin)	2–6 year: 2 mg bid >6 year: 4 mg bid
Megestrol acetate (Megace)	7.5–10 mg/kg/day in 1–4 divided doses Maximum 800 mg/day or 15 mg/kg/day
Dronabinol (Marinol)	2.5 mg/m^2/dose every 4–6 hours Use with caution in children with depression; avoid in children with sensitivity to sesame oil

Support for emotional distress
Discontinue medications that might be causing anorexia

Step 3: more aggressive therapies (if consistent with plan of care)

Medications (see Table 29.3)

Nutritional supplementation

If acceptable to patient and family, enteral feeding with a nasogastrostomy (NG) or gastrostomy tube is often reasonably well tolerated unless the patient has a GI obstruction or is chronically nauseated.

Total parenteral nutrition (TPN) is rarely useful in the end-of-life setting except for short-term use in the patient with GI obstruction.

Fatigue

The National Comprehensive Cancer Network defines cancer-related fatigue as "a distressing persistent, subjective sense of physical, emotional and/or cognitive tiredness or exhaustion related to cancer or cancer treatment that is not proportional to recent activity and interferes with usual functioning." It is pervasive, multidimensional, and incapacitating; as such it significantly decreases health-related quality of life in children. While it can exist throughout the entire period of cancer treatment, fatigue is most often seen as significant as the child's disease progresses. In several studies, parents have identified fatigue as the most significant symptom that moderately or severely impacted their child's well-being toward the end of life. These same studies have also demonstrated that it is the symptom most likely to be missed by care providers; fewer than 50% of children whose parents described them as suffering highly from fatigue had this documented in their medical record.

Cancer-related fatigue is more common and more severe in children with brain tumors than in those with other cancers. Pediatric patients tend more often to associate their feelings of fatigue to sleep disturbance or side effects of therapy whereas parents are more likely to include emotions and nutritional status as potential causes. A recent study suggested that pain and dyspnea were frequently associated with fatigue; the authors postulated that opioids and benzodiazepines, common therapies for pain and dyspnea, might have significantly contributed to their patients' fatigue.

In a recent review on the assessment and management of fatigue and dyspnea in pediatric palliative care, Dr. Christina Ulrich defined a conceptual model for understanding fatigue in this population. This framework is outlined in Figure 29.2.

Data are very limited regarding effective treatments for cancer-related fatigue in children, although a number of interventions

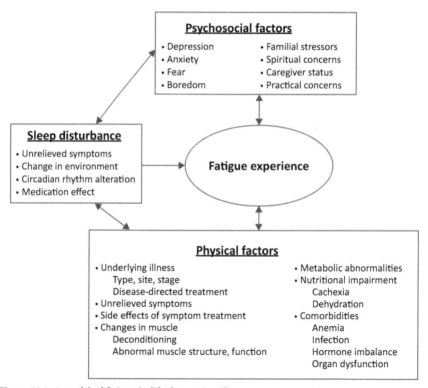

Figure 29.2 A model of fatigue in life-threatening illness.

Table 29.4 Treatments for cancer-related fatigue.

Nonpharmacologic interventions	Pharmacologic interventions
Psychosocial	Stimulants
• Education	• Methylphenidate
• Support groups	• Modafinil
• Individual counseling	Antidepressants
• Coping strategies	• SSRIs
• Stress management training	Paroxetine
• Individualized behavioral intervention	Sertraline
Exercise	• Other antidepressants
Sleep therapy	Bupropion
• Behavioral therapy	Steroids
• Stimulus control	
• Sleep restriction	
• Sleep hygiene	
Acupuncture	

Abbreviation: SSRI, selective serotonin reuptake inhibitor.

have been shown to be effective in adults. These are outlined in Table 29.4.

Psychosocial and activity-based interventions have been shown to be quite effective in adults with cancer-related fatigue; data in children are lacking. Exercise has the strongest data regarding its value, but this is largely in adult cancer survivors suffering from fatigue after the completion of curative therapy. Its utility in ameliorating fatigue in patients near the end of life is less well established.

Dyspnea

Dyspnea is the term used to describe the feeling of breathlessness that occurs when the respiratory system fails to meet the body's need for oxygen uptake or carbon dioxide removal. It occurs under normal circumstances such as after brisk exercise, but in pathological conditions it can cause severe distress. It occurs very frequently at the end of life, as respiratory failure occurs very commonly as a terminal event. Therefore, recognition of dyspnea and its effective treatment is a key component of end-of-life care.

Dyspnea can result from either an increased metabolic demand or an inability to maintain a normal minute ventilation. The former can be caused by complications of the disease or its treatment, such as infection, metabolic acidosis, or increased metabolic demands caused by extensive tumor burden. The latter can result from conditions such as decreased lung compliance due to tumor, infection, or fluid, or by other conditions such as interstitial lung disease, anemia, or fatigue.

It follows that treatment of dyspnea would involve steps to decrease metabolic demand or improve the efficiency of respiration. However, this can prove to be quite challenging in practice. It is often difficult to determine whether the cause of dyspnea is in fact respiratory or metabolic, and once discovered, the unwillingness of the patient or family to accept certain interventions can create additional challenges for the treatment team.

Appropriate therapies to decrease metabolic demand depend on the cause of the increased demand. For the patient who becomes dyspneic with activity, it may be as simple as recommending that the patient use a wheelchair instead of walking or decrease physical activity in other ways. Increased metabolic demand caused by infection or inflammation can be treated with aggressive use of antibiotics or anti-inflammatory agents, as long as such therapies are in keeping with the patient's and family's wishes.

Respiratory failure can result from two general causes: lung parenchymal dysfunction and respiratory muscle fatigue or failure. It is important to distinguish between these, as the treatments are different. An algorithm for distinguishing between these causes is presented in Table 29.5. It is important to note that hypercarbia can be a late finding in parenchymal dysfunction as well.

Treatment

Treatment for dyspnea can be divided into three general categories: mechanical support of respiration, support of gas exchange, and therapies to decrease the sensation of dyspnea.

Support of respiration

When intubation and mechanical ventilation are not appropriate or acceptable to the patient and family, noninvasive positive pressure ventilation (NIPPV) can be useful in supporting respiration. However, the use of NIPPV in adult patients who have elected to forgo intubation or other aggressive respiratory support is controversial. Its use in children with cancer is unstudied; there have been a handful of papers published regarding its use in children with neuromuscular disorders.

From the adult literature, it appears clear that the most important issue when deciding on the use of NIPPV to support respiration is a clear understanding of the goals of therapy among all involved. In 2007, the Society of Critical Care Medicine Palliative Noninvasive Positive Pressure Ventilation Task Force published its recommendations on the use of NIPPV in the palliative care setting. While intended for adults, the concepts can be applied to the pediatric care setting as well. The Task Force proposed a three-category approach to assist in decision making regarding this technology. An overview of this approach is presented in Table 29.6.

The key areas of distinction in this model are goals of care, determination of success, appropriate endpoints, and response to

Table 29.5 Classification and features of respiratory failure.

	Parenchymal dysfunction	Muscle failure/fatigue
Causes	Airway obstruction • Interstitial, bronchial inflammation • Excessive secretions External compression • Pleural fluid • Pleural-based nodules • Infiltration of interstitium by metastases	Neuromuscular disease • Weak musculature • Lowered fatigue threshold • Prolonged recovery time Abnormal load on respiratory system Weakness caused by systemic disease
Blood gas findings	Hypoxemia	Hypoxemia, hypercarbia

Table 29.6 Approach to decision making regarding noninvasive positive pressure ventilation.

Approach	Category 1	Category 2	Category 3
Definition	Life support; no preset limits	Life support; do not intubate	Comfort measures only
Primary goals of care	Assist ventilation and/or oxygenation	Includes same as category 1 except intubation declined	Palliation of symptoms (relief of dyspnea)
	Alleviate dyspnea	Also could include briefly	
	Achieve comfort	prolonging life for a specific	
	Reduce risk of intubation	purpose (e.g., arrival of family	
	Reduce risk of mortality	member)	
	Avoidance of intubation		
Main goals to communicate with patient and family	Goal is to restore health and use intubation if necessary and indicated	Goal is to restore health without using endotracheal intubation and without causing unacceptable discomfort	Goal is to maximize comfort while minimizing adverse effects of opiates
Determination of success	Improved oxygenation and/or ventilation	Improved oxygenation and/or ventilation	Improved symptoms
	Tolerance of NIPPV or minor discomfort that is outweighed by potential benefit	Tolerance of NIPPV or minor discomfort that is outweighed by potential benefit	Tolerance of NIPPV

(Continued)

Table 29.6 (*Continued*)

Approach	Category 1	Category 2	Category 3
Endpoint for NIPPV	Unassisted ventilation adequately supporting life Intolerance of NIPPV	Unassisted ventilation adequately supporting life Intolerance of NIPPV	Patient is not more comfortable having NIPPV on or wants NIPPV stopped Patient becomes unable to communicate
Response to failure	Intubation and mechanical ventilation (if indicated)	Change to comfort measures only and palliate symptoms without NIPPV	Palliate symptoms without NIPPV
Likely location of NIPPV	ICU but may include stepdown unit or acute care bed in some hospitals with appropriately monitored setting and trained personnel	Variable but may include ICU, stepdown unit, or acute care bed	Acute care bed but could be applied in hospice by appropriately trained personnel

Abbreviations: NIPPV, noninvasive positive pressure ventilation; ICU, intensive care unit.

failure. It is imperative that each member of the care team agrees on each of these components to avoid confusion and conflict later in the course.

Support of gas exchange

NIPPV can also be used to augment gas exchange in patients with low lung volumes in whom the surface area for gas exchange is reduced and the caliber of the airways is decreased, increasing the likelihood of obstruction. Continuous positive airway pressure and bilevel positive airway pressure are useful in situations in which the pressure necessary to maintain airway patency is too high to allow for efficient exhalation.

In the setting of respiratory failure without hypercapnia, supplemental oxygen is the most appropriate intervention to facilitate gas exchange. It is often better tolerated than NIPPV devices, especially by young children, facilitating pulmonary vasculature dilatation and inhibiting cerebral artery dilatation, a frequent cause of headaches. It is important to remember, however, that patients with hypercapnic respiratory failure frequently rely on a "hypoxic drive" to maintain respiration. Provision of supplemental oxygen to these patients can lead to hypopnea or apnea.

Therapies to decrease the sensation of dyspnea

In end-of-life settings respiratory failure is often the ultimate cause of death and the main goal of therapy is minimizing the distress resulting from the sensation of dyspnea as this occurs. This goal can be achieved with a combination of pharmacologic and nonpharmacologic therapies.

The two most effective classes of drugs for minimizing the perception of dyspnea are opioids and benzodiazepines. Morphine is the opioid used most often for this purpose, but fentanyl and hydromorphone (Dilaudid) have been shown to be effective

as well. The dose that is required is lower than what is commonly used for pain; a morphine dose of 0.025 mg/kg, or an equivalent dose of fentanyl or Dilaudid, is often effective in the narcotic-naïve child, and an increase in the dose by 25% will often be effective in the child already receiving morphine. The dose should then be titrated to achieve symptom relief, with no set upper limit. Benzodiazepines can help with the anxiety associated with dyspnea; lorazepam 0.05 mg/kg (maximum 2 mg) can be given every 4 to 8 hours for this purpose.

A variety of nonpharmacologic interventions have been shown to decrease the distress associated with dyspnea. These include:

1. Cool air blown on the face
2. Chest wall percussion
3. Relaxation therapy and counseling
4. Proper positioning
5. Limitation of activities
6. Cooler room temperature
7. Avoidance of respiratory irritants (tobacco smoke and cleaning fluids)

Most experts agree that these work best as an adjunct to pharmacologic therapy; they are rarely effective alone.

Conclusion

Unfortunately, many questions remain about how to best care for children who are destined to die before they reach adulthood. These include practical issues such as how to best manage distressing symptoms such as those listed above, how to best communicate with children about the dying process and involve them in decisions regarding their care, and how to avoid aggressive end-of-life therapies that only delay death and prolong suffering instead of extending life. After the child's death, families must continue to move forward, raising questions about how best to help them deal with the bereavement that inevitably accompanies such an event. It is fortunate that research into these questions has expanded greatly over the past few years, and it is likely that answers to these questions will soon be available in the medical literature. The children we care for, but cannot save, deserve no less.

Case study for review

Julie, a 13-year-old girl with widely metastatic alveolar rhabdomyosarcoma diagnosed 6 months earlier continues to have extensive bony disease, including possible new metastatic lung lesions. Julie's treatment has been complicated by chronic pain and a challenging family situation. Although Julie lives with her mother, her father oversees her care. Her parents do not get along with one another. They frequently argue and scream in her presence, which clearly upsets her.

Since diagnosis, her father has adamantly refused to let caregivers have one-on-one conversations with Julie. He insists on remaining the only one to relate to Julie any disease-related information, as he knows her best and can gauge how she will react. He has stated that Julie need not know that she will likely die of her disease and he has forbidden the medical team from discussing issues related to prognosis.

Julie is to undergo a CT-guided lung biopsy to determine the nature of the lung lesions. Her parents state that she is already anxious enough and do not want the medical team to tell her about the biopsy or the possibility that her disease has progressed. Instead, they ask that Julie be told that she is to be sedated only for a "scan." Moreover, should she prove to have new disease, they do not want Julie to be informed and ask that her caregivers not discuss end-of-life matters with her.

Questions

- As Julie's physician, are you comfortable with her parents' approach?
- Should Julie's parents prevent her from knowing information relevant to her disease?
- How do you reconcile your responsibility to be forthright with Julie while simultaneously being respectful of her parents' request?
- If you believe that her parents' approach is not in Julie's best interest, how might you proceed?
- Should children with life-limiting illnesses be involved in end-of-life decisions?

Understanding familial adaptation toward the dying process is imperative. As healthcare providers, our goal is to anticipate and identify problems and to assist dying children and their families as they adjust to and cope with the emotional responses, which are part of the dying process.

Many children, parents, and physicians are hesitant to discuss death and dying so that opportunities for planning how to cope are often missed. Failure to prepare adequately for death can deprive families of the chance to enjoy what time they have left with one another.

Each child and family grieve in their own unique way, determined by personal experiences with death, religious and cultural backgrounds, and individual makeup.

Dying is a *process* and all parties need to learn to live with dying or, as stated by the American Academy of Pediatrics, "the goal [of palliative care] is to add life to the child's years, not simply years to the child's life" [1].

Parents' natural tendency to protect their children influences the amount of information children receive and the degree to which they are involved in decision making about their care [2]. Some parents feel that by giving their child a choice their responsibilities are being usurped, while others perceive including their sick child in decisions as overly burdensome. For many parents, the sicker their child, the more they assume decisional priority and attempt to minimize, veto, or even preclude their child from having a role in decisions at all. Seemingly, such an approach is understandable; however, parents need to be aware of the consequences of not preparing their children for medical outcomes that are inevitable, such as anxiety, stress, and confusion.

Children frequently know more about their disease than for which they are credited. Even when kept in the dark by parents and providers, children often know that the endpoint of a life-threatening illness is death [3–5]. As children appreciate certain facts about their diseases and know that they are dying, it stands to reason that they should be involved in decisions about their care so that they can voice their preferences [6,7]. Therefore, the question we ask ourselves should not be "*should I tell*," rather it should be "*how do I tell?*" Increasingly, research supports the need for direct communication between parents, physicians, and children with life-limiting illnesses. This includes discussions relating to prognosis and even death [1,2,8,9]. Hinds et al. [10] found that children with life-limiting cancer between ages 10 to 20 years were capable of participating in end-of-life decision making.

Physicians must be aware of the unique barriers to a child's ability to participate in decision making as it relates to the dying process. The first question we must ask is, "*does* **this** *child have the ability to understand that he/she is dying and what dying entails.*"

As children mature, their intellectual and emotional understanding of serious illness and the prospect of death matures too. Discussions about death should be honest and take into consideration the child's emotional and developmental level. It is important to follow the child's lead [11]. In other words, answer what children ask and on their terms. Often, rather than being direct, a child's question or statement may be suggestive of something they are uncomfortable asking and therefore it is vital to determine what their underlying intention is and not to give too much or too little information or answer the wrong question. Finally, failure to inform and involve children can lead to feelings of isolation and distress [12].

Ideally, discussions should occur early and routinely and physicians should reassess how the child and parents understand the plan and goals of care. This helps the dying child and parents make appropriate decisions. Discussions should be in language that parents *and* children can understand and be presented gently, accurately, and repeatedly. Doing so will help minimize misunderstandings and defuse conflicts. The challenge is to do so in a way that is both sensitive and respectful of the child's, parents', and providers' needs, needs that are often in conflict with one another.

According to the Institute of Medicine (IOM), "conflicts may . . . be productive or beneficial" [11]. Confronted with a disagreement, parties tend to engage in a more in-depth discussion allowing for a greater appreciation of each other's position, and, in the process, each side may become more sensitive to the other's values and concerns.

Mack et al. [13] surveyed parents of children with cancer and found that parents rated the quality of care provided by physicians more favorably when physicians communicated directly with children (when appropriate). Similarly, in a survey of more than 400 Swedish parents of children who died of cancer, Kreicbergs et al. [14] found that none of the parents who spoke with their child about death regretted doing so, whereas more than one-quarter of parents who did not speak with their child regretted not doing so. The latter parent group had higher levels of anxiety and depression than parents who did speak to their children.

Parents are not alone in valuing the importance of direct communication between children and physicians. Recent research has shown that children with cancer consider direct communication between doctors and children more important than any other aspect [15]. Nearly 40 years ago, following parental approval, Nitschke et al. [4] began including children aged 5 years and older who were near death from cancer in end-of-life discussions. They found that the majority of children and parents found the child's inclusion a positive experience. They also reported that some children from whom information was withheld experienced fear and isolation prior to dying.

Conclusions and practical suggestions

Situations like Julie's do not lend themselves to easy solutions. Dishonesty, evading the question at hand, inconsistencies, and white lies are to be avoided at all costs. Deception is difficult to maintain. When the truth is ultimately discovered, the patient–parent–physician relationship is often irrevocably damaged, an unfortunate circumstance in any situation, but particularly for a child like Julie who is nearing the end of life. Such action may lead Julie to withdraw and even to experience feelings of isolation and fear, let alone profoundly disrespect her developing autonomy.

By helping to facilitate, clarify, and resolve areas of contention, pediatricians can be extremely helpful. As appreciated by the IOM, the following steps may be useful: (1) postpone decisions to allow for time to think about concerns and to discuss goals, (2) rather than making definitive decisions that offer no room for compromise,

consider temporary steps that accommodate each party's goals, and (3) periodically reevaluate each party's views concerning the goals of care and the options to achieve those goals [11].

Case resolution

Since Julie's diagnosis, her father has periodically sought the guidance of the unit's social worker. Prior to the lung biopsy, Julie's father agreed to meet with her oncologist and the social worker in the latter's office, a place where he is comfortable speaking. Following a brief update by the oncologist of Julie's current medical status, the social worker asked her father to share his concerns about Julie not being included in disease-related discussions. Her father stated that Julie is "*just a kid,*" and that it was "*his job to protect, and to decide what is best for her.*" He recounted his limited parental role in Julie's life prior to her cancer diagnosis and blamed himself for not being more present in her life, admitting that Julie's illness and likely death "*terrify*" him and that he is resolute not to abandon her again.

The social worker asked Julie's father what he believes she knows of her disease and its prognosis. He replied that Julie knows she has cancer and that it is "treatable," and nothing more. She then asked if he would allow Julie to join them, which would permit the oncologist (in his presence) to answer any questions she may have about the "scan" and to clarify what she indeed knows. Hesitant at first, he ultimately agreed. After greeting and thanking her for joining them, the oncologist asked Julie if she has any questions about the upcoming CT scan. Julie asked why she has to have another CT when reevaluation scans, including a chest CT, were just completed 1 week ago. Directing her words to the oncologist, Julie asked, *"is something wrong?"* Before the oncologist or her father could reply, Julie stated, *"I've been online talking to other kids with cancer. A few of them said that the only reason to repeat a scan so soon is to see if the disease is back."* Without hesitation and still speaking to her oncologist, Julie said, *"I know that most kids with my kind of cancer die."*

The social worker encouraged Julie and her father to speak openly and freely. Tentatively, and with the support of the oncologist and social worker, they began to speak to one another and share their respective concerns and goals. Following their conversation, Julie's father cautiously agreed to include Julie in future discussions. The oncologist assured both Julie and her father that although he remains hopeful, her disease is difficult to cure and that she might indeed die of her cancer. However, the medical team would continue to treat both her cancer and her pain, all along adhering to her and her parents' wishes.

Successful care of the dying child requires that healthcare providers acknowledge families' emotions, assure families that their responses are normal, provide a balanced and honest perspective, and communicate frequently and consistently.

We would like to acknowledge and thank Yoram Unguru, MD, MS, MA, for writing this case and instructor guide. Dr. Unguru is an attending physician in the Division of Pediatric Hematology/Oncology, The Herman and Walter Samuelson Children's Hospital at Sinai, and Berman Institute of Bioethics, Johns Hopkins University.

Suggested Reading

Feudtner C. Collaborative communication in pediatric palliative care: a foundation for problem-solving and decision-making. Pediatr Clin N Am 54:583–607, 2007.

Freyer DR. Care of the dying adolescent: special considerations. Pediatrics 113:381–388, 2004.

Himelstein BP, Hilden JM, Boldt AM, Weissman D. Pediatric palliative care. N Engl J Med 350:1752–1762, 2004.

Kazak AE, Rourke MT, Alderfer MA, et al. Evidence-based assessment, intervention and psychosocial care in pediatric oncology: a blueprint for comprehensive services across treatment. J Pediatr Psychol 32:1099–1110, 2007.

Liben S, Papadatou D, Wolfe J. Paediatric palliative care: challenges and emerging ideas. Lancet 371:852–864, 2008.

Wolfe J, Grier HE, Klar N, et al. Symptoms and suffering at the end of life in children with cancer. N Engl J Med 342:326–333, 2000.

References

1. American Academy of Pediatrics. Committee on Bioethics and Committee on Hospital Care. Palliative care for children. Pediatrics 106:351–357, 2000.

2. Bluebond-Langer M. The Private Worlds of Dying Children. Princeton, NJ: Princeton University Press, 1978.

3. Hilden JM, Watterson J, Chrastek J. Tell the children. J Clin Oncol 18:3193–3195, 2000.

4. Nitschke R, Meyer WH, Sexauer CL, et al. Care of terminally ill children with cancer. Med Pediatr Oncol 34:268–270, 2000.

5. McConnell Y, Frager G, Levetown M. Decision making in pediatric palliative care. In: Carter B, Levetown M (eds), Palliative Care for Infants, Children, and Adolescents: A Practical Handbook. Baltimore: JHU Press, 2004.

6. Informed consent, parental permission, and assent in pediatric practice. Committee on Bioethics, American Academy of Pediatrics. Pediatrics 95:314–317, 1995.

7. Spinetta JJ, Masera G, Jankovic M, et al. Valid informed consent and participative decision-making in children with cancer and their parents: a report of the SIOP working committee on psychosocial issues in pediatric oncology. Med Pediatr Oncol 40:244–246, 2003.

8. Wolfe J, Hinds P, Sourkes B (eds). Textbook of Interdisciplinary Pediatric Palliative Care. Philadelphia: Elsevier, 2011.

9. Himelstein BP, Hilden JM, Morstad Boldt A, Weissman D. Pediatric palliative care. N Engl J Med 350:1752–1762, 2004.

10. Hinds PS, Drew D, Oakes LL, et al. End-of-life care preferences of pediatric patients with cancer. J Clin Oncol 23:9146–9154, 2005.

11. Field MJ, Behrman RE (eds). When children die: improving palliative and end-of-life care for children and their families. Committee on Palliative and End-of-Life Care for Children and Their Families. Board on Health Sciences Policy, Institute of Medicine. Washington, DC: National Academies Press, 2003.

12. Sourkes B. Armfuls of Time: The Psychological Experience of the Child with a Life-Threatening Illness. Pittsburgh: University of Pittsburgh Press, 1995.

13. Mack JW, Hilden JM, Watterson J, et al. Parent and physician perspectives on quality of care at the end of life in children with cancer. J Clin Oncol 23:9155–9161, 2005.

14. Kreicbergs U, Valdimarsdottir U, Onelov E, et al. Talking about death with children who have severe malignant disease. N Engl J Med 351:1175–1186, 2004.

15. Unguru Y, Sill A, Kamani N. The experiences of children enrolled in pediatric oncology research: implications for assent. Pediatrics 125:e876–e883, 2010.

30 Chemotherapy Basics

Chemotherapeutic agents have multiple mechanisms of action and many potential side effects. In order to be prepared for the potential complications, we discuss the most common pediatric agents, their mechanisms of action, the types of malignancies for which they are utilized, and finally, the most likely side effects. We discuss how best to monitor for these adverse events, and how to manage them should they occur. Note that side effects from chemotherapy are numerous and we detail some of the more common ones rather than provide a comprehensive list; further reading may be required in appropriately diagnosing and managing a patient. Emetogenic potential of common pediatric agents is included in Chapter 25. The majority of agents are dosed depending on the patient's body surface area (BSA) rather than weight, especially for patients older than 1 year of age. Multiple formulas exist for the calculation of BSA; we prefer the Mosteller formula:

$$BSA = \sqrt{\frac{Height(cm) \times Weight(kg)}{3600}}$$

Asparaginase

Asparaginase comes in three forms: L-asparaginase (Elspar®), polyethylene glycol (PEG)-asparaginase (Oncaspar®), and Erwinia (Erwinase®). Asparaginase is a naturally occurring enzyme produced by many microorganisms. In the L- and PEG-asparaginase forms, the enzyme is produced by *Escherichia coli*, whereas the Erwinia form is produced by *Erwinia chrysanthemi*. PEG-asparaginase is a modified form of L-asparaginase with a much longer half-life resulting from its covalent binding to PEG, allowing the same therapeutic effect from fewer doses. Intramuscular asparaginase is the current standard of care due to concerns about severe anaphylaxis with intravenous (IV) use; however, two current Children's Oncology Group (COG) protocols are investigating the safety and efficacy of IV PEG-asparginase. Less frequent dosing with PEG-asparaginase is important for patient comfort and convenience until intravenous asparaginase becomes more widely accepted. Since Erwinia is produced by a different microorganism, it is immunologically distinct and can be utilized in patients that have had a hypersensitivity reaction to the *E. coli* forms.

Mechanism of action

L-asparagine is a nonessential amino acid that cannot be synthesized by malignant cells of lymphoid and myeloid origin. Asparaginase depletes L-asparagine from leukemic cells by catalyzing the conversion of L-asparagine to aspartic acid and ammonia.

Handbook of Pediatric Hematology and Oncology: Children's Hospital & Research Center Oakland, Second Edition. Caroline A. Hastings, Joseph C. Torkildson, and Anurag K. Agrawal.
© 2012 John Wiley & Sons, Ltd. Published 2012 by John Wiley & Sons, Ltd.

Utilized in

Acute lymphoblastic leukemia
Acute myelogenous leukemia
Non-Hodgkin lymphoma

Side effects, monitoring, and treatment

The most immediate side effect from asparaginase compounds is an allergic reaction that can range from local irritation to anaphylaxis. Patients should be monitored closely for at least 1 hour after Elspar injection, and 2 hours following Oncaspar injection. Based on the level of allergic symptoms, treatment can range from an antihistamine such as diphenhydramine to treatment of anaphylaxis with steroids, an antihistamine, an H_2 blocker (i.e., ranitidine), and epinephrine. A common later side effect is coagulopathy secondary to decreased synthesis of antithrombin III (ATIII), fibrinogen, and other clotting factors. Currently, routine monitoring of ATIII and fibrinogen and repletion of low levels are not recommended without clinical symptoms. Rare side effects that should be considered include pancreatitis, thrombosis, and seizures.

Bleomycin

Bleomycin is obtained as a mixture of antibiotics isolated from *Streptomyces verticillus*.

Mechanism of action

Bleomycin leads to the formation of oxygen-free radicals that cause single-strand and double-strand DNA breaks. In addition, bleomycin leads to cellular degradation of cellular RNA. Bleomycin is cell cycle specific, targeting the G2 and M phases, thus inhibiting cell growth and division, especially in rapidly dividing cells.

Utilized in

Germ cell tumors
Hodgkin lymphoma

Side effects, monitoring, and treatment

Bleomycin can cause infusional fever and chills followed later by mucositis, as well as pruritus and excoriation leading to hyperpigmentation. Raynaud's phenomenon can also commonly occur later, especially with combination chemotherapy. Patients may occasionally complain of rash, dysgeusia, and anorexia. Due to the formation of oxygen-free radicals, patients are at risk for dose-dependent pneumonitis and rarely pulmonary fibrosis and therefore should be monitored with pulmonary function testing, especially carbon monoxide-diffusing capacity (PFT/DLCO). An anaphylactoid-type reaction may also rarely occur.

Cisplatin/Carboplatin

Cisplatin was the first of the platinum-based chemotherapeutic agents. Carboplatin has less severe side effects, in particular decreased nephrotoxicity and ototoxicity. It is more myelosuppressive, however.

Mechanism of action

The platinum agents, like the alkylators, cause interstrand DNA cross-linking. In addition, they bind to replicating DNA causing single-strand breaks.

Utilized in

Brain tumors
Germ cell tumors
Hepatoblastoma
Hodgkin lymphoma
Neuroblastoma
Osteogenic sarcoma
Soft tissue sarcomas
Wilms tumor

Side effects, monitoring, and treatment

Infusional nausea and vomiting are common as platinum agents have an extremely high emetogenic potential. This is followed later by myelosuppression. Electrolyte abnormalities including hypokalemia, hypomagnesemia, hypocalcemia, and hyponatremia are common and the patient may develop Fanconi syndrome (diminished reabsorption of solutes by the proximal tubule resulting in hypophosphatemia, metabolic acidosis, and secondary hypokalemia). Nephrotoxicity and ototoxicity (high-frequency sensorineural hearing loss) occur occasionally with carboplatin but are more common and severe with cisplatin.

Ototoxicity must be monitored with serial audiograms during therapy. Due to the risk of electrolyte abnormalities, chemistry panels including magnesium should be followed daily while receiving platinum-based therapy. In addition, due to the risk of nephrotoxicity, the patient's intake and output should be followed closely and be well-matched. If it appears the patient is developing a negative fluid balance, additional fluids should be provided. If the patient develops a positive fluid balance, mannitol should be used to increase urine output. Renal function should be monitored closely, as a reduction in the glomerular filtration rate will necessitate a dose reduction. In general, for pediatric patients with no previous history of nephrotoxicity, serum creatinine can serve as a measure of renal function utilizing the Cockcroft-Gault equation:

Estimated creatinine clearance
$$= \frac{(140 - \text{Age[years]}) \times \text{Mass(kg)} \times [0.85(\text{if female})]}{72 \times \text{serum creatinine(mg/dL)}}$$

Decrease in the estimated creatinine clearance should lead to more formal measurements of the glomerular filtration rate and likely platinum dose reduction.

Cyclophosphamide/Ifosfamide

Cyclophosphamide (Cytoxan) and ifosfamide are alkylating agents and structural analogues. They are related to nitrogen mustard.

Mechanism of action

Cyclophosphamide and ifosfamide require conversion by the hepatic P450 system to their active form that ultimately leads to the intracellular release of two compounds, acrolein and phosphoramide mustard. Phosphoramide mustard causes interstrand DNA cross-linking.

Utilized in

Acute lymphoblastic leukemia
Acute myelogenous leukemia
Brain tumors
Ewing sarcoma
Germ cell tumors
Hodgkin and non-Hodgkin lymphoma
Neuroblastoma
Osteogenic sarcoma
Soft tissue sarcomas
Wilms tumor

Side effects, monitoring, and treatment

Cyclophosphamide and ifosfamide commonly cause nausea, vomiting, and anorexia with drug infusion. Myelosuppression, immunosuppression, and alopecia are common later adverse effects. Sterility is dose dependent (greatest with cumulative doses of cyclophosphamide $>7.5\,\text{g/m}^2$) and occurs more commonly in pubertal males (though prepubertal males and females are also at risk). Due to the risk of nephrotoxicity, particularly with ifosfamide, patients should be well-hydrated prior to and after infusion. Though the syndrome of inappropriate diuretic hormone (SIADH) is rare, patients should be monitored for appropriate urine output by following their intake and output as well as urine specific gravity. Electrolytes are also routinely followed for hyponatremia. If there are signs of fluid retention, the patient should initially be given increased hydration followed by diuresis with furosemide or mannitol if hydration is ineffective.

Excretion of acrolein into the urine can cause hemorrhagic cystitis. The addition of MESNA for bladder protection when the cyclophosphamide dose exceeds $1.0\,g/m^2/day$ has significantly decreased the frequency of this adverse event. MESNA specifically binds to acrolein and other toxic metabolites in the urine to detoxify them and protect the bladder wall. The urine should be monitored for the presence of occult blood during and after infusion and, if positive, should be examined microscopically. If red blood cells are noted on microscopy, hydration should be increased. Of note, MESNA can cause a false positive test for ketones on urine dipstick. Finally, metabolism of ifosfamide leads to formation of chloroacetaldehyde, a byproduct thought responsible for nephrotoxicity as well as the neurotoxicity seen occasionally with ifosfamide (somnolence, depressive psychosis, and confusion). Thiamine prophylaxis may have benefit in a patient with prior neurotoxicity.

Cytarabine (Ara-C)

Cytarabine, also known as cytosine arabinoside or Ara-C (arabinofuranosyl cytidine), is utilized in the treatment of hematologic malignancies.

Mechanism of action
Cytarabine is an antimetabolite that inhibits DNA polymerase. In addition, it is cell cycle specific, killing cells during synthesis (S phase); it therefore specifically targets rapidly dividing cells.

Utilized in
Acute lymphoblastic leukemia
Acute myelogenous leukemia
Hodgkin and non-Hodgkin lymphoma

Side effects, monitoring, and treatment
Cytarabine commonly causes nausea, vomiting, and anorexia immediately after infusion. Later, myelosuppression, stomatitis, and alopecia are common. Although not common, the patient should be monitored for Ara-C syndrome that includes fever, myalgias, bone pain, malaise, conjunctivitis, maculopapular rash, and occasionally chest pain. High-dose IV cytarabine requires prophylaxis with dexamethasone eye drops to prevent conjunctivitis. A flu-like syndrome with fever, chills, and rash occurs occasionally with cytarabine; infection must still be ruled out with bacterial cultures. *Streptococcus viridans* sepsis and acute respiratory distress syndrome are possible after high-dose cytarabine, therefore the addition of vancomycin with fever or clinical deterioration should be strongly considered. Intrathecal (IT) cytarabine similarly can cause fever, nausea, and vomiting in addition to headache. More serious and immediate side effects including arachnoiditis, somnolence, meningismus, convulsions, and paresis are rare but should be considered as clinically indicated.

Dactinomycin (Actinomycin-D)

Dactinomycin is an antibiotic compound isolated from *Streptomyces parvullus*, similar to the anthracycline class.

Mechanism of action

Dactinomycin intercalates with DNA, inhibiting RNA and DNA synthesis. In addition, dactinomycin interacts with topoisomerase, which is required for DNA replication, and leads to single-strand DNA breaks.

Utilized in

Soft tissue sarcomas
Wilms tumor

Side effects, monitoring, and treatment

Infusional nausea and vomiting are common, followed later by alopecia and myelosuppression. Anorexia, fatigue, diarrhea, and mucositis also occur occasionally. Radiation recall can occur in patients who previously received radiation therapy.

Daunorubicin/Doxorubicin/ Idarubicin

Daunorubicin and doxorubicin are both anthracycline antibiotics isolated from *Streptomyces* species (*S. coeruleorubidus* and *S. peucetius*, respectively). Idarubicin is an analogue of daunorubicin used less commonly in pediatric oncology.

Mechanism of action

Anthracyclines as a group are cytotoxic to malignant cells due to nucleotide base intercalation and cell membrane lipid-binding activity. Nucleotide intercalation inhibits replication as well as DNA and RNA polymerases. The anthracyclines also interact with topoisomerase II, which is vital for DNA replication. Cell membrane binding affects a variety of cellular functions. In addition, electron reduction of the anthracyclines produces free radicals leading to DNA damage and lipid peroxidation. Daunorubicin differs from doxorubicin structurally as the side chain terminates in a methyl group

rather than an alcohol. Idarubicin lacks a methoxy group which increases its lipophilicity as compared with other anthracyclines.

Utilized in

Acute lymphoblastic leukemia
Acute myelogenous leukemia
Hepatoblastoma
Hodgkin and non-Hodgkin lymphoma
Neuroblastoma
Osteogenic sarcoma
Soft tissue sarcomas
Wilms tumor

Side effects, monitoring, and treatment

Anthracyclines commonly cause nausea and vomiting with treatment. Due to the color of the infusion, the patient should be warned that urine, saliva, tears, and sweat may all have a pink or red coloring. After treatment, myelosuppression, alopecia, and mucositis commonly occur. Due to the production of free radicals during electron reduction of anthracyclines, patients are at risk for dose-dependent cardiotoxicity occurring as a late finding. Echocardiographic monitoring is required during and after treatment at regular intervals based on the total anthracycline dose received as well as concomitant radiation therapy to the chest. Cardioprotection with continuous versus rapid infusion as well as agents such as dexrazoxane remains controversial and is not yet routinely recommended. Dexrazoxane may have benefit when patients receive high cumulative doses of anthracyclines (i.e., $\geq 300 \, mg/m^2$). Additionally, anthracyclines provide different cumulative toxicity, and dose conversion based on doxorubicin isotoxic dose equivalents must be performed as below:

Doxorubicin: multiply total dose × 1
Daunorubicin: multiply total dose × 0.833
Epirubicin: multiply total dose × 0.67
Idarubicin: multiply total dose × 5
Mitoxantrone: multiply total dose × 4

Radiation recall is also a potential rare complication of anthracyclines when given after radiation therapy.

Etoposide

Etoposide is derived from podophyllotoxin, a toxin found in the American mayapple.

Mechanism of action

Etoposide binds to topoisomerase II, which is vital for DNA replication, leading to DNA strand breakage. Etoposide is cell cycle specific and appears to act mainly on the G2 and S (synthesis) phases, thus targeting rapidly dividing cells.

Utilized in

Acute myelogenous leukemia
Brain tumors
Ewing sarcoma
Germ cell tumors
Hodgkin and non-Hodgkin lymphoma
Hemophagocytic lymphohistiocytosis
Neuroblastoma
Osteogenic sarcoma
Soft tissue sarcomas
Wilms tumor

Side effects, monitoring, and treatment

Infusional nausea and vomiting is common followed by myelosuppression and alopecia. Although rare, the patient should be monitored closely for hypotension and anaphylaxis during the infusion. In addition to fluid support, the infusional rate can be slowed if the patient develops hypotension.

Imatinib (Gleevec®)

Imatinib was the first successful targeted drug therapy for oncology patients.

Mechanism of action

Imatinib is a selective inhibitor of the tyrosine kinase activity of the BCR-ABL fusion protein, a product of the Philadelphia chromosome (reciprocal translocation of chromosome 9 and 22) seen mainly in chronic myeloid leukemia and rarely with acute lymphoblastic leukemia.

Utilized in

Acute lymphoblastic leukemia (Philadelphia chromosome-positive)
Chronic myelogenous leukemia

Side effects, monitoring, and treatment

Imatinib has multiple potential side effects. Common immediate effects include fluid retention, nausea, and diarrhea. Later common effects include fatigue, muscle cramps, rash, arthralgias, and myelosuppression.

Irinotecan

Irinotecan is a semisynthetic analog isolated from the plant alkaloid *Camptotheca acuminata.*

Mechanism of action

Irinotecan in its active form is a potent inhibitor of topoisomerase I which is vital for DNA replication. Inhibition of topoisomerase inhibits replication and also leads to DNA damage.

Utilized in

Brain tumors
Hepatoblastoma
Soft tissue sarcomas

Side effects, monitoring, and treatment

Patients receiving irinotecan can suffer from cholinergic symptoms including intestinal hyperperistalsis that can lead to abdominal cramping and early diarrhea. Patients should be monitored closely for early diarrhea; if it occurs loperamide should be given prior to an anticholinergic (e.g., atropine). Other cholinergic symptoms that may occur with drug administration include rhinitis, increased salivation, miosis, lacrimation, diaphoresis, and flushing. Common later side effects include diarrhea, alopecia, transaminitis, neutropenia, mucositis, and hyperbilirubinemia.

Mercaptopurine (6-MP)

Mercaptopurine is a purine analog.

Mechanism of action
Mercaptopurine is converted into several active metabolites that inhibit RNA and DNA synthesis. As a purine analog it can also interfere with purine biosynthesis. Mercaptopurine is converted to nucleotide metabolites, some of which can lead to DNA toxicity.

Utilized in
Acute lymphoblastic leukemia
Non-Hodgkin lymphoma

Side effects, monitoring, and treatment
Mercaptopurine is generally well tolerated, although myelosuppression occurs commonly. Mercaptopurine is usually administered at night as patients may occasionally complain of anorexia, nausea, and vomiting. Many foods can decrease absorption and therefore administration should be separated from meals. Diarrhea and an erythematous rash may also occasionally occur.

Methotrexate

Methotrexate was the first successful chemotherapeutic agent utilized in children after the observation that folic acid worsened leukemia and dietary deficiency of folic acid could improve leukemia symptoms.

Mechanism of action
Methotrexate inhibits folic acid by preventing the reduction of folic acid by the enzyme dihydrofolate reductase. This inhibition subsequently limits the synthesis of purines and DNA. Some of the methotrexate metabolites also lead to DNA damage.

Utilized in
Acute lymphoblastic leukemia
Acute myelogenous leukemia
Brain tumors
Non-Hodgkin lymphoma
Osteogenic sarcoma

Side effects, monitoring, and treatment
Because of significant enterohepatic circulation of methotrexate, transaminitis is common. Nausea, vomiting, and anorexia may also occur; therefore, oral doses are generally given at bedtime. Many side effects of methotrexate are due to delayed clearance after high-dose IV treatment. Aggressive hydration and alkalinization of fluids can improve renal clearance. Drugs including trimethoprim-sulfamethoxazole, penicillin, nonsteroidal anti-inflammatories (NSAIDs), and proton pump inhibitors (PPIs) can competitively inhibit renal clearance and must be held during high-dose therapy. Leucovorin (folinic acid) is used to decrease many of the toxic effects of folic acid antagonists such as methotrexate. Leucovorin can participate in metabolic reactions requiring folic acid without the necessity of reduction by dihydrofolate reductase which is inhibited by methotrexate. This mechanism of action can also counteract the therapeutic effect of methotrexate; therefore, leucovorin should not be started until 18 to 24 hours after the methotrexate infusion has been completed. For this reason, patients should be advised to not

take folic acid supplements during methotrexate therapy as this may similarly reduce efficacy.

Urine pH should be monitored closely and kept above 7.5 during high-dose therapy to facilitate renal excretion of methotrexate. The patient's intake and output should also be followed. Methotrexate levels are usually drawn starting 24 hours after the infusion is started. Leukemia protocols provide a methotrexate nomogram that allows the practitioner to determine if methotrexate levels are declining appropriately or are in a toxic range requiring an increase in hydration and leucovorin frequency or dose. Rarely, renal failure occurs and can be managed with carboxypeptidase G2. Toxicity is typically worse after delayed clearance and includes severe mucositis and myelosuppression. IT methotrexate often causes nausea and headache. Arachnoiditis occasionally occurs and the patient should be monitored for symptoms including fever, vomiting, and meningismus. Long-term cognitive dysfunction and learning disabilities occasionally occur. Leukoencephalopathy and progressive cognitive deterioration rarely occur, especially in adolescents and adults, with high-dose IV methotrexate and accentuated by cranial radiation therapy. Management of patients with neurotoxicity including seizures, confusion, ataxia, cranial nerve palsies, speech disorders, and paraparesis is controversial. Practitioners may recommend leucovorin rescue after future IT doses or replacement with IT cytarabine, with or without hydrocortisone. Conclusive evidence is lacking on the use of dextromethorphan as a neuroprotectant.

Steroids

Dexamethasone and prednisone are the steroids used most commonly as chemotherapeutic agents.

Mechanism of action

Steroids have a variety of actions on the body. Although not completely understood, steroids are thought to destroy lymphoblasts by binding to the cortisol receptor found on lymphoid cells and specifically in large number on lymphoblasts. Steroids are immunosuppressive and target T-lymphocytes, monocytes, and eosinophils. Steroids may also function by halting DNA synthesis. Dexamethasone has better central nervous system (CNS) penetration than prednisone and has benefit in preventing CNS relapse in ALL.

Utilized in

Acute lymphoblastic leukemia
Hemophagocytic lymphohistiocytosis
Hodgkin and non-Hodgkin lymphoma
Langerhans cell histiocytosis

Side effects, monitoring, and treatment

Steroid treatment results in a multitude of side effects. Common ones include hyperphagia, insomnia, personality changes, adrenal suppression, acne, immunosuppression, and Cushing's syndrome. Occasional side effects include gastritis, hyperglycemia, poor wound healing, facial erythema, striae, thinning of the skin, muscle weakness, osteopenia, and cataracts. Avascular necrosis of various joints, most commonly hips, knees, and ankles, occurs rarely. It is more common in adolescents, and females are at higher risk. It appears to occur more commonly with dexamethasone than with prednisone. Hypertension occurs rarely; blood pressure should be monitored closely in addition to blood glucose. Patients should be on an H_2 blocker (i.e., ranitidine) while receiving daily steroids to prevent gastritis and peptic ulcer disease.

Temozolomide

Temozolomide (Temodar®) is an oral alkylating agent.

Mechanism of action
As with other alkylators, temozolomide leads to DNA interstrand cross-linking.

Utilized in
Brain tumors

Side effects, monitoring, and treatment
Temozolomide commonly causes anorexia, nausea, vomiting, and constipation followed by myelosuppression. Occasionally, temozolomide may cause abdominal pain, diarrhea, headache, and mucositis. Continuous low-dose (metronomic) therapy may be effective in some patients with a decreased side effect profile.

Thioguanine (6-TG)

Like mercaptopurine, thioguanine is an oral antimetabolite and purine analog.

Mechanism of action
Metabolites of thioguanine interfere with purine synthesis and DNA replication. The intercalation of nucleotide metabolites into DNA also leads to DNA strand breaks.

Utilized in
Acute lymphoblastic leukemia
Acute myelogenous leukemia
Non-Hodgkin lymphoma

Side effects, monitoring, and treatment
Thioguanine commonly leads to myelosuppression and occasionally causes fatigue, nausea, vomiting, diarrhea, and anorexia.

Although rare, the patient should be monitored for transaminitis as well as signs of venoocclusive disease (now termed sinusoidal obstructive syndrome) and hepatic fibrosis.

Topotecan

Like irinotecan, topotecan is a semisynthetic analog isolated from the plant alkaloid *C. acuminata*.

Mechanism of action
Topotecan is a potent inhibitor of topoisomerase I that is vital for DNA replication. Inhibition of topoisomerase inhibits replication and also leads to DNA damage.

Utilized in
Brain tumors
Neuroblastoma

Side effects, monitoring, and treatment
Topotecan can commonly cause nausea, vomiting, diarrhea or constipation, fever, pain and later myelosuppression, fatigue, and alopecia. The patient should also be monitored for the occasional findings of headache, rash, hypotension, transaminitis, and mucositis.

Vincristine/Vinblastine

Vincristine and vinblastine are alkaloids isolated from the Madagascar periwinkle plant (*Vinca rosea*, now *Catharanthus roseus*) and therefore often referred to as vinca alkaloids. Vincristine and vinblastine are structurally identical except for a single substitution (a formyl group in vincristine is replaced by a methyl group in vinblastine), which leads to significant differences in their cytotoxic effects.

Mechanism of action

The vinca alkaloids bind to microtubules especially in the mitotic spindle leading to metaphase arrest, thus targeting rapidly dividing cells. They have other disruptive cellular functions that may or may not be related to their effects on tubulin and microtubules.

Utilized in

Acute lymphoblastic leukemia
Brain tumors
Ewing sarcoma
Hepatoblastoma
Hodgkin and non-Hodgkin lymphoma
Langerhans cell histiocytosis
Neuroblastoma
Soft tissue sarcomas
Wilms tumor

Side effects, monitoring, and treatment

Vinblastine more commonly causes myelosuppression, whereas vincristine more commonly causes neurotoxicity including constipation and loss of deep tendon reflexes. Both can lead to alopecia. Jaw pain, peripheral paresthesias, wrist and foot drop, and abnormal gait occasionally occur, especially with vincristine. Ptosis, vocal cord dysfunction, and damage to the eighth cranial nerve (clinically with dizziness, nystagmus, vertigo, and hearing loss) are rare findings. Vinca alkaloids are vesicants; therefore, extravasation, if it occurs, can lead to local ulceration (see Chapter 32 for management of extravasation).

Suggested Reading

Committee on Shortening the Time Line for New Cancer Treatments. National Cancer Policy Board. In: Adamson PC, Weiner SL, Simone JV, Gelband H (eds), Making Better Drugs for Children with Cancer. Washington, DC: National Academies Press, 2005.

31 Guide to Procedures

Patients with suspected or known oncologic or hematologic disease undergo procedures to obtain valuable diagnostic information and receive certain therapies. Traditionally, tumor biopsies are performed under general anesthesia by pediatric surgeons, pediatric orthopedic oncologists, and pediatric interventional radiologists. Pediatric hematology/oncology physicians and their trained staff perform lumbar punctures (LPs) to look for involvement of the cerebral spinal fluid (CSF) by malignancy and to administer intrathecal (IT) chemotherapy. Intrathecal refers to the administration of a drug directly into the subarachnoid space of the spinal column. Drugs are administered in this manner to bypass the blood–brain barrier and therefore be more available for central nervous system (CNS) directed therapy. Currently, there are only three agents licensed for intrathecal chemotherapy: methotrexate, cytarabine (Ara-C), and hydrocortisone. Other common procedures include bone marrow aspiration (BMA) and biopsy and administration of chemotherapy via a peripheral vein or Ommaya reservoir.

Bone marrow examination is required for the diagnosis of leukemia, lymphoma, bone marrow failure states, evaluation of pancytopenia of unknown etiology, suspected storage diseases, and certain cases of anemia. The bone marrow produces the cellular elements of the blood including platelets, red blood cells, and white blood cells in addition to the supporting matrix to allow for cell growth and maturation. Aspirates are routinely obtained for morphologic as well as immunohistochemical and flow cytometric evaluation in patients with suspected leukemia. Those with suspected or known solid tumors, storage diseases, aplastic anemia, or other marrow failure states require evaluation by bone marrow biopsy as well. A core section of the marrow matrix is obtained in order to assess the suitability of the marrow environment for growth of normal cellular elements, the cellularity of the marrow, and the presence of abnormal cells that may be adherent to the trabeculae. Samples are typically taken from more than one site when looking for evidence of marrow involvement by solid tumors in order to increase the sensitivity of the test.

Basic principles for performing such procedures include: (1) ensuring the procedure is indicated for diagnosis, assessment of response to therapy, or for possible relapse; (2) ensuring the proper medication is being administered at the proper time; (3) providing a safe and sterile environment; and, (4) obtaining informed consent with proper documentation. The patient's medical record should be carefully reviewed prior to the procedure and the purpose and nature of the procedure be reviewed with the patient and family. A discussion should be held to review anticipated risks and

Handbook of Pediatric Hematology and Oncology: Children's Hospital & Research Center Oakland,
Second Edition. Caroline A. Hastings, Joseph C. Torkildson, and Anurag K. Agrawal.
© 2012 John Wiley & Sons, Ltd. Published 2012 by John Wiley & Sons, Ltd.

benefits and documented in the medical record with the signed informed consent.

All procedures should be performed or supervised by practitioners with technical expertise. For patients undergoing anesthesia, a skilled caregiver (i.e., anesthesiologist, nurse anesthetist, or critical care physician) should administer the sedation and monitor the patient. In addition to the practitioners performing the procedure and sedation, another skilled caregiver (i.e., nurse or physician) should be present to assist with positioning, sterile transfer of chemotherapy, and general patient care and monitoring. Many centers perform all LPs and BMAs under deep sedation or anesthesia; however, some patients prefer to have these procedures performed awake, or possibly with mild sedation.

Prior to initiation of the procedure, a **time out** should be done to properly identify the patient (hospital wrist band, medical record, and labels on medications) and acknowledge the procedure and informed consent. All materials and medications should be brought into the room and checked by at least two practitioners. If multiple medications are to be administered, care should be taken to avoid an error in administration by bringing in one drug at a time. Standardized procedures should be followed to minimize error. Procedures may be performed in an outpatient or inpatient setting by individuals who have been properly trained and supervised. Many teaching hospitals will also provide a training opportunity for procedures and close supervision by an experienced practitioner is mandatory.

Lumbar puncture/intrathecal chemotherapy

Indications

Patients with suspected leukemia or lymphoma (staging), history of leukemia or CNS lymphoma (treatment or assessment of relapse), CNS malignancy, and therapy complications related to the CNS, specifically infection or neurotoxicity (patients with suspected meningitis, encephalitis, or change in mental status without evidence of increased intracranial pressure).

Pretreatment evaluation

1. Review patient history for use of anticoagulants (should be discontinued with appropriate time interval prior to procedure), seizures, or other CNS concerns including prior complications with LPs or intrathecal chemotherapy. Review of systems to include history of headaches, altered mental status, fevers, bleeding, back pain, or lower extremity weakness.

2. Physical examination should be performed prior to the procedure with special attention to a focused neurologic evaluation with assessment for papilledema or other evidence of increased intracranial pressure such as high blood pressure, widened pulse pressure, or altered level of consciousness. Evaluate vitals and assess for any evidence of infection or metabolic abnormalities to ensure safety for anesthesia. Evaluate site of procedure to assure no localized infection or skin breakdown.

3. Laboratory parameters must be checked to confirm that the chemotherapy should be given (platelet count, absolute neutrophil count, and hemoglobin). A current metabolic panel and coagulation tests should be checked as indicated. Patients with moderate thrombocytopenia (platelet count $< 50 \times 10^9$/L) may need a platelet transfusion, although this varies with the skill of the practitioner and the purpose of the procedure (many practitioners prefer a platelet count $\geq 100 \times 10^9$/L for a diagnostic LP in suspected or newly diagnosed leukemia).

4. The chemotherapy to be administered should be checked on the label to ensure the correct drug, dose, mode of infusion, and patient identification. This should be compared to the patient's medical record and schema sheet to ensure appropriate timing as well.

Materials

1. Standard LP tray, 10 mL sterile syringe for chemotherapy transfer, 22 g spinal needle (1.5 in. for infants, 2.5 in. for older children, longer needles available as needed for larger patients), 25 gauge needle for lidocaine injection if needed, providone iodine and alcohol, mask, and sterile gloves. A Quincke needle is the standard needle used for an LP; however, the pencil point Whitacre needle may be indicated in patients with prior history of severe spinal headache (see below under Post-procedure monitoring).

2. Chemotherapy agent(s) to be administered. Errors have occurred in the past with vincristine being inadvertently administered intrathecally. This is almost uniformly fatal. This drug should never be brought into the room of a patient undergoing an LP with IT chemotherapy.

Procedure

1. Proper positioning is the key to a successful procedure. The lateral decubitus position may be used for a sedated or small patient. The patient should be placed on a firm bed, head flexed with chin to chest, and legs maximally flexed toward the head. Ensure the hips and shoulders are aligned and the back is straight. Alternatively, an awake patient may prefer the sitting position, flexed forward, and supported by the assistant.

2. Identify the landmark with palpation of the interspaces. The L4–5 interspace is located by a perpendicular line at the top of the iliac crests; either this space or the one above (L3–4) may be used.

3. Some centers require the person performing the procedure to wear a mask to prevent infection. Put on sterile gloves and set up the tray.

4. Prepare the skin surface in a sterile manner with providone iodine solution beginning at the site of puncture, working outward with friction. Repeat for a total of three scrubs. The skin may then be cleansed with alcohol. Place a fenestrated drape over the site and ensure an adequate sterile field with additional drapes as desired.

5. Have the assistant transfer the chemotherapy in a sterile manner to the sterile syringe on the tray. Open all CSF collection tubes.

6. Administer local anesthetic with preservative-free 1% lidocaine with a 25 gauge needle, if desired. Awake patients may prefer application of a topical lidocaine anesthetic (LMX or EMLA) or ethyl chloride cold spray. Local anesthesia is not necessary in the anesthetized patient.

7. Insert the spinal needle into the midline of the interspace with the bevel up, directed at a slight (10–20°) angle toward the umbilicus. Ensure the needle is perpendicular to the surface. Advance the needle; if bony resistance is noted, draw back and reposition. The less experienced practitioner should check for CSF flow every 2 to 3 mm by withdrawing the stylet and looking at the translucent window hub for visualization of CSF. If blood is returned, the needle should be removed and the procedure be reattempted one interspace higher. The most experienced practitioner should assume responsibility for subsequent LPs.

8. Once clear CSF return is established, rotate the needle 90° counterclockwise (bevel in transverse plane) for patients in the lateral decubitus position to increase rapidity of CSF flow and allow for easier administration of the chemotherapy. Patients in the sitting forward position do not usually need repositioning of the needle. Obtain the desired amount of CSF in 2 or 3 collection tubes. Traditionally the volume of CSF withdrawn should approximate the volume of medication

administered. CSF should be collected in one tube for a chamber count (red blood cell and white blood cell counts) and a second tube for cytology (assessment of morphology). Additional tubes may be necessary for culture, immunohistochemistry, or any special studies such as myelin basic protein, tumor markers, or research studies. Glucose and protein are checked initially for all patients, though not routinely for leukemia patients receiving intrathecal chemotherapy.

9. For intrathecal administration of chemotherapy, attach the chemotherapy syringe to the spinal needle, ensuring no advancement or withdrawal of the spinal needle and a tight fit to avoid leakage. One can attempt to withdraw CSF to assure proper placement (will see a mix in the syringe) but this may not be possible and is not necessary. Slowly inject the chemotherapy over 1 to 2 minutes. There should be no resistance.

10. Chemotherapy should not be administered when any of the following situations exist: the spinal fluid is bloody indicating puncture of a vessel; the patient is moving not allowing for a safe procedure; the chemotherapy does not advance easily and when the syringe is removed, the flow of CSF has stopped or greatly diminished; the chemotherapy drug or dose is incorrect; or the awake patient experiences pain with injection.

11. Remove the needle. Apply gentle pressure, cleanse as necessary with alcohol, and place a dry sterile dressing.

12. Assess patient for any adverse effect of the procedure. Have the patient in the supine position.

13. Label all CSF tubes and send to the lab.

14. Document the procedure in the medical record.

15. Follow up with the patient and family as to the results of the procedure, including interpretation of the CSF specimens.

Post-procedure monitoring and complications

1. Observe the patient for 1 hour or until fully recovered from anesthesia with appropriate postanesthesia monitoring. Most centers direct that patients remain in a supine position (without head pillow, mild Trendelenburg position) for 1 hour post-procedure to minimize spinal headache and assist with dilution and flow of chemotherapy in the CSF.

2. Patients should be monitored for signs of bleeding, pain at site, headache, nausea, vomiting, or change in neurologic status. In addition to monitoring for post-procedure complications, the patient's cardiovascular and respiratory status should be monitored along with frequent vital signs until recovered from anesthesia.

3. Headache occurs following lumbar puncture in a small percentage of patients, primarily adolescents and females. Typically, onset of headache is within 12 hours to 5 days of the procedure and is due to a slow leakage of CSF from the puncture site (though may not be visible externally). Other symptoms include nausea, vomiting, dizziness, neck stiffness, light sensitivity, and diminished hearing or vision. These symptoms may be worse in a standing position.

   a. Patients are instructed to take fluids liberally in addition to caffeine (highly caffeinated sodas or coffee) with onset of symptoms and after subsequent LPs.

   b. Patients with severe headache or neurologic symptoms should be evaluated immediately. If a postdural puncture headache is suspected, treatment is initiated with caffeine, fluids, and narcotics. If these steps are ineffective, a dural blood patch may be performed by an anesthesiologist to provide immediate relief.

   c. Use of a pencil point spinal needle (Whitacre) for subsequent LPs should be considered for these patients. These needles are designed to spread the dural fibers and help reduce the frequency and severity of postdural headaches. They can be more difficult to use and may require an introducer to puncture the skin and soft tissues.

4. Fever may occur following administration of intrathecal chemotherapy. Some drugs (e.g., cytarabine) have been implicated in causing fever; however, the patient should be assessed for presumed infection. Frequently patients have indwelling central venous catheters and are receiving other immunosuppressive therapy. Evaluation should be comprehensive and may include hospitalization for observation and administration of intravenous antibiotics.

5. Patients may experience pain or bleeding at the LP site for several days. The patient should be evaluated and if experiencing minor bleeding, be treated with local therapy (dry sterile bandaging) and pain medication as needed. Prolonged or heavy bleeding requires immediate evaluation including physical examination and imaging.

6. Neurotoxicity may occur related to the intrathecal medication or related to nerve damage secondary to the procedure. Patients should be evaluated immediately and intervention be taken as appropriate.

Intra-Ommaya reservoir tap and injection of chemotherapy

Indications

See *Lumbar puncture/intrathecal chemotherapy*. The Ommaya reservoir is an intraventricular catheter with a reservoir implanted under the scalp that allows for administration of chemotherapy or other medication directly into the ventricular system, in addition to facilitating sampling the CSF. Although they are placed infrequently, they are useful in the management of patients for whom it is difficult to perform LPs for any reason. They are also used in patients who suffer a CNS relapse of their leukemia and require frequent administration of intrathecal chemotherapy. Practitioners may opt to administer chemotherapy in reduced dosing compared to standard intrathecal dosing (50% to 100% of IT dosing) or give small daily dosing for up to 4 days (based on the concept of concentration × time to optimize therapeutic benefit).

Pretreatment evaluation

The same principles apply as in *Lumbar puncture/intrathecal chemotherapy*. Patients are not sedated for this procedure.

Materials

1. Standard LP tray, two 5 mL sterile syringes for chemotherapy transfer and CSF collection, 25 g butterfly needle, mask, razor, antibacterial soap, 4 × 4 sterile gauze, providone iodine and alcohol, and two sets of sterile gloves.

2. Chemotherapy agent(s) to be administered. *Do not bring vincristine into the room.*

Procedure

1. The patient is placed in a supine or sitting position. If needed, the reservoir area is shaved.

2. Topical anesthesia may be achieved with lidocaine gels (EMLA or LMX) prior to the procedure.

3. While wearing a mask and sterile gloves, the LP tray is set up.

4. Prepare the skin surface overlying the reservoir site by cleansing with sterile gauze moistened with an antibacterial soap in a circular fashion, three times. Change gloves. Continue with a routine sterile prep with three providone iodine scrubs and alcohol wipes. Place a fenestrated drape over the site and ensure an adequate sterile field with additional drapes as desired.

5. Have the assistant transfer the chemotherapy in a sterile manner to the sterile syringe on the tray. Open all CSF collection tubes.

6. Holding the reservoir firmly with one hand, puncture the reservoir site with a 25 g butterfly needle. The CSF is allowed to drip (or is slowly withdrawn) from the butterfly into a sterile tube. The total volume collected should approximate the total volume of chemotherapy and normal saline flush to be delivered. CSF should be collected in one tube for a chamber count and a second tube for cytology. Additional tubes may be necessary for culture, immunohistochemistry, or any special studies such as myelin basic protein, tumor markers, or research studies. Glucose and protein are checked initially for all patients, though not routinely for leukemia patients receiving intra-Ommaya chemotherapy.

7. The chemotherapy is injected over 2 to 3 minutes. Do not give the chemotherapy if the CSF is blood tinged.

8. The needle is removed and firm pressure is applied to the site for several minutes. A spot bandage is applied.

9. Assess the patient for any adverse effects from the procedure.

10. Label all CSF tubes and send to the lab.

11. Follow up with the patient and family as to the results of the procedure, including interpretation of the CSF specimens.

Post-procedure monitoring and complications

1. Document in the patient's chart details of the procedure, chemotherapy administered, specimens collected, and the patient's status after the procedure.

2. See *Post-procedure monitoring for LP* regarding complications such as headache, fever, bleeding, or neurologic changes.

Bone marrow aspiration and biopsy

Indications

The purpose of bone marrow aspiration or biopsy is to obtain tissue for diagnostic and staging evaluation of malignancies, marrow infiltrative diseases, or marrow failure states.

Pretreatment evaluation

1. Review of systems including recent illnesses or back pain.

2. Physical examination should be performed prior to the procedure, with vitals and assessment for any evidence of infection or metabolic abnormalities to assure safety for anesthesia. Evaluate site of procedure to assure no localized infection or skin breakdown.

3. Routine laboratory studies may include a complete blood count, chemistries, and coagulation studies. No specific platelet count is necessary for the procedure. The anesthesiologist will want to ensure an adequate hemoglobin level and be aware of any metabolic abnormalities.

4. The technician to assist with the marrow slide preparation should be present at the start of the procedure with appropriate materials.

Materials

1. Biopsy tray with providone iodine, alcohol, 4×4 gauze, 20 mL syringes (2 to 4 depending on samples to be collected), 16 gauge bone marrow aspirate needle, 11 gauge 4 in. or 13 gauge 3.5 in. Jamshidi biopsy needle (or similar), 22 to 25 gauge needles, sterile gloves, and Elastoplast adhesive or other pressure dressing.

2. EDTA and heparin to anticoagulate samples, lidocaine 1% for local anesthesia.

Procedure

1. Position patient in a prone or lateral decubitus position with a small lift under the hip to accentuate the posterior iliac crests. Identify the posterior superior iliac spine. Have assistant secure patient's position. At times, other locations for bone marrow specimen collection are necessary (infants, children on ventilators, and so on) and may include the anterior iliac spine, tibia, sternum, or other sites.

2. Put on gloves and set up sterile tray.

3. Scrub the site with providone iodine, applying some friction, beginning at the site and moving outward, and repeating for a total of three scrubs. Repeat procedure with alcohol swabs. Allow to dry and apply sterile drapes.

4. Administer local anesthetic with a 22 to 25 gauge needle. This is often done in the sedated patient to minimize post-procedure discomfort. Local anesthesia is achieved with lidocaine 1% (2 to 3 mL depending on size of the patient) injected down to and including the periosteum.

5. Prepare marrow aspirate and/or biopsy needles, ensuring the stylets are freely removable. Prime syringes as per institutional protocol with heparin, EDTA, etc. Ensure inner side of syringe is coated with anticoagulant, if being used.

6. Holding skin taught with outstretched fingers, insert the bone marrow aspiration needle (with stylet in place) initially at an angle to the skin and then perpendicular to the iliac spine once through the skin. With gradual, controlled pressure and a gentle twisting motion, insert the needle into the iliac spine. Once through the cortex, the needle will "give" as it enters the marrow space and a crunching sound or feeling may be appreciated. The stylet should then be removed, and the needle should remain firmly in place. A 20 mL syringe is then firmly attached to the hub of the aspiration needle. Holding onto both the needle and syringe, constant and strong pressure should be applied to draw up marrow into the syringe. If awake, the patient may experience a shooting sensation down the legs at the time of aspiration. Aspirate approximately 1 to 2 mL of marrow, detach the syringe carefully, and hand the specimen immediately to the technician for quick visual inspection for marrow tissue (fat, spicules). Once this has been confirmed, obtain additional marrow as needed with the other primed syringes. Once complete, remove the needle. If marrow is not visible and the sample is thought to represent peripheral blood, reposition the needle and reattempt an aspirate.

7. A bone marrow biopsy may be obtained from the same side and skin puncture site as the aspirate. The needle should be inserted into a fresh spot on the iliac spine (although should utilize the same skin puncture site). Holding the skin tight, insert the bone marrow (trephine) biopsy needle (with cutting trocar in place) holding at an angle until through the skin, then placing perpendicular to the spine and inserting with strong, controlled pressure until the needle is firmly anchored into the cortex. Remove the trocar and holding the forefinger along the needle at the desired depth of the core biopsy (5 to 20 mm depending on size of the patient), insert the needle with a firm twisting pressure. The needle is then rocked in four angles (i.e., sideways as well as up and down) to break off the core marrow biopsy sample at the base and then the needle is removed. The provided push rod (no sharp edge) is inserted into the sharp end of the needle and the biopsy is pushed out gently onto sterile gauze. It is then examined to ensure that adequate marrow tissue is present. If so, it is given to the technician.

8. Apply pressure for several minutes, cleanse the site with alcohol swabs, and apply a Band-Aid. If needed, a dry 4 × 4 folded into quarters may be applied over the

Band-Aid with an elastic tape such as Elastoplast.

9. Assess the patient for any adverse effect of the procedure.

10. Document procedure(s) in the medical record.

11. Follow up with the patient and family to ensure completion of procedure, explanation of any complications, review care of wound, and follow up on results of studies done on specimens obtained.

Post-procedure monitoring and complications

1. Patients may be discharged from the recovery area after appropriate monitoring postanesthesia.

2. The pressure dressing, if used, should be removed after 6 hours and the Band-Aid after 24 hours. The parents should inspect the site for evidence of infection, bleeding, or other drainage. If noted, a practitioner should be contacted and the site be evaluated. Pain medications including acetaminophen, acetaminophen with codeine, or occasionally an intravenous narcotic may be administered for local pain (especially following biopsy). Patients may feel achy or bruised for several days following the procedure. Discomfort can also be alleviated with a warm pack.

3. Patients may resume normal activities as desired.

Administration of peripheral chemotherapy

Indications

Intravenous (IV) chemotherapy may be given into a central venous catheter (CVC) or by peripheral vein administration in patients without a CVC. Many patients may have had their catheters removed due to infection, thrombosis, or electively in order for the patient to resume more normal activities. In the hands of experienced practitioners, administration of push intravenous chemotherapy is a safe alternative to the use of a CVC. Vincristine is frequently administered via peripheral vein in the outpatient setting during maintenance phases of treatment for acute lymphoblastic leukemia. Peripheral access should not be used routinely for infusional chemotherapy due to the difficulty in monitoring and ensuring continued patency of the IV during infusion. Many chemotherapeutic drugs are vesicants and may cause significant injury with extravasation (see Chapter 32).

Pretreatment evaluation

1. Review the patient's chemotherapy regimen to determine what medications are to be administered and at what dose. The patient's height, weight, and total body surface area are verified with the dosage calculations.

2. Ensure that required laboratory criteria have been met (e.g., absolute neutrophil count, platelet count, and transaminases) as directed by the treatment protocol.

3. Complete a physical examination on the patient and assess the adequacy of venipuncture sites.

4. Verify the labels on the syringe(s) of the drug(s) against the patient's chart and orders to ensure accuracy.

5. Prepare the patient for the procedure. Explain the procedure, taking into account the patient's age, developmental status, and prior experience with the procedure. Elicit the patient's help by encouraging him/her to hold as still as possible. Enlist the assistance of the parent(s) and staff (including child life) as needed. Explain each step as you go; be honest, thorough, and patient. Establish a routine with each patient; many also like to have the same practitioner if possible (confidence boosting).

6. Patients desiring topical anesthesia should have a topical lidocaine gel (EMLA or LMX) applied 30 to 60 minutes in

advance of the procedure. This may result in vasoconstriction and increase difficulty of access in some patients.

Materials

1. Chemotherapy (premixed by pharmacy in enclosed syringe).
2. 25 g butterfly needle, stopcock, alcohol wipes, gauze (2 × 2), tourniquet, 10 mL saline flush, bandage, and gloves.

Procedure

1. Assemble equipment; attach butterfly tubing to stopcock, attach chemotherapy syringe to right side of stopcock, attach saline flush syringe to remaining junction of stopcock, and flush stopcock and butterfly with saline.
2. Select an appropriate vein, preferably on the dorsum of the hand or foot. Ask the child to assume a comfortable position that also allows for easy access to the desired vein. Avoid the antecubital fossae or joint spaces due to the possibility of deep extravasation of chemotherapy with resultant injury.
3. Clean the venipuncture site with alcohol and apply tourniquet. Let air dry or wipe dry with clean gauze. Insert butterfly needle with bevel pointed up. Advance needle until blood returns. When blood returns, remove tourniquet, connect stopcock, and flush line with 2 to 3 mL of saline.
4. If no sign of infiltration occurs (e.g., pain or swelling) and blood return continues, administer chemotherapy slowly via IV push, checking intermittently every 5 to 10 seconds for blood return or swelling. When chemotherapy administration is completed, flush with remaining saline.
5. Remove butterfly and apply pressure for 1 to 2 minutes with clean gauze. Apply bandage.
6. Document in the patient's chart the indication for and details of the procedure, medication, dosage, site, and any complications.

Post-procedure monitoring and complications

If infiltration has occurred, see Chapter 32. Areas that may have sustained tissue damage should not be used for future administration of chemotherapy. At times, subclinical burns and scarring may occur and can appear as hyperpigmented areas.

32 Treatment of Chemotherapy Extravasations

Extravasation is the leakage of an intravenous (IV) drug into the surrounding tissues. Local reactions from extravasation of a vesicant chemotherapy agent can range from mild pain and erythema to tissue necrosis, ulceration, and damage to tendons and nerves. Cytotoxic drugs are classified as irritants or vesicants (causing blisters), depending on their potential for local toxicity.

• Extravasation of an **irritant** drug may cause an inflammatory reaction, with pain, burning, tightness, or phlebitis at the needle insertion site or along the vein. Clinical signs include warmth, erythema, and tenderness in the area of extravasation, but there is no tissue sloughing or necrosis. Symptoms are typically of short duration (days) and there are no long-lasting sequelae. An irritant may cause a soft tissue ulcer if a large amount of concentrated drug solution is inadvertently extravasated causing an inflammatory reaction; again, this will not result in persistent tissue damage.

• Extravasation of a **vesicant** drug may cause tissue necrosis with a more severe or lasting injury. Clinical signs and symptoms may be similar to extravasated irritants. Vesicant extravasation may result in loss of the full thickness of the skin and, if severe, underlying structures.

The incidence of vesicant extravasation injury ranges from 0.5% to 6% in peripheral IV infusions and 0.3% to 4.7% in implanted venous access port infusions, although realistically the incidence is likely higher as many milder events may not be reported by patients. Treatment of an extravasation is determined by the particular chemotherapy agent involved, although the efficacy of such therapy may be modest. Prevention is the key, and every possible measure should be taken to avoid such a complication. If it is anticipated that a patient will need frequent or prolonged infusions of vesicants, it is advisable to place a central venous catheter for safer drug administration. Rarely, extravasation may occur even with such a device.

The causes of extravasation are multiple and largely preventable. Factors that place children at risk for peripheral IV extravasation include poor vein selection, multiple venous punctures to establish a patent IV, obesity, dehydration, inability to report pain at the injection site, a moving patient, and inexperience of the individual

Handbook of Pediatric Hematology and Oncology: Children's Hospital & Research Center Oakland, Second edition. Caroline A. Hastings, Joseph C. Torkildson, and Anurag K. Agrawal. © 2012 John Wiley & Sons, Ltd. Published 2012 by John Wiley & Sons, Ltd.

administering the chemotherapy. Risk factors for extravasation from central venous catheters include needle displacement, catheter migration, or fibrin sheath formation and thrombosis. Mechanical occlusions may be due to thrombus formation, drug precipitation, and positional catheter occlusion or kinking of the line. Avoidance of extravasation depends on proper placement and maintenance of IV access and frequent monitoring. Recommendations to **prevent extravasation** are:

- Venipuncture and placement of the cannula or other intravenous access performed by experienced personnel.
- Vesicants should be administered in accordance with the manufacturers' recommendations (e.g., proper dilution and specified administration time) with proper verification and identification (patient and protocol specific).
- Avoid multiple venipunctures in the same area. Do not use a vein distal to a recent venipuncture site as the vesicant may leak from one of these proximal sites.
- Instruct the patient to avoid movement. In young children, this may require additional physical assistance for holding or coaxing with diversion techniques.
- Never use a previously placed IV access device; a new IV cannula should be placed immediately prior to delivery of the medication.
- Choose a large, intact visible vein with good blood flow.
- Use the smallest needle or cannula possible for venipuncture. Check the patency of the device by aspirating blood, as well as patency of the vein by flushing with the carrier solution (normal saline), before administering the medication. Obtain a blood return prior to, and during, vesicant administration.
- The intravenous infusion should flow freely without pressure. The local area should not swell, become erythematous, or cause pain. If this occurs, immediately stop the infusion and attempt to withdraw any medication in the needle/cannula.
- After infusing the medication, flush the vein with 3 to 10 mL of the carrier solution. Do not continue to flush if resistance is met or a local reaction suggesting a blown vein occurs.

Each incident of extravasation should be documented and reported.

Although this complication is frequently encountered with antineoplastic agents, a number of other drugs can also act as vesicants if extravasated into the surrounding tissues. These noncytotoxic drugs include alcohol, aminophylline, digoxin, nafcillin, phenytoin, tetracycline, and total parenteral nutrition. Among cytotoxic drugs that cause extravasation injury, the anthracyclines are among the most important, both because of their widespread use in various chemotherapeutic protocols and because of their ability to produce severe tissue damage and necrosis. The extent of tissue damage depends on the chemotherapeutic agent's binding capacity to DNA.

DNA-binding agents include anthracyclines, antitumor antibiotics, platinum analogues, and some alkylating agents. These drugs cause tissue damage by propagating lethal DNA crosslinking or strand breaks caused by free radicals, which lead to cell apoptosis. As the cells die, the drug is released and enters undamaged cells. This further increases the area of damage and slows healing. Injuries from doxorubicin may continue for weeks.

Non-DNA-binding antineoplastics (vinca alkaloids, taxanes, and topoisomerase inhibitors) also function as vesicants by interfering with mitosis. These agents clear more easily from extravasation sites and cause less damage than the DNA-binding agents. The tissue often resembles a chemical burn and heals more quickly.

Table 32.1 Extravasation treatment.

Drug	Local care	Pharmacologic treatment
DNA-binding vesicants		
Anthracyclines	Cold pack, 20 minutes	Dexrazoxane 1000 mg/m^2 IV within
Doxorubicin	4 times/day × 48–72 hours	6 hour on day 1, repeat day 2;
Daunomycin	Elevate	500 mg/m^2 day 3 *or*
		DMSO 50% topical 1–2 mL within
		10–25 minutes, then q8 hour
		× 7–14 days; allow to dry, then
		apply nonocclusive dressing*
		Do not use Dexrazoxane and DMSO
		concurrently
Alkylating agents	Cold pack, 20 minutes	None
Nitrogen mustard	4 times/day × 48–72 hours	
	Elevate	
Other	Cold pack, 20 minutes	Sodium thiosulfate
Dactinomycin	4 times/day × 48–72 hours	10% 2 mL in 6 mL sterile water for
Mitomycin C	Elevate	IV/SC injection*
Dacarbazine		None
		DMSO as above*
		Hydrocortisone 1% cream topically
Non-DNA binding vesicants		
Vinca alkaloids	Warm pack, 20 minutes	None
Vinblastine	4 times/day × 48–72 hours	Hyaluronidase 150 units in 1 mL
Vincristine	Elevate	injected SC in multiple sites with
Vendesine		small gauge needle*
Taxanes	Cold pack, 20 minutes	Hyaluronidase as above*
Docetaxel	4 times/day × 48–72 hours	
Paclitaxel	Elevate	
Irritants		
Alkylating agents		
Carboplatin, cisplatin	Cold pack as above	Hydrocortisone 1% cream topically
Topotecan		
Ifosfamide, cyclophosphamide	No local care	None
Melphalan	No local care	None
Antimetabolites		
Cytarabine, fludarabine	None	None
Methotrexate, 5-fluorouracil	Cold pack as above	Hydrocortisone 1% cream topically
Gemcitabine	None	None
Other		
Bleomycin	None	None
Etoposide, irinotecan	Cold pack	Hydrocortisone 1% cream topically

*Suggested as possible antidote in the literature; lack of prospective studies to currently advocate as treatment. Abbreviation: SC, subcutaneous.

The **signs and symptoms** of extravasation may be readily apparent with pain and erythema although it may take days for the full extent of the epithelial damage to be evident. Discoloration and skin induration may progress with the development of blisters or necrosis and possibly ulceration or deep tissue injury. Patients may develop scarring or permanent hyperpigmentation at the site of drug extravasation. These sites should not be utilized for subsequent administration of chemotherapy or placement of an IV device.

Treatment should begin immediately with discontinuation of the chemotherapy and cooling or dilution of the site. Initial treatment includes an attempt to aspirate the vesicant with a 10 mL syringe. Clinicians should work quickly to reduce morbidity and avoid further patient harm. Management of nonvesicant extravasation includes elevation and cooling and does not usually include the use of pharmacologic therapy. An exception to the cooling technique is extravasation with vinca alkaloids (see Table 32.1) for which local heat is applied. For other vesicant extravasations, including anthracyclines, initial treatment is geared toward localizing and neutralizing the agent with cold compresses, thus limiting its uptake into cells. The placement of extravasation kits that contain syringes and cannulas, cold and hot packs, gauze pads, sterile and chemoprotective gloves, and medications to treat extravasation in locations where chemotherapy is administered will facilitate early treatment (see Table 32.1). In addition to local care and possible pharmacologic antidotes, topical hydrocortisone 1% and pain medications may alleviate local discomfort.

Suggested Reading

Goolsby TV, Lombardo FA. Extravasation of chemotherapeutic agents: prevention and treatment. Semin Oncol 33:139–143, 2006.

Schulmeister L. Extravasation management. Semin Oncol Nurs 23:184–190, 2007.

Formulary

Sample entry:

Generic name
Trade and other names
Drug category
How supplied
Pregnancy category (see explanation below)
Indications
Dosage
Notes, including adverse events, monitoring, and dose modification

Pregnancy categories:

A. Adequate studies in pregnant women have not demonstrated a risk to the fetus in the first trimester of pregnancy and there is no evidence of risk in later trimesters.

B. Animal studies have not demonstrated a risk to the fetus, but there are no adequate studies in pregnant women; or animal studies have shown an adverse effect, but adequate studies in pregnant women have not demonstrated a risk to the fetus during the first trimester of pregnancy, and there is no evidence of risk in later trimesters.

C. Animal studies have shown an adverse effect on the fetus, but there are no adequate studies in humans; or there are no animal reproduction studies and no adequate studies in humans.

D. There is evidence of human fetal risk, but the potential benefits from the use of the drug in pregnant women may be acceptable despite its potential risk.

X. Studies in animals or humans demonstrate fetal abnormalities or adverse reaction; reports indicate evidence of fetal risk. The risk of use in a pregnant woman clearly outweighs any possible benefit.

ACYCLOVIR

Zovirax
Antiviral
Capsules: 200 mg
Tablets: 400, 800 mg
Suspension: 200 mg/5 mL
Injection: 500 mg vial

Pregnancy category B

Indications:

Treatment of initial, and prophylaxis for recurrent, mucosal and cutaneous herpes simplex virus (HSV-1 and HSV-2) infections, herpes simplex encephalitis, herpes zoster infections, and varicella zoster infections.

Dosage:

Children and neonates:

Mucocutaneous HSV: 750 mg/m^2/day IV divided q8h or 15 to 25 mg/kg/day IV divided q8h for 5 to 10 days

Handbook of Pediatric Hematology and Oncology: Children's Hospital & Research Center Oakland, Second Edition. Caroline A. Hastings, Joseph C. Torkildson, and Anurag K. Agrawal.
© 2012 John Wiley & Sons, Ltd. Published 2012 by John Wiley & Sons, Ltd.

HSV encephalitis: 1500 mg/m²/day IV divided q8h or 30 to 50 mg/kg/day IV divided q8h for 10 days

Neonatal HSV: 1500 mg/m²/day IV divided q8h or 30 to 50 mg/kg/day IV divided q8h for 10 to 14 days

Varicella zoster: 1500 mg/m²/day IV divided q8h or 30 to 50 mg/kg/day IV divided q8h for 7 to 10 days

HSV prophylaxis: 750 mg/m²/day IV divided q8h during risk period or 600 to 1000 mg/day divided q6–8h during risk period

Notes:

Adjust dose in renal impairment. Adequate hydration and slow IV (1 hour) administration are essential to prevent crystallization in the renal tubules. Oral absorption is unpredictable (15% to 30%). Use ideal body weight for obese patients when calculating dosage.

ALLOPURINOL

Zyloprim, Alloprim
Uric acid lowering agent, xanthine oxidase inhibitor, antigout agent
Tablets: 100, 300 mg
Suspension: 20 mg/mL
Injection (Alloprim): 500 mg vial

Pregnancy category C

Indications:

Prevention of uric acid nephropathy in myeloproliferative neoplastic disorders that may occur as a result of tumor lysis syndrome (beginning 1 to 2 days prior to initiation of chemotherapy); prevention of recurrent calcium oxalate calculi; prevention of gouty arthritis and nephropathy.

Dosage:

Children ≤10 years of age:

10 mg/kg/day PO divided q6–8h; maximum dose 800 mg/day or 200 to 300 mg/ m²/day IV q8–24h; maximum 600 mg/day, 300 mg/dose

Children >10 years of age to adult:

600 to 800 mg/day PO q8–12h for the prevention of acute uric acid nephropathy; maximum 800 mg/day, 300 mg/dose *or* 200 to 400 mg/m²/day IV divided q8–24h; maximum 600 mg/day, 300 mg/dose

Notes:

Reduce dosage in renal impairment; discontinue with rash (may be exacerbated with ampicillin or amoxicillin). Risk of hypersensitivity may be increased in patients receiving thiazides/angiotensin-converting enzyme inhibitors. May cause fever, neuritis, gastrointestinal disturbance, hepatotoxicity, bone marrow suppression, and drowsiness. Avoid concomitant use of amoxicillin, ampicillin, mercaptopurine, cyclophosphamide, theophylline derivatives, and vitamin K antagonists.

ALTEPLASE

Tissue plasminogen activator (TPA)
Activase, Cathflo Activase
Thrombolytic
Injection:
Cathflo Activase: 2 mg/2 mL vial
Activase: 50 mg (29 million units), 100 mg (58 million units)

Pregnancy category C

Indications:

Treatment of recent severe or massive deep vein thrombosis (DVT) or arterial thrombosis, pulmonary embolus, or occluded central venous catheter (CVC).

Dosage:

Pulmonary embolus, DVT, central venous thrombosis, superior vena cava syndrome:

Systemic thrombolytic therapy should be given in consultation with a hematologist.

Under 3 months of age: 0.06 mg/kg/hour for 6 to 24 hours

Over 3 months of age: 0.03 mg/kg/hour (max 2 mg/hour)

If no clinical improvement in 24 hours, double the dose to 0.06 to 0.12 mg/kg/hour.

Systemic TPA can be given for up to 96 hours.

In the case of a pulmonary embolus, bolus dosing of 1 mg/kg up to a maximum of 50 mg may be given.

Maximum duration of therapy is 96 hours or based on the patient's clinical course.

Preferable to infuse thrombolytic agent distal to (and as close to) the site of thrombus as possible.

Occluded CVC:
Under 3 months of age: 0.25 mg IV (in 0.5 mL)
Over 3 months of age: 0.5 mg IV (in 1 mL)
Instill a dose in each lumen of the central venous catheter; allow to dwell for 30 minutes. If unsuccessful, repeat dose. If the catheter remains obstructed, begin systemic thrombolytic therapy as outlined above.

Purpura fulminans:
0.5 mg/kg IV infusion over 1 hour, followed by 0.25 mg/kg/hour over 3 hours (total dose 1.25 mg/kg over 4 hours)

Notes:

Avoid central venous puncture and non-compressible arterial sticks during infusion. Avoid use in excessive hypertension, within 10 days of a cerebral vascular accident, with gastrointestinal bleeding or trauma, within 1 week of surgery, in patients with a bleeding diathesis, or with suspicion of a subarachnoid hemorrhage. Plasminogen levels should be followed daily and fresh frozen plasma be given for replenishment if level <50%.

AMIFOSTINE

Ethyol
Antidote for cisplatin, cytoprotective agent
Injection: 500 mg vial

Pregnancy category C

Indications:

A cytoprotective drug that scavenges free radicals and binds to reactive drug derivatives reducing toxicity of radiation and platinum-containing and alkylating agents such as cisplatin, carboplatin, ifosfamide, carmustine, melphalan, mechlorethamine, and cyclophosphamide.

Dosage:

Refer to individual protocol.

Usual dosage is 740 to 910 mg/m^2 IV daily over 15 minutes prior to the dose of a platinum or alkylating agent. Infusions over less than 15 minutes are associated with a higher incidence of adverse reactions.

Notes:

Avoid in hypotension or dehydration. Can cause severe nausea and vomiting and usually requires antiemetic premedication.

AMINOCAPROIC ACID

Amicar
Hemostatic agent
Tablet: 500, 1000 mg
Syrup: 250 mg/mL
Injection: 250 mg/mL (20 mL)

Pregnancy category C

Indications:

Treatment of bleeding resulting from excessive activity of the fibrinolytic system. Typically used to treat mucosal-type bleeding in patients with bleeding diatheses (von

Willebrand disease, mild hemophilia, immune thrombocytopenia purpura).

Dosage:

100 to 200 mg/kg IV/PO loading dose (maximum 10 g), followed by 50 to 100 mg/kg q4–6h maintenance dose; maximum 30 g/24 hour. Treat until symptoms resolve (1 to 14 days).

Low doses (10 mg/kg) have been reported to control bleeding in patients with thrombocytopenia for long periods of time (weeks to months).

Continuous IV infusion:

Loading dose of 100 mg/kg, then 10 to 33 mg/kg/hour in 5% dextrose in water (maximum 1.25 g/hour)

Notes:

May accumulate in patients with decreased renal function and require decreased dosing. Avoid in patients with disseminated intravascular coagulation or hematuria. Increased risk of thrombosis with oral contraceptives, estrogens, and factor IX or prothrombin complex concentrates. May cause nausea, diarrhea, malaise, headache, decreased platelet function, and false increase in urinary amino acids.

AMPHOTERICIN B

Fungizone, Amphocin
Polyene antifungal
Injection: 50 mg vial

Pregnancy category B

Indications:

Treatment of severe systemic infections and meningitis caused by susceptible fungi such as *Candida* species, *Histoplasma capsulatum*, *Cryptococcus neoformans*, *Aspergillus* species, *Blastomyces dermatitidis*, *Torulopsis glabrata*, *Coccidioides immitis*, *Mucormycoses*, and *Rhizopus*. Also used empirically to treat suspected invasive fungal disease in immunocompromised hosts with prolonged fever and neutropenia. May be given intrathecally or via bladder irrigation for localized therapy.

Dosage:

Optional test dose: 0.1 mg/kg to a maximum of 1 mg IV over 20 to 60 minutes

Initial dose: 0.5 to 1.0 mg/kg/day

The daily dose is increased by 0.25 mg/kg until the desired daily dose is reached. In critically ill patients, rapid escalation of dosing may be needed.

Empiric dose is 0.6 mg/kg/day

Therapeutic dose for confirmed invasive fungal infection is 0.6 to 1 mg/kg/day. Daily infusion is over 2 to 6 hours, depending on the infusion tolerability. Salt loading with 10 to 15 mL/kg of normal saline prior to each infusion may prevent hypokalemia and nephrotoxicity. Premedication is frequently needed with acetaminophen and/or diphenhydramine, and if the patient experiences rigors, meperidine hydrochloride may be given. Once therapy has been established, alternate-day dosing may be administered at a dose of 1 to 1.5 mg/kg/every other day.

Notes:

Because of the nephrotoxic potential of this drug, avoidance of other nephrotoxic medications is advised, if possible. Monitor daily electrolytes, renal and hepatic studies, and urine output. Common metabolic abnormalities include hypokalemia, hypomagnesemia, and hypocalcemia. Other problems that may occur are thrombocytopenia, hyperglycemia, diarrhea, dyspnea, back pain, and increases in transaminases and bilirubin. Common *infusion-related toxicities* are fever, chills, rigors, nausea, vomiting, hypotension, and headache. Imidazole derivatives (e.g., miconazole, fluconazole, and ketoconazole) may antagonize the effect and induce fungal resistance to amphotericin.

AMPHOTERICIN B CHOLESTERYL SULFATE

Amphotec
Polyene antifungal
Injection: 50,100 mg vial

Pregnancy category B

Indications:

Treatment of invasive fungal disease in patients who are refractory to or intolerant of conventional amphotericin B.

Dosage:

Start at 3 to 4 mg/kg/day and increase to 6 mg/kg/day if necessary. A test dose of 10 mL of the diluted solution over 15 to 30 minutes is recommended. Give first dose at 1 mg/kg/hour; if well tolerated, the infusion time can be gradually decreased to 2 hours.

Notes:

See Amphotericin B.

AMPHOTERICIN B LIPID COMPLEX

Abelcet
Polyene antifungal
Injection: 5 mg/mL (10, 20 mL)

Pregnancy category B

Indications:

Treatment of aspergillosis or invasive fungal infection in patients who are refractory to or intolerant of conventional amphotericin B therapy. Patients with acute or preexisting renal toxicity (serum creatinine level double that of baseline) should receive this product in lieu of conventional amphotericin B. Higher concentrations are achieved in the spleen, lung and liver, and therefore may be more beneficial in the treatment of hepatosplenic candidiasis. Cerebrospinal fluid (CSF) levels may be lower than with amphotericin B or the liposomal compound.

Dosage:

Usual dose is 2.5 to 5 mg/kg IV once daily over 2 hours. Rate should not exceed 2.5 mg/kg/hour.

Notes:

See Amphotericin B.

AMPHOTERICIN B, LIPOSOMAL

AmBisome
Polyene antifungal
Injection: 50 mg vial

Pregnancy category B

Indications:

Treatment of systemic or invasive fungal infection in patients refractory to or intolerant of conventional amphotericin B. Cerebrospinal fluid concentrations are higher than with other amphotericin products. Higher concentrations in the liver and spleen than with conventional amphotericin B.

Dosage:

Systemic fungal infections: 3 to 5 mg/kg/day IV over 2 hours. Doses as high as 10 mg/kg/day have been used in patients with *Aspergillus* species.

Empiric therapy for fever and neutropenia: 3 mg/kg/day

Infusion may be shortened to 1 hour if well tolerated.

Notes:

See Amphotericin B.

ASPARAGINASE

L-Asparaginase, (Elspar [native or *Escherichia coli*], Erwinase [*Erwinia chrysanthemia*])
PEG-asparaginase (polyethylene glycol asparaginase; Oncaspar)
Antineoplastic, results in asparagine depletion in malignant cells
Injection: 10,000 unit vial (Elspar)
   10,000 unit vial (Erwinase)
   3,750 unit vial (Oncaspar)

Pregnancy category C

Indications:

Treatment of acute lymphoblastic leukemia (ALL). Current and future trials for ALL treatment largely incorporate PEG-asparagase during induction therapy due to an increased rapid early response compared to the native form, prolonged half-life, and decreased likelihood of developing neutralizing antibodies during later phases of therapy. Due to the longer half-life of the pegylated form (5.8 days in children compared to 1.24 days with native and 0.65 days with Erwinase), longer intervals for therapy are suggested. Recent studies have established safety of the intravenous preparation, thereby decreasing the pain associated with intramuscular injection of the drug. Erwinase has traditionally been utilized if hypersensitivity develops to the native or pegylated forms, although its availability may be limited.

Dosage:

Refer to individual protocol.

Usual dose in ALL of PEG-asparagase is 2500 IU/m^2 IV/IM every 2 to 4 weeks (induction, delayed intensification, and interim maintenance phases).

Dose for native (*E. coli*) L-asparaginase is 6000 units/m^2 IM three times a week for nine doses. High-dose protocols may give 15,000 to 20,000 IU/m^2/dose.

Dose for Erwinia L-asparaginase is per protocol.

Maximum 2 mL volume per injection site. Many patients require multiple injections.

IM administration results in delayed peak plasma concentration compared with IV administration.

Patients should be observed in a clinic or hospital setting for at least 1 hour after administration to monitor for a hypersensitivity reaction. Appropriate agents for treatment of hypersensitivity should be readily available (oxygen, epinephrine, antihistamines, intravenous steroids) in addition to resuscitative equipment.

Notes:

Do not give to patients with prior significant pancreatitis associated with asparaginase. Hypersensitivity to *E. coli* or pegylated asparaginase necessitates a switch to the Erwinia form or omission of future doses. Patients who have had a significant hemorrhagic or thrombotic event should have levels of fibrinogen and antithrombin III checked and may be rechallenged with future doses if with improvement in their symptoms and normalization of their laboratory parameters. Use with caution in patients with hepatic impairment or in those receiving other hepatotoxic drugs. Use with caution in patients receiving anticoagulation or nonsteroidal anti-inflammatory agents (NSAIDs). Asparaginase may cause hyperglycemia, hyperuricemia, hyperammonemia, hypofibrinogenemia, thrombosis, hemorrhage, anaphylaxis, and hemorrhagic cystitis. Dexamethasone may alleviate allergic symptoms.

BEVACIZUMAB

Avastin
Angiogenesis inhibitor; monoclonal antibody to vascular endothelial growth factor
Injection: 25 mg/mL

Pregnancy category C

Indications:

Treatment of metastatic colon cancer, lung cancer, and glioblastoma multiforme. Currently being investigated in pediatric protocols for the treatment of brain tumors, refractory or recurrent solid tumors, and neurofibromatosis.

Dosage:

Refer to individual protocol.

15 mg/kg q2 weeks in 28-day cycles as a single agent *or*

5 to 10 mg/kg q2 weeks in combination regimens.

Notes:

Avoid use in patients with recent surgery, hemoptysis, gastrointestinal or central nervous system bleeding, or any other serious bleeding. The interval required between surgery and drug administration to avoid impairment in wound healing has not been determined. General recommendation is to allow 28 days prior to and following major surgery. Use with caution in patients with thrombocytopenia. An increased risk of thromboembolic events have been reported in combination regimens. May impair fertility and have adverse effects on fetal development; adequate contraception must be used during therapy. May cause infusional toxicity (discontinue infusion until symptoms abate) or proteinuria. May potentiate cardiac effects of anthracyclines. Discontinue therapy in patients who develop fistulas, hypertensive crisis, encephalopathy, or nephrotic syndrome.

BLEOMYCIN SULFATE

Blenoxane, generic
Antineoplastic antibiotic
Injection: 15 unit vial (1 unit = 1 mg)

Pregnancy category D

Indications:

Treatment of Hodgkin and non-Hodgkin lymphoma, soft tissue sarcoma, renal cell carcinoma, and germ cell tumor. Used as a sclerosing agent to control malignant effusions.

Dosage:

Refer to individual protocol.

10 to 20 IU/m^2 IV one to two times per week or once every 2 to 4 weeks.

Test dose recommended for lymphoma patients (1 to 2 units for the first 2 doses; if well tolerated, give remainder of dose 1 hour later). Administer over at least 10 minutes, not to exceed 1 IU/minute.

May be given as continuous IV infusion 15 to 20 IU/m^2/day over 24 hours for 3 to 5 days in some protocols.

Notes:

Do not give to patients with known hypersensitivity to bleomycin. Premedication with acetaminophen, hydrocortisone, and antihistamine may decrease infusional toxicity. Dose may need to be modified for renal or pulmonary toxicity. Monitor renal function studies and pulmonary function, including forced expiratory volume in 1 minute, forced vital capacity, and carbon monoxide diffusion in lungs.

BUSULFAN

Myleran, Busulfex
Antineoplastic
Tablet: 2 mg
Injection: 6 mg/ml

Pregnancy category D

Indications:

Treatment of chronic myelogenous leukemia (CML) and for marrow-ablative conditioning regimens prior to bone marrow transplant.

Dosage:

Refer to individual protocol.

For CML induction:

0.06 to 0.12 mg/kg once daily PO (or 1.8 to 4.6 mg/m^2/day); titrate dose to maintain a leukocyte count $>40 \times 10^9$/L and discontinue if the leukocyte count drops to $\leq 20 \times 10^9$/L.

Hematopoietic stem cell transplant regimen: (dose based on actual body weight; adjustments based on therapeutic drug monitoring per protocol)

$\leq$12 kg: 1.1 mg/kg/dose q6h for 16 doses over 4 consecutive days

$>$12 kg: 0.8 mg/kg/dose q6h for 16 doses over 4 consecutive days

Notes:

Do not give to patients with known hypersensitivity to busulfan; should not be used in pregnancy or while nursing. May cause severe bone marrow suppression. Use with caution with other myelosuppressive drugs or radiation. May cause hemorrhagic cystitis. Use with thioguanine may increase hepatic toxicity. Patients with a known seizure history or those at risk for seizures (e.g., sickle cell disease) should be placed on a prophylactic antiepileptic drug while receiving busulfan.

Metabolism of busulfan may be inhibited by antifungal agents (azoles), CYP3A4 inhibitors, dasatinib, and metronidazole leading to increased levels and effect.

Busulfan metabolism may be potentiated by CYP3A4 inducers, deferasirox, and Echinacea, leading to decreased levels and effect.

CARBOPLATIN

Paraplatin-AQ, generic
Antineoplastic, alkylating agent
Injection: 50, 150, and 450 mg vials

Pregnancy category D

Indications:

Treatment of pediatric brain tumors, neuroblastoma, testicular tumors, relapsed leukemia, and solid tumors.

Dosage:

Refer to individual protocol. Many require dose calculation using the modified Calvert formula to achieve the appropriate area under the curve for concentration over time rather than dosing by body surface area. IV administration over 15 minutes to 1 hour is less toxic than bolus dosing.

Solid tumors:

400 to 560 mg/m^2 every 3 to 4 weeks or per protocol

Brain tumor protocols:

175 mg/m^2 weekly for 4 weeks, then 2 week recovery

Dose is adjusted based on suppression of neutrophil and platelet counts or renal toxicity

Bone marrow transplant preparative regimen:

500 mg/m^2/day for 3 days

Notes:

Do not give to patients with known hypersensitivity to carboplatin, cisplatin, or other platinum-containing compounds. Anaphylaxis may occur within minutes of administration. May cause hypotension, electrolyte abnormalities, nausea, hearing loss, and peripheral neuropathy. Severe marrow suppression or vomiting may occur. Reduce dose in impaired renal function (creatinine clearance <60 mL/min) utilizing the modified Calvert formula. Aminoglycosides may increase serum levels/effects of carboplatin and augment ototoxicity and nephrotoxicity; nephrotoxic drugs may increase renal toxicity of carboplatin. Avoid concomitant administration of topotecan and taxanes.

All patients should receive hydration prior to and following administration with sodium chloride containing solution, with or without mannitol and/or furosemide, to ensure good urine output and decrease risk of nephrotoxicity. Reduce dose for young children (<6 months) and with renal impairment. Electrolytes and magnesium should be monitored. Acute leukemia has been reported as a second malignant neoplasm.

CARMUSTINE

BCNU
BiCNU, Gliadel
Antineoplastic, alkylating agent
Injection: 100 mg vial

Pregnancy category D

Indications:

Treatment of brain tumors and Hodgkin and non-Hodgkin lymphoma. Wafer implant (Gliadel) may be an adjunct to surgery and radiation for glioblastoma multiforme and high-grade glioma.

Dosage:

Refer to individual protocol.

Typical dose may be 200 to 250 mg/m^2/dose IV every 4 to 6 weeks.

Bone marrow transplant conditioning regimen: 300 to 600 mg/m^2 divided into 1 to 6 doses, infused over 2 hours and administered 12 hours apart.

Notes:

Do not give to patients with known hypersensitivity to carmustine. Severe, prolonged (6 weeks) marrow suppression may necessitate change in dosing for subsequent cycles. Toxicity is cumulative and delayed pulmonary fibrosis may occur in patients receiving 770 to 1800 mg/m^2. Cimetidine potentiates myelosuppressive effects.

CASPOFUNGIN

Cancidas
Antifungal agent, echinocandin
Injection: 50, 70 mg

Pregnancy category C

Indications:

Treatment of invasive aspergillosis in patients refractory or intolerant to amphotericin B (including lipid formulations) or itraconzaole; candidemia, candidal intra-abdominal abscess, or esophageal candidiasis; empiric therapy of presumed fungal infection in febrile neutropenic patients.

Dosage:

Preterm neonates to infants <3 months: 25 mg/m^2/dose IV once daily

Infants ≥3 months to adults: 70 mg/m^2 loading dose IV, followed by 50 mg/m^2/dose IV once daily

Patients may benefit from increased daily dosing to 70 mg/m^2 once daily dependent on clinical status and response.

Empiric therapy should be given until neutropenia resolves. In neutropenic patients, continue treatment for at least 7 days after signs and symptoms of infection and neutropenia have resolved and at least 14 days following a positive culture in patients with documented fungal infection.

Notes:

Modify dose in patients with hepatic impairment. Drug interactions exist with cyclosporine, tacrolimus, and rifampin and may require dose modification.

CISPLATIN

Platinol, generic
Antineoplastic, alkylating agent
Injection: 50, 100, 150 mg vials

Pregnancy category D

Indications:

Treatment of soft tissue sarcoma, osteosarcoma, Hodgkin and non-Hodgkin lymphoma, brain tumors, germ cell tumor, and neuroblastoma.

Dosage:

Refer to individual protocol. Verify any dosing schedule in which the cisplatin dose exceeds 120 mg/m^2 per course.

Intermittent dosing schedule: 37.5 to 100 mg/m^2 every 2 to 3 weeks

Daily dosing schedule: 15 to 20 mg/m^2/day for 5 days every 3 to 4 weeks

Osteosarcoma and neuroblastoma: 60 to 100 mg/m^2 once every 3 to 4 weeks

Bone marrow transplant: 55 mg/m^2/day continuous infusion for 72 hours (total dose 165 mg/m^2)

The rate of intravenous infusion is dose dependent and ranges from a 15- to 20-minute infusion to a 6- to 8-hour infusion; 24-hour continuous infusions are also used.

Notes:

Do not give to patients with known hypersensitivity to cisplatin or platinum-containing compounds, preexisting renal impairment, hearing impairment, and myelosuppression. Increased risk of nephrotoxicity when given with other nephrotoxic drugs (aminoglycosides and amphotericin B). Reduces renal elimination of methotrexate. Cisplatin may increase the levels/effects of aminoglycosides, taxane derivatives, topotecan, and vinorelbine. Effects or levels of cisplatin may be increased with concomitant administration of loop diuretics.

All patients should receive hydration prior to and for 24 hours after administration with a sodium chloride containing solution (with or without mannitol and/or furosemide), to ensure good urine output and decrease risk of nephrotoxicity. Reduce dose for young children (<6 months) and with renal impairment. Electrolytes and magnesium should be monitored. Acute leukemia has been reported as a second malignant neoplasm.

CLOFARABINE

Clolar
Antineoplastic, antimetabolite
Injection: 1 mg/mL

Pregnancy category D

Indications:

Treatment of relapsed or refractory acute lymphoblastic leukemia, acute myelogenous leukemia, myelodysplastic syndrome.

Dosage:

Children (≥1 year) to adults: 40 mg/m^2/day for 5 days every 28 days or per protocol

Notes:

Cytokine release may develop into a systemic inflammatory response with resultant capillary leak syndrome and organ failure. If this occurs, discontinue clofarabine and initiate therapy with diuretics, corticosteroids, and albumin. If hypotension resolves without pharmacologic intervention, clofarabine may be resumed. The risk for hepatic toxicity and veno-occlusive disease is increased in patients who have previously undergone hematopoietic stem cell transplantion. Avoid concomitant use of nephrotoxic and hepatotoxic drugs.

CYCLOPHOSPHAMIDE

Cytoxan, generic
Antineoplastic, alkylating agent
Tablets: 25, 50 mg
Injection: 500 mg, 1 g, 2 g vials

Pregnancy category D

Indications:

Treatment of Hodgkin and non-Hodgkin lymphoma, acute leukemia, and neuroblastoma. Conditioning therapy for bone marrow transplant. Treatment of nephrotic syndrome, systemic lupus erythematosus, and other rheumatic diseases.

Dosage:

Refer to individual protocol.

Acute lymphoblastic leukemia: 1000 to 1200 mg/m^2/dose, in consolidation and delayed intensification phases

Bone marrow transplant conditioning: 50 mg/kg/day IV for 3 to 4 days

Nephrotic syndrome: 2 to 3 mg/kg/day orally for up to 12 weeks

Systemic lupus erythematosus: 500 to 750 mg/m^2 IV monthly; maximum dose 1 g/m^2

Juvenile idiopathic arthritis/vasculitis: 10 mg/kg IV every 2 weeks

Notes:

Do not give to patients with known hypersensitivity to cyclophosphamide. Dose may need to be adjusted for myelosuppression or impaired renal function. Mesna should be given with high-dose therapy (>1 g/m^2/day) to reduce potential of hemorrhagic cystitis. Allopurinol may increase the myelotoxicity of cyclophosphamide by inhibiting its metabolism. Ensure aggressive hydration with sodium chloride containing fluids and frequent bladder emptying.

CYCLOSPORINE

Sandimmune, Neoral, Gengraf
Immunosuppressant
Capsules: 25, 50, 100 mg
Solution: 100 mg/mL
Injection: 50 mg/mL

Pregnancy category C

Indications:

Used with corticosteroids to prolong organ and patient survival in kidney, liver, heart, and bone marrow transplants; treatment of aplastic anemia and other bone marrow failure syndromes.

Dosage (Sandimmune):

Due to better absorption, lower doses of Neoral and Gengraf may be required compared to Sandimmune.

Oral:

Initial: 15 mg/kg single oral dose, beginning 4 to 12 hours pretransplant

Maintenance: 15 mg/kg/day PO for 1 to 2 weeks posttransplant, decrease by 5% per week to 3 to 10 mg/kg/day

Intravenous:

Initial: 5 to 6 mg/kg IV single dose, administered over 2 to 6 hours, beginning 4 to 12 hours pretransplant. Continue same IV dose posttransplant until patient able to tolerate oral form.

Conversion from IV to PO dose (1:3 ratio): Multiply total daily IV dose by 3 and administer in two divided oral doses per day.

Notes:

Do not give to patients with known hypersensitivity to cyclosporine (castor oil is an ingredient in the preparation). May cause nephrotoxicity, hepatotoxicity, hypomagnesemia, hyperkalemia, hyperuricemia, hypertension, hursuitism, acne, gastrointestinal symptoms, tremor, leukopenia, headache, and gingival hyperplasia. Use with caution with concomitant administration of other nephrotoxic drugs (e.g. amphotericin B, aminoglycosides, tacrolimus, acyclovir, NSAIDs). Requires close monitoring of renal and hepatic function and frequent determination of trough levels (drawn just prior to dose at steady state).

Cyclosporine is a substrate for the cytochrome P450 3A4 oxidase system. Drug interactions include ketoconazole, itraconazole, fluconazole, erythromycin, and methylprednisolone, which increase the cyclosporine concentration by inhibiting hepatic metabolism. Cimetidine may increase cyclosporine concentration. Refer to the Physicians' Desk Reference for more extensive drug interaction information.

CYTARABINE HYDROCHLORIDE

Ara-C
Cytosar-U, generic
Antineoplastic, antimetabolite
Injection: 100 and 500 mg, 1 and 2 g vials

Pregnancy category D

Indications:

Treatment of acute lymphoblastic and myelogenous leukemia (ALL and AML), refractory non-Hodgkin lymphoma, and may be used in conditioning regimens for bone marrow transplantation. High doses penetrate the blood–brain barrier into the cerebrospinal fluid.

Dosage:

Refer to individual protocol.

Infants under 3 years:

3.3 mg/kg/day IV/SC for 4 days (dose reduced in children with Down syndrome)

Children and adults:

Remission induction:

200 mg/m^2/day for 5 days at 2-week intervals as a single agent; 100 to 200 mg/m^2/day (or 2 to 6 mg/kg/day) for 5 to 10 days or every day until remission (as a part of combination chemotherapy). Give IV continuous infusion or every 12 hours.

Maintenance:

1 to 1.5 mg/kg IM/SC as a single dose at 1- to 4-week intervals or 70 to 200 mg/m^2/day for 2 to 5 days at monthly intervals

High-dose cytarabine: (AML, relapsed or refractory ALL, non-Hodgkin lymphoma) 3 g/m^2/dose q12h for up to 12 doses

For central nervous system (CNS) treatment and prophylaxis (intrathecal dose): Dosing per age

Drug may be combined with other intrathecal agents such as hydrocortisone and methotrexate per protocol

Children <1 year: 20 mg

Children 1 to <2 years: 30 mg

Children 2 to <3 years: 50 mg

Children ≥3 years and adults: 70 mg

Notes:

Do not give to patients with known hypersensitivity to cytarabine. May need to reduce dose with myelosuppression or hepatic dysfunction. Causes significant bone marrow suppression. High doses have been associated with gastrointestinal, CNS, pulmonary, and ocular toxicities as well as cardiomyopathy. May cause nausea, vomiting, mucositis, fever, headache, somnolence, anorexia, alopecia, conjunctivitis, ataxia, diarrhea, hepatic dysfunction, and peripheral neuropathy. Prophylaxis with dexamethasone ophthalmic drops may decrease effects of conjunctivitis.

When prepared for intrathecal use, added precautions should be taken when other medications are also being delivered to ensure appropriate labeling and handling such that only medications intended for administration in the CNS are with the patient for the procedure.

DACARBAZINE

DTIC
Antineoplastic
Injection: 100, 200 mg

Pregnancy category C

Indications:

Treatment of Hodgkin lymphoma and solid tumors.

Dosage:

Refer to individual protocol.

Solid tumors:

200 to 470 mg/m²/day IV over 5 days every 3-4 weeks

Neuroblastoma:

800 to 900 mg/m² IV as a single dose on day 1 of the cycle every 3 to 4 weeks

Hodgkin lymphoma:

375 mg/m² on days 1 and 15 of each course, repeated every 28 days

Notes:

Do not give to patients with known hypersensitivity to dacarbazine. Dosage reduction may be necessary in patients with renal or hepatic insufficiency. Drug extravasation may result in tissue damage and severe pain.

DACTINOMYCIN

Actinomycin D
Cosmegen
Antineoplastic antibiotic
Injection: 500 mg vial

Pregnancy category D

Indications:

Treatment of Wilms tumor, rhabdomyosarcoma, Ewing sarcoma, ovarian germ cell tumor, and gestational trophoblastic neoplasm.

Dosage:

Refer to individual protocol. *Note that medication orders for dactinomycin may be written in micrograms (mcg) or milligrams (mg).*

Children over 6 months to adult:

15 mcg/kg/day or 400 to 600 mcg/m²/day once daily for 5 days; repeat every 3 to 6 weeks. Higher doses are given in some protocols.

Notes:

Do not give to patients with known hypersensitivity to dactinomycin. Avoid in infants <6 months of age because of increased adverse events. Use with caution in patients with hepatobiliary dysfunction or who have received radiation (radiation recall effect). Reduce dosage in patients receiving concurrent radiation. Avoid extravasation. May cause myelosuppression, anorexia, vomiting, diarrhea, and stomatitis.

DAPSONE

Generic
Antibacterial
Tablet: 25, 100 mg

Pregnancy category C

Indications:

Prevention and treatment of *Pneumocystis jiroveci* pneumonia (PCP) in immunocompromised hosts; treatment of *Toxoplasma gondii* and *Mycobacterium leprae.*

Dosage:

Children 1 month to <12 years: 2 mg/kg/day or 4 mg/kg/dose once weekly (maximum 100 mg/dose daily or 200 mg/dose weekly)

Children >12 years and adults: 100 mg/day or 200 mg once weekly

Notes:

Do not give to patients with known hypersensitivity to dapsone. Dapsone is a strong oxidizing agent and may cause hemolysis in susceptible individuals. Screening for glucose-6-phosphate dehydrogenase (G6PD) deficiency is suggested in high-risk populations (e.g., Mediterranean) and should not be used if positive. May be safe to use in the African-American variant of G6PD deficiency though some degree of hemolysis may occur. May also cause marrow suppression or methemoglobinemia. Drug interactions occur, primarily with rifampin. May be given to immunosuppressed patients who cannot tolerate or are allergic to cotrimoxazole.

DAUNORUBICIN HYDROCHLORIDE

Cerubidine
Antineoplastic antibiotic, anthracycline
Injection: 20 mg vial

Pregnancy category D

Indications:

Treatment of acute lymphoblastic and acute myelogenous leukemia (ALL and AML); used in combination with other chemotherapeutic agents during ALL and AML induction therapy.

Dosage:

Refer to individual protocol.

Infants <2 years or <0.5 m² should have dosing based on body weight:

0.67 mg/kg/day IV with frequency dependent on protocol

Children ≥2 years:

25 to 60 mg/m² IV with frequency dependent on protocol

Notes:

Do not give to patients with known hypersensitivity to daunorubicin, congestive heart failure, arrhythmias, or preexisting bone marrow suppression. Reduce dosage in patients with hepatic, biliary, or renal impairment. May cause myelosuppression, nausea, vomiting, alopecia, stomatitis, and pigmentation of nail beds. Irreversible myocardial toxicity may occur as the cumulative dosage approaches 550 mg/m² (or 400 mg/m² with chest irradiation or concomitant cyclophosphamide administration; based on anthracycline dose equivalents, see

Chapter 30). This may be an acute or late effect and monitoring with ECHO or MUGA and ECG is required per protocol. Secondary leukemia has been reported.

Extravasation may result in severe local tissue necrosis and require intervention. A transient red-orange discoloration of the urine, sweat, saliva, and tears may occur for up to 48 hours after a dose.

DEFEROXAMINE MESYLATE

Desferal
Chelating agent; antidote, iron toxicity
Injection: 500, 2000 mg

Pregnancy category C

Indications:

Treatment of acute iron intoxication and chronic transfusional iron overload.

Dosage:

Chronic iron overload:

25 to 60 mg/kg/day SC/IV over 8 to 24 hours; maximum 2 g/24 hours

Notes:

Avoid in severe renal disease, anuria, or primary hemochromatosis. Prolonged use can result in cataracts, decreased visual acuity, impaired peripheral, night, and color vision, and neurotoxicity-related auditory abnormalities (i.e., high-frequency hearing loss). Periodic hearing and vision exams should be performed. High doses (>60 mg/kg) especially in children ≤3 years have been associated with growth retardation; reduction in dosage may increase growth velocity.

Discontinue use in febrile patients because of increased susceptibility to infection with *Yersinia enterocolitica*. Avoid rapid IV administration as flushing, urticaria, hypotension, and shock have been reported.

DEFERASIROX

Exjade

Chelating agent, iron; antidote, iron toxicity

Tablet, for oral suspension: 125, 250, 500 mg

Pregnancy category C

Indications:

Treatment of chronic iron overload due to blood transfusions.

Dosage:

Children ≥2 years to adults: 20 to 40 mg/kg daily (round to nearest whole tablet)

Initiate therapy at 20 mg/kg/day. Adjust dose every 3 to 6 months based on serum ferritin levels or other measurement of iron overload; increase by 5 to 10 mg/kg/day (round to nearest whole tablet). Consider higher doses for ferritin >2500 ng/mL. Consider holding dose or discontinuing for ferritin <500 ng/mL. Maintenance range: 20 to 40 mg/kg/day.

Consider giving daily dose divided BID to patients experiencing abdominal discomfort or nausea and vomiting.

Do not chew or swallow whole tablets. Disperse tablets in water, apple juice, or orange juice (use 3.5 ounces for doses <1 g; 7 ounces for doses ≥1 g); stir to form suspension and drink entire contents. Rinse remaining residue in glass and drink. Administer at the same time every day, at least 30 minutes prior to food ingestion.

Notes:

Do not give to patients with known hypersensitivity to deferasirox, low platelet counts ($<50 \times 10^9$/L), creatinine clearance <40 mL/min, or serum creatinine >2× age-appropriate upper limit of normal. Assess patients for renal impairment and concurrent nephrotoxic drugs. May cause intermittent proteinuria. Monitor serum electrolytes and urinalysis. Use with caution in patients with hepatic disease as well as in patients with concomitant anticoagulant, NSAID, or corticosteroid use. Monitor transaminases and liver function. May cause ocular or auditory disturbances, skin rash, gastrointestinal pain, headache, diarrhea, sore throat, nausea, and vomiting. Interruption or dose modification may be necessary for evidence of renal, hepatic, or gastrointestinal dysfunction.

DESMOPRESSION ACETATE

DDAVP, Stimate

Antihemophilic, hemostatic agent

Injection: 4 mg/mL (1 mL)

Tablets: 0.1, 0.2 mg

Solution: 1500 mcg/mL, 150 mcg/spray (25 sprays, 2.5 mL) (Stimate)

100 mcg/mL, 10 mcg/spray (50 sprays, 5 mL, with rhinal tube) (DDAVP)

Pregnancy category B

Indications:

Intranasal Stimate or IV DDAVP are indicated for maintenance of hemostasis in patients with mild or moderate hemophilia A during surgery and postoperatively as well as treatment of mucosal bleeds in patients with von Willebrand disease and mild hemophilia A. DDAVP is indicated for the treatment of central diabetes insipidus and primary nocturnal enuresis.

Dosage:

Von Willebrand disease, hemophilia A, bleeding diathesis:

IV: 0.3 mcg/kg, dilute in normal saline (10 mL for patients <10 kg and 50 mL for ≥10 kg), infuse slowly over 15 to 30 minutes

or

Intranasal spray (Stimate): one puff (150 mcg) for children under 50 kg and 2 puffs (300 mcg) for children over 50 kg

Peak effect is 1 to 5 hours with intranasal route, 1.5 to 3 hours with IV route, and 2 to 7 hours with PO route. Duration of effect is 5 to 24 hours. Tachyphylaxis may occur with repeated dosing within 72 hours.

Diabetes insipidus:

Children ≤12 years: Start with 0.05 mg/dose BID and titrate to effect (i.e., control of excessive thirst and urination); usual dose range is 0.1 to 0.8 mg/24 hours.

Children >12 years and adults: Start with 0.05 mg/dose BID and titrate to effect; usual dose range is 0.1 to 1.2 mg/24 hours divided BID or TID or

Children 3 months to 12 years: 5 to 30 mcg/24 hours intranasally divided BID.

Children >12 years and adults: 10 to 40 mcg/24 hours intranasally divided daily to TID; titrate dose to effect.

Nocturnal enuresis (≥6 years):

0.2 mg PO at bedtime, titrate to effect (maximum dose 0.6 mg) or

20 mcg intranasal at bedtime; divide and administer 10 mcg in each nostril.

Notes:

Do not give to patients with known hypersensitivity to desmopressin. Avoid in patients with severe type I, type IIB, or platelet-type von Willebrand disease, hemophilia B, and severe hemophilia A (<1% factor VIII activity). Patients with moderate hemophilia A may not demonstrate an adequate response. Use cautiously in patients with a predisposition to thrombophilia, electrolyte imbalance, and hypertensive cardiovascular disease. May cause headache, nausea, emesis, seizures, blood pressure changes, hyponatremia, nasal congestion, abdominal cramps, and hypertension. Avoid in young children <2 years due to hyponatremia and seizures. Not FDA approved in <6 years for treatment of nocturnal enuresis.

A desmopressin challenge to document responsiveness to these agents is indicated in patients with bleeding disorders to document benefit prior to emergent use.

Note: intranasal forms come in two concentrations, use as specifically indicated.

DEXAMETHASONE

Decadron, generic
Corticosteroid, anti-inflammatory, immunosuppressant
Tablets: 0.25, 0.5, 0.75, 1.5, 2, 4, 6 mg
Solution: 1 mg/mL
Ophthalmic solution: 0.1% (5 mL)
Injection: 4 mg/mL

Pregnancy category C

Indications:

Used systemically for chronic inflammation, allergic, hematologic, neoplastic (e.g., leukemia), autoimmune disease, cerebral edema and increased intracranial pressure, and septic shock. Utilized as an antiemetic for chemotherapy-induced nausea and vomiting and as an ophthalmic solution for control of chemical conjunctivitis from concomitant administrations of agents such as high-dose cytarabine.

Dosage:

Antiemetic:

0.2 mg/kg/dose (5 mg/m^2/dose) IV 30 minutes prior to and every 6 hours after chemotherapy

Brain tumor associated cerebral edema:

Loading dose: 1 to 2 mg/kg IV as a single dose; *maintenance:* 1 to 2 mg/kg/day IV in 4 to 6 divided doses for 1 to 5 days, or longer; maximum dose 16 mg/24 hours

Spinal cord compression with neurologic abnormalities:

2 mg/kg/24 hours IV divided q6 hours

Chemotherapy:

Refer to individual protocol.

Doses range from 6 to 20 mg/m^2/day for 5 to 7 days (may be longer in induction therapy for acute lymphoblastic leukemia).

Ophthalmic use:

Instill 1 to 2 drops into the conjunctival sac bilaterally. May use q1–2 hours as needed to prevent and control symptoms.

Notes:

Do not administer during active, untreated infections with viral, fungal, or bacterial organisms. Prolonged use may cause bone pain, glucose intolerance, hypertension, fat redistribution and striae, and avascular necrosis of bone.

DEXRAZOXANE

Zinecard, generic
Antidote, anthracycline; antidote (anthracycline extravasation)
Injection: 250, 500 mg

Pregnancy category C/D

Indications:

Reduction of anthracycline-induced cardiotoxicity. Treatment for local tissue extravasation of anthracyclines. Currently, FDA approved in adults only.

Dosage:

Refer to individual protocol.

Children and adults: 10:1 dose ratio with doxorubicin for acute lymphoblastic leukemia (ALL; i.e., 300 mg/m^2 dexrazoxane for 30 mg/m^2 doxorubicin). Complete anthracycline administration within 30 minutes of start of dexrazoxane.

Treatment for extravasation: Adolescents ≥18 years to adults: 1000 mg/m^2/dose within 6 hours on days 1 and 2; maximum dose

2000 mg; followed by 500 mg/m^2/dose on days 3; maximum dose 1000 mg.

Do not use dimethylsulfoxide (DMSO) in patients receiving dexrazoxane for anthracycline-induced extravasation.

Notes:

Limited experience in pediatrics (high risk acute lymphoblastic leukemia). Use only in patients with a cumulative doxorubicin dose of 300 mg/m^2 who are continuing to receive anthracyclines or as directed by protocol. Dose-limiting toxicity is myelosuppression, which may be additive to chemotherapy. May chelate heavy metals, leading to increases in calcium, iron, and triglycerides and decreases in sodium and zinc. May have antitumor effects.

DIMETHYL SULFOXIDE

DMSO
Antidote (anthracycline extravasation)
Topical: 50% solution

Pregnancy category C

Indications:

Used after cooling for local control of extravasation of anthracyclines. May also be indicated for extravasation of ifosfamide, cisplatin, fluorouracil, and carboplatin.

Dosage:

Apply 1 to 2 mL within 10 to 25 minutes to affected area, then every 4 to 8 hours for 7 to 14 days, until resolution. Allow to dry and apply clean, dry dressing. Vitamin E or aloe vera have been used topically following the first application to alleviate local burning or stinging (ensure DMSO has dried).

Notes:

The role of DMSO in the treatment of anthracycline extravasation remains controversial. *Do not use with dexrazoxane. Use with local cooling of tissues.*

DIMERCAPROL

British anti-Lewisite (BAL)
Chelating agent (antidote for gold, mercury, lead, and arsenic toxicity)
Injection: 100 mg/mL

Pregnancy category C

Indications:

Antidote to gold, mercury, and arsenic poisoning; used in conjunction with edetate calcium disodium to treat severe lead poisoning.

Dosage:

For severe lead poisoning (lead level ≥70 mcg/dL) or encephalopathy:

25 mg/kg/day divided q4h *deep IM* for a minimum of 72 hours, may give up to 5 days in severely symptomatic patients. Calcium sodium EDTA should be started at a dose of 50 mg/kg/day continuous IV infusion immediately after the second dimercaprol dose. If symptoms of encephalopathy persist, a second course of treatment can begin after a minimum of 2 days of rest following the initial 5-day course. Therapy should be continued until the patient is clinically stable. Once this occurs, a 10- to 14-day period of equilibration should occur before again measuring the lead level. If the level remains ≥70 mcg/dL, another course of double therapy should be provided.

Less severe lead poisoning (45 to <70 mcg/dL):

Treatment with dimercaprol is not recommended in this situation due to toxicity; patients should be treated with succimer or calcium disodium EDTA instead.

Notes:

Do not give to patients with hepatic or renal insufficiency. Do not use in iron, selenium, or cadmium poisoning. *Use with caution* in patients with G6PD deficiency (may cause hemolysis) and peanut sensitivity. Hydrate and alkalinize urine to protect the kidneys. May cause hypertension, tachycardia, gastrointestinal disturbance, headache, fever, transient neutropenia, and nephrotoxicity. Symptoms may be relieved by antihistamines. *Ensure calcium salt is given if edetate calcium disodium is used in conjunction with BAL.*

DIPHENHYDRAMINE

Benadryl, generic
Antihistamine
Capsules/tablets (OTC): 25, 50 mg
Chewable tablets: 12.5 mg
Elixir: 12.5 mg/5 mL
Injection: 50 mg/mL

Pregnancy category B

Indications:

Treatment of allergic symptoms, anaphylaxis, medication and transfusion reactions, chemotherapy and other induced nausea and vomiting, and motion sickness; used as an antitussive or for mild sedation. Prevents or treats metocloperamide- and phenothiazine-induced dystonic reactions.

Dosage:

Antiemetic and antivertigo:

0.5 to 1 mg/kg/dose q6h PO, IM, or IV

Pruritus:

0.5 to 1 mg/kg/dose q6h PO, IM, or IV

Notes:

Do not give to patients with known hypersensitivity to diphenhydramine. Do not use with concurrent MAO inhibitors, in acute attacks of asthma, or in patients with GI or urinary obstruction. Use with caution in patients with glaucoma, peptic ulcer disease, urinary tract obstruction, and hyperthyroidism. Avoid alcohol. Note: many preparations contain alcohol. May cause sedation, nausea, vomiting, xerostomia, blurred vision, and central nervous system effects. May cause paradoxical activation in children.

DOXORUBICIN HYDROCHLORIDE

Adriamycin, Doxil (liposomal formulation)
Antineoplastic antibiotic, anthracycline
Injection: 10, 50 mg vials (protect from light)

Pregnancy category D

Indications:

Treatment of acute lymphoblastic leukemia, acute myelogenous leukemia, lymphoma, Wilms tumor, and sarcoma.

Dosage:

Refer to individual protocol.

20 to 90 mg/m^2 IV in repeated doses (may be weekly or monthly or per phase of therapy). Infusions may be over 15 minutes, several hours, or as a continuous infusion over 24 to 48 hours. Although controversial, longer infusions may be more cardioprotective, especially when high cumulative doses (i.e., >450 mg/m^2) are anticipated. Children <12 kg and infants are dosed based on weight rather than body surface area. The use of cardioprotective agents such as dexrazoxane is being studied in pediatric trials.

Notes:

Do not give to patients with known hypersensitivity to doxorubicin, severe congestive heart failure or cardiomyopathy, or preexisting myelosuppression. Use with caution in patients who have received very high cumulative doses of anthracyclines (i.e., ≥550 mg/m^2 or ≥400 mg/m^2 with concomitant use of cyclophosphamide or chest radiation; based on anthracycline dose equivalents, see Chapter 30). Monitor

ECHO or MUGA and ECG after every 75 to 100 mg/m^2 of anthracycline given. Cardiac toxicity may be acute or delayed and long-term monitoring is essential.

Modify dosage in renal impairment. May cause severe bone marrow suppression, alopecia, mucositis, and transient (48 hour) red-orange discoloration of the urine, sweat, saliva, and tears. Extravasation may result in severe local tissue necrosis. May cause photosensitivity reactions and patients should be instructed to avoid excessive exposure to sunlight and utilize sunblock (SPF ≥ 15).

DRONABINOL

Marinol, tetrahydrocannabinol
Cannabinoid
Capsules: 2.5, 5, and 10 mg

Pregnancy category C

Indications:

Treatment of nausea and vomiting associated with chemotherapy in patients who have failed to respond to conventional antiemetic therapy; treatment of anorexia associated with weight loss in patients with human immunodeficiency virus (HIV). Evidence of benefit in chemotherapy-induced anorexia is mixed; no well-controlled studies have been performed in children.

Dosage:

Antiemetic:

5 mg/m^2/dose 1 to 3 hours prior to chemotherapy, then q2–4h; maximum 6 doses/24 hour, 15 mg/m^2/dose in adults. Titrate dose to effect.

Appetite stimulant:

Adult dosing: 2.5 mg BID 1 hour prior to lunch/dinner; if not tolerated, reduce dose to 2.5 mg qhs; maximum dose 20 mg/24 hour.

Notes:

Do not give to patients with known hypersensitivity to any cannabinoid or sesame oil. Do not use in patients with history of substance abuse or mental illness. Use with caution in heart disease, seizures, and hepatic disease. A dose-related "high" (easy laughing, elation, or heightened awareness) is reported in one-quarter of patients using cannabinoids as antiemetics. Other side effects include dizziness, anxiety, difficulty concentrating, hypotension, and increased appetite. Psychological and physiologic dependence may occur, but addiction is uncommon. It is a controlled (Schedule III) substance.

EDETATE CALCIUM DISODIUM

Calcium EDTA, CaNa$_2$EDTA
Calcium disodium versenate
Heavy metal antagonist; antidote, lead toxicity
Injection: 200 mg/L

Pregnancy category B

Indications:

Used as an adjunct in the treatment of acute and chronic lead poisoning.

Dosage:

For severe lead poisoning (lead level ≥70 mcg/ dL) and/or encephalopathy:

50 mg/kg/day (continuous IV infusion) given in combination with dimercaprol (BAL). *Give at a separate site starting with the second dimercaprol dose.*

Less severe lead poisoning (45 to <70 mcg/dL):

25 mg/kg/day as a continuous or intermittent IV infusion

Notes:

Do not give to patients with severe renal disease or anuria. Requires inpatient admission with aggressive intravenous hydration and frequent monitoring of serum electrolytes including calcium and phosphorus, renal function, and urinalyses. Establish urine flow prior to administration and maintain hydration/urine output throughout course of therapy. Dose reduction is recommended for mild renal disease. Monitor with continuous ECG due to risk for arrhythmias. Rapid IV infusion can result in sudden increase in intracranial pressure in patients with cerebral edema. May cause zinc and copper deficiency. May be administered IM; give with 0.5% prilocaine. *Ensure calcium salt is given.*

ENOXAPARIN

Lovenox
Anticoagulant, low-molecular-weight heparin (LMWH)
Injection (prefilled syringe): 30 mg/0.3 mL, 40 mg/0.4 mL, 60 mg/0.6 mL, 80 mg/0.8 mL, 100 mg/mL
Approximate anti-factor Xa activity: 100 IU/mg

Pregnancy category B

Indications:

Prophylaxis and treatment of thromboembolic disorders such as deep vein thrombosis (DVT) following surgery or trauma and pulmonary embolus.

Dosage:

Treatment of DVT or thromboembolus (TE):

Infants <1 month: 1.625 mg/kg q12h SC

Infants 1 to 12 months: 1.5 mg/kg q12h SC

Children 1 to 6 years: 1.375 mg/kg q12h SC

Children 6 to 21 years: 1.25 mg/kg q12h SC

Titrate dose to achieve peak anti-factor Xa levels of 0.5 to 1.0 U/mL. Peak anti-factor Xa levels should be drawn 4 hours after administration of a steady state dose (minimum 2 to 3 prior doses).

See Chapter 10 for further guidelines. Some centers advocate that TPA be given concomitantly with enoxaparin in high risk situations (i.e., large central embolism). Prophylaxis or treatment with enoxaparin may continue for prolonged periods dependent on the underlying risks for thrombophilia and response to therapy. For those patients that will be maintained with oral anticoagulation (e.g., warfarin), 4 to 5 days of overlap with enoxaparin should be given in order to achieve a therapeutic international normalized ratio (INR).

DVT/TE prophylaxis:

0.5 mg/kg q12h SC

Anti-factor Xa levels do not need to be followed in patients on prophylactic dosing. Data is limited but 1 mg/kg once daily dosing can be considered in patients with compliance issues and in those with difficulty giving twice daily SC injections. An insuflon catheter should also be considered.

Note: LMWH may be given IV at the same dose as SC.

Notes:

Do not give to patients with known hypersensitivity to enoxaparin or pork products (derived from porcine intestinal mucosa), active major bleeding, prosthetic heart valves, acute heparin-induced (or LMWH-induced) thrombocytopenia, and recent major surgery or cerebral hemorrhage. Use of the medication should be discussed in patients with religious beliefs which prohibit the consumption of pork products. Do not give to patients with drug-induced thrombocytopenia. Use with caution in patients with recurrent gastrointestinal ulcers, bleeding diathesis, and severe renal dysfunction; lower initial doses should be given to patients with renal insufficiency and failure. Do not use with concurrent spinal or epidural anesthesia or lumbar puncture for chemotherapy. May cause fever, confusion, edema, nausea, hemorrhage,

hypochromic anemia, thrombocytopenia, and pain/erythema at the injection site.

In case of overdose, protamine sulfate can be given although the reversal is not complete as with unfractionated heparin. 1 mg of protamine sulfate neutralizes approximately 0.6 to 0.7 mg of enoxaparin.

EPOETIN ALFA

Recombinant human erythropoietin
Epogen, Procrit
Blood formation
Injection: 2000, 3000, 4000, 10,000, 20,000 U/mL (1 mL)

Pregnancy category C

Indications:

Treatment of anemia associated with chronic renal failure, anemia related to therapy with zidovudine (AZT) in HIV-infected patients, and anemia of prematurity. Usage in cancer patients remains controversial. May be considered as an adjunct for anemia treatment in patients with religious beliefs against utilization of blood transfusion.

Dosage:

Anemia in chronic renal failure:

50 to 150 U/kg administered SC/IV three times a week; higher doses may be needed. Dose is individualized to achieve and maintain the lowest hemoglobin sufficient to avoid transfusion, not to exceed 12 g/dL.

Anemia in AZT-treated HIV patients:

100 U/kg SC three times a week; dose range 50 to 4000 U/kg two to three times per week

Anemia in cancer patients:

600 U/kg IV once weekly; dose titrated to effect (maximum 40,000 U). Do not initiate therapy at Hgb $\geq$ 10 g/dL; adjust dose to maintain the lowest Hgb level needed to avoid transfusions. Adult dose 150 U/kg

SC three times a week or 40,000 U SC once weekly.

Anemia of prematurity:

No FDA-approved dosing regimen, a variety of different doses and schedules have been used. Utility in decreasing need for transfusion in VLBW and ELBW infants is not well-proven.

Notes:

Do not give to patients with known hypersensitivity to albumin, uncontrolled hypertension, and in newborns with neutropenia. Use with caution in patients with porphyria or a history of seizures. May cause headache and elevated blood pressure. Meta-analyses have shown that usage leads to a significant increased risk of death, thrombosis, and serious cardiovascular events in cancer patients.

Evaluate iron stores (ferritin and total iron binding capacity [TIBC]) before therapy initiation. Iron supplementation is recommended unless iron stores are already in excess.

ETOPOSIDE

VP-16
VePesid, Toposar
Antineoplastic, mitotic inhibitor
Capsule, softgel: 50 mg
Injection: 20 mg/mL

Pregnancy category D

Indications:

Treatment of germ cell tumors, lymphoma, brain tumors, acute myelogenous leukemia (AML), neuroblastoma, rhabdomyosarcoma, histiocytosis, and conditioning for bone marrow transplantion (BMT).

Dosage:

Refer to individual protocol.

AML remission induction:

$150 \, mg/m^2$/day for 2 to 3 days for 2 to 3 cycles in induction, followed by $250 \, mg/m^2$/day for 3 days in consolidation and intensification courses. Dose per body weight in infants.

Brain tumors:

$150 \, mg/m^2$/day for 2 days; may also be given long term orally (using injection for oral administration); has good central nervous system penetration

Neuroblastoma:

$100 \, mg/m^2$/day over 1 hour days 1 to 5 or alternate day for 3 doses q3–4 weeks for 3 to 4 courses

BMT conditioning regimen:

$160 \, mg/m^2$/day for 4 days

Notes:

Do not give to patients with known hypersensitivity to etoposide. Use with caution and consider dose reduction in patients with renal or hepatic impairment. May cause facial flushing, fever, fatigue, nausea, vomiting, bone marrow suppression, and peripheral neuropathy. Associated with second malignant neoplasms, likely dose and frequency related.

Give IV infusions over at least 1 hour due to associated hypotension with rapid infusion. Infusion should be stopped or infusion rate be decreased with hypotension. After fluid resuscitation, the infusion may be restarted at a slower rate if stopped and the hypotension resolved.

EUTECTIC MIXTURE OF LIDOCAINE AND PRILOCAINE

EMLA, LMX
Local anesthetic, topical anesthetic
Cream: 5, 30 g tubes

Pregnancy category B

Indications:

Used as a topical anesthetic applied to normal intact skin to provide local anesthesia for minor procedures such as venipuncture, placement of peripheral venous access line, lumbar puncture, and minor dermatologic procedures.

Dosage:

Apply 2.5 g per site to normal intact skin and cover with occlusive dressing for 30 to 60 minutes prior to procedure.

Notes:

Do not give to patients with known hypersensitivity to lidocaine, prilocaine, or other local anesthetic or methemoglobinemia. Do not use in neonates <37 weeks gestation or in infants <12 months of age who are receiving concurrent treatment with methemoglobin producing agents (e.g., sulfa drugs, dapsone, phenobarbital, benzocaine).

FERROUS GLUCONATE

Fergon
Iron (12% elemental Fe)
Tablets (OTC): 240 mg (29 mg Fe), 300 mg (36 mg Fe), 325 mg (39 mg Fe)

Pregnancy category A

Indications:

Prevention and treatment of iron deficiency anemia.

Dosage:

Dose is expressed in terms of elemental iron

Severe iron deficiency anemia:

4 to 6 mg/kg/day PO in two to three divided doses

Mild to moderate iron deficiency anemia:

3 mg/kg/day PO in 1 to 2 divided doses

Prophylaxis:

Premature infant: 2 mg/kg/day, maximum dose 15 mg/24 hour

Term infant: 1 to 2 mg/kg/day, maximum dose 15 mg/24 hour

Notes:

Do not give to patients with known hypersensitivity to iron salts, hemochromatosis, and transfusional iron overload. Absorption of iron is decreased when given with tetracycline, antacids, or milk. Less gastrointestinal irritation when given with food. Concurrent administration of 200 mg or more of vitamin C per 30 mg elemental iron increases absorption of oral iron; iron replacement products should be given with orange juice. May cause constipation, dark stools, nausea, and epigastric pain.

FERROUS SULFATE

Feosol, Fer-In-Sol
Iron (20% elemental Fe)
Tablet OTC: 300 mg (60 mg Fe), 324 mg (65 mg Fe), 325 mg (65 mg Fe)
Drops (Fer-in-sol) OTC: 75 mg (15 mg Fe)/0.6 mL
Elixir OTC: 220 mg (44 mg Fe)/5 mL
Oral liquid OTC: 300 mg (60 mg Fe)/5 mL

Pregnancy category A

Indications:

Prevention and treatment of iron deficiency anemia.

Dosage:

See Ferrous Gluconate.

Notes:

See Ferrous Gluconate.

FERROUS FUMARATE

Iron salt (33% elemental Fe)

Tablet OTC: 90 mg (29.5 mg Fe), 200 mg (66 mg Fe), 324 mg (106 mg Fe), 325 mg (106 mg Fe), 350 mg (115 mg Fe)
Chewable tablets: 100 mg (33 mg Fe)
Timed-release tablet OTC: 150 mg (50 mg Fe)

Pregnancy category A

Indications:

Prevention and treatment of iron deficiency anemia.

Dosage:

See Ferrous Gluconate.

Notes:

See Ferrous Gluconate.

FILGRASTIM

G-CSF
Neupogen
Blood formation, colony-stimulating factor
Injection: 300 mcg/mL (1, 1.6 mL)

Pregnancy category C

Indications:

Used to decrease the period of neutropenia and the associated risk of infection in patients with malignancies receiving myelosuppressive chemotherapy associated with a significant incidence (i.e., >20%) of severe neutropenia. Has been used in zidovudine-associated neutropenia in human immunodeficiency virus infected patients and in patients with nonchemotherapy-induced neutropenia (acquired and congenital). Should be considered in patients with complicated infection with underlying neutropenia.

Dosage:

Neonates: 5 to 10 mcg/kg IV/SC daily for 3 to 5 days in neutropenia with sepsis

Children and adults: 5 to 10 mcg/kg IV/SC once daily until absolute neutrophil count (ANC) is greater than 2 to 10×10^9/L (per protocol; given beyond nadir period 7 to 10 days after chemotherapy administration).

Peripheral blood progenitor cell mobilization:

10 mcg/kg SC daily for 4 days before the first leukapheresis procedure and continued until the last leukapheresis.

Congenital neutropenia:

2.5 to 6 mcg/kg/day SC; titrate dose to desired ANC to prevent infection.

Idiopathic or cyclic neutropenia:

5 mcg/kg SC once daily; titrate dose to desired ANC to prevent infection.

Elevation of ANC is usually within 24 hours, though it may be delayed in severe myelosuppression. Transient increase in ANC may occur when granulocyte colony-stimulating factor (G-CSF) is begun shortly after completion of chemotherapy; avoid premature discontinuation.

SC route of administration is preferred due to prolonged serum levels over IV route. If used IV and the G-CSF concentration >15 mcg/mL, add 2 mg albumin/1 mL of IV fluid to prevent drug absorption in the IV administration set.

Notes:

Avoid in patients with hypersensitivity to *Escherichia coli* derived proteins or G-CSF. May cause bone pain and increases in uric acid and lactate dehydrogenase. Do not administer 24 hours before or after administration of chemotherapy.

FLUCONAZOLE

Diflucan
Antifungal
Tablet: 50, 100, 150, 200 mg
Injection: 2 mg/mL
Suspension: 10, 40 mg/mL

Pregnancy category C

Indications:

Prophylaxis and treatment of susceptible fungal infections, including oropharyngeal, esophageal, and vaginal candidiasis and systemic fungal infections with *Candida* sp. as well as treatment and suppression of cryptococcal meningitis. Species of *Candida* with decreased *in vitro* susceptibility to fluconazole are being isolated. Fluconazole is more active against candidal species such as *C. albicans* than species such as *C. parapsilosis*, *C. glabrata*, and *C. tropicalis*.

Dosage:

Oropharnygeal candidiasis:

6 mg/kg loading dose PO/IV followed by 3 mg/kg/day (dependent on severity of infection) for 2 to 4 weeks (dependent on clinical response and immune status of the patient). Neonates under 14 days of age are dosed every 24 to 72 hours.

Esophageal candidiasis:

12 mg/kg loading dose PO/IV, followed by 6 mg/kg/day for 2 to 4 weeks; maximum dose 400 mg/day

Invasive systemic candidiasis and cryptococcal meningitis:

12 mg/kg loading dose PO/IV, followed by 6 to 12 mg/kg/day for 2 to 4 weeks or longer

Prophylaxis in immunocompromised hosts:

3 to 6 mg/kg/dose PO/IV; maximum dose 400 mg/day

Notes:

Do not give to patients with known hypersensitivity to fluconazole or other azoles. May cause nausea, headache, rash, vomiting, abdominal pain, hepatitis, cholestasis, and diarrhea. Antagonism may occur if amphotericin B and fluconazole are used concurrently. Many drug interactions exist. May increase effects, toxicity, and/or levels of cyclosporine, midazolam, tacrolimus, and many other drugs. Rifampin increases fluconazole metabolism. Consult the Physicians' Desk Reference or a pharmacist when ordering fluconazole in a patient receiving many medications.

FOLIC ACID

Folate
Folvite
Blood formation, water-soluble vitamin
Tablet OTC: 0.4, 0.8, 1 mg
Solution: 50 mcg/mL
Injection: 5 mg/mL

Pregnancy category A/C

Indications:

Treatment of megaloblastic anemia resulting from folate deficiency; supplementation for patients with chronic hemolytic anemia (e.g., sickle cell disease, hereditary spherocytosis).

Dosage:

Infants to children <12 months: 15 mcg/kg daily; maximum 50 mcg/day

Children 1 to 11 years: initial dose 1 mg/day; maintenance dose 0.1 to 0.4 mg/day

Children >11 years and adults: initial dose 1 mg/day; maintenance dose 0.5 mg/day

Notes:

May mask hematologic effects of vitamin B_{12} deficiency but will not prevent progression of neurologic abnormalities.

FOSCARNET

Foscavir, generic
Antiviral
Injection: 24 mg/mL

Pregnancy category C

Indications:

Alternative to ganciclovir for treatment of CMV infection; treatment of acyclovir-resistant HSV infections in immunocompromised hosts.

Dosage:

Children and adults:

CMV retinitis: 180 mg/kg/day IV divided q8–12h for 14 to 21 days followed by daily IV maintenance of 90 mg/kg/day

Acyclovir-resistant HSV infection: 40 mg/kg/dose IV q8–12h up to 3 weeks or until lesions heal; repeat treatment may lead to resistance.

Notes:

May cause renal impairment, adjust dose for renal dysfunction. Assure adequate hydration. May adversely affect tooth and bone growth in children, safety and efficacy not fully evaluated. May cause electrolyte imbalances and symptoms of hypocalcemia. May cause seizures; risk factors include renal impairment, low serum calcium, and underlying central nervous system condition. Foscarnet is a vesicant; only infuse into veins with adequate blood flow.

GANCICLOVIR

Cytovene-IV
Antiviral
Injection: 500 mg (can be prepared into oral suspension)

Pregnancy category C

Indications:

Treatment of CMV retinitis, pneumonitis, encephalitis, and gastrointestinal infection in immunocompromised patients. Prevention of symptomatic CMV disease in transplant patients with reactivation of latent disease. Has antiviral activity against HSV-1 and HSV-2.

Dosage:

Congenital CMV infections, neonates and infants: 12 mg/kg/day slow IV infusion q12h for 6 weeks

CMV Retinitis, children >3 years and adults: 10 mg/kg/day divided q12h as a 1-hour infusion for 14 to 21 days followed by maintenance 5 mg/kg/day as a single daily dose for 7 days/week or 6 mg/kg/day for 5 days/week

Treatment of CMV reactivation in transplant recipients, children and adults: 10 mg/kg/day divided q12h for 1 to 2 weeks followed by maintenance 5 mg/kg/day once daily for 7 days/week or 6 mg/kg/day for 5 days/week until 100 days posttransplant

Other CMV infections, children and adults: 10 mg/kg/day divided q12h for 14 to 21 days or 7.5 mg/kg/day divided q8h followed by maintenance 5 mg/kg/day once daily for 7 days/week or 6 mg/kg/day once daily for 5 days/week

Notes:

Do not give to patients with known hypersensitivity to ganciclovir, acyclovir, or any component. Patients must use appropriate contraception due to teratogenic effects for at least 90 days after therapy completion. Cytopenias may occur; do not administer if ANC $< 0.5 \times 10^9$/L or platelets $<25 \times 10^9$/L. Use with caution in patients with renal impairment.

GEMTUZUMAB OZOGAMICIN

Mylotarg
Antineoplastic, monoclonal antibody
Injection: 5 mg

Pregnancy category D

Indications:

Treatment of acute myelogenous leukemia.

Dosage:

Children with body surface area (BSA) <0.6 m²: 0.1 mg/kg/dose

Children with BSA ≥0.6 m²: 3 mg/m²/dose

Notes:

Do not give to patients with known hypersensitivity to gemtuzumab. Severe hypersensitivity reactions and infusion-related reactions may occur including pulmonary edema, acute respiratory distress syndrome, and anaphylaxis. Patients should be premedicated with acetaminophen and diphenhydramine. Administer by slow infusion over 2 hours. Severe hepatic toxicity including veno-occlusive disease (sinusoidal obstructive syndrome) has been reported. Use with caution in patients with renal or hepatic impairment or pulmonary disease. May cause fetal harm; appropriate contraception is advised.

GRANISETRON

Kytril
Antiemetic agent, serotonin (5-HT$_3$)
 antagonist
Tablet: 1 mg
Solution: 0.2 mg/mL
Injection: 1 mg/mL

Pregnancy category B

Indications:

Prevention and treatment of nausea and vomiting associated with chemotherapy. Has also been utilized in prevention of postoperative and radiation-induced nausea and vomiting.

Dosage:

Chemotherapy-induced   nausea   and vomiting:

Children ≥2 years to adults: 10 to 20 mcg/kg/dose IV 15 to 60 minutes before chemotherapy; may be repeated two to thee times following chemotherapy over 24 hours; maximum dose 3 mg/dose or 9 mg/24 hour. Alternatively, a single dose of 40 mcg/kg 15 to 60 minutes before chemotherapy has been used.

Adults: 2 mg/24 hours PO divided q6–12h; initiate first dose before chemotherapy.

Postoperative   nausea   and   vomiting prevention:

Children ≥4 years to adults: 20 to 40 mcg/kg IV dosed prior to anesthesia or immediately before anesthesia reversal; maximum dose 1 mg once

Radiation-induced   nausea   and   vomiting prevention:

Adults: 2 mg PO daily administered 1 hour prior to radiation

Notes:

Inducers or inhibitors of the cytochrome P450 drug-metabolizing enzymes may increase or decrease, respectively, the drug's clearance. Use with caution in liver disease. May cause hypertension, hypotension, arrhythmias, agitation, and insomnia.

HEPARIN SODIUM

Lipo-Hepin, Hep-Lock
Anticoagulant
Injection: many vial sizes, porcine based origin; preservative free
Lock flush solution: 1, 10, 100 U/mL (porcine based, some products may be preservative free or contain benzyl alcohol)
Injection for IV infusion: (porcine based, D$_5$W: 40 U/mL, 50 U/mL, 100 U/mL; 0.9% NaCl: 2 U/mL; 0.45% NaCl: 50 U/mL, 100 U/mL, contains EDTA)
120 U = approximately 1 mg

Pregnancy category C

Indications:

Prophylaxis and treatment of thromboembolic disorders; thrombus prophylaxis for central venous access devices.

Dosage:

Anticoagulation in infants and children:

Initial: 75 U/kg IV bolus over 10 minutes

Maintenance IV continuous infusion:

  <1 year: 28 U/kg/hour

  ≥1 year: 18 to 20 U/kg/hour

or

Maintenance intermittent dosing: 75 to 100 U/kg/dose IV q4h

Adjust dose to keep APTT 1.5 to 2.5 times upper limit of control reference range (best measure 6 to 8 hour after initiation or after change in dosing).

Heparin flush:

Peripheral IV: 1 to 2 mL of 10 U/mL solution q4h

Central lines: 2 to 3 mL of 10 U/mL solution q24h and after access. Dosing often established by institutional policy.

Arterial lines and TPN lines (central lines): add heparin to make a final concentration of 0.5 to 1 U/mL.

Notes:

Do not give to patients with known hypersensitivity to heparin or pork products, severe thrombocytopenia, suspected intracranial hemorrhage, shock, severe hypotension, and uncontrolled bleeding (unless secondary to disseminated intravascular coagulation). Should discuss usage in patients with religious beliefs which prohibit the consumption of pork products. Use preservative free heparin in neonates and consider more dilute heparin.

Antidote: protamine sulfate 1 mg per 100 U heparin in previous 4 hour

HYALURONIDASE

Amphdase, Hydase (bovine source, may contain thimersol)
Hylenex (recombinant human source)
Vitrase (ovine source, preservative free)
Antidote (extravasation)
Injection: 150 U/mL (Vitrase 200 U/mL)

Pregnancy category C

Indications:

Used to influence the dispersion and absorption of other drugs and increase rate of absorption of parenteral fluids given by hypodermoclysis (subcutaneously); treatment of IV extravasations.

Dosage:

Infants and children:

Dilute 150 unit vial in 10 mL normal saline (15 U/mL). Give 1 mL (15 U) by administering five separate injections of 0.2 mL (3 U) at borders of extravasation site SC or intradermal using a 25- or 26-gauge needle. Administer as early as possible after extravasation (minutes to 1 hour).

Notes:

Do not give to patients with known hypersensitivity to hyaluronidase or respective sources (bovine, ovine). Do not inject in or around infected, inflamed, or cancerous lesions; do not use with dopamine or alpha-agonist extravasation. May cause urticaria.

HYDROCORTISONE

Solu-Cortef, Cortef, and others
Corticosteroid
Tablet (Cortef): 5, 10, and 20 mg
Suspension: 2.5 mg/mL
Injection, as sodium succinate (Solu-Cortef): 100, 250, 500, 1000 mg vial

Pregnancy category C

Indications:

Treatment of inflammatory dermatoses and adrenal insufficiency; also used as a chemotherapeutic agent for intrathecal administration.

Dosage:

Physiologic replacement:

12 to 18 mg/m^2/day PO divided q6–8h

Stress dosing (consider for >2 weeks on glucocorticoid therapy or patients in shock):

Solu-Cortef, 25 to 100 mg/m^2/day

Intrathecal chemotherapy with methotrexate and/or cytarabine:

Dose per protocol, range 15 to 30 mg

Notes:

Do not give to patients with known hypersensitivity to hydrocortisone, polymyxin B sulfate, or neomycin sulfate. Avoid in patients with infections from herpes simplex, vaccinia, and varicella.

HYDROMORPHONE HYDROCHLORIDE

Dilaudid, Dilaudid-HP, generics
Narcotic, analgesic
Tablets: 2, 4, 8 mg
Solution: 1 mg/mL
Suppository: 3 mg
Injection: 1, 2, 3, 4, 10 mg/mL

Pregnancy category C/D

Indications:

Management of moderate to severe pain.

Dosage:

Children (not for use in neonates):

PO: 0.03 to 0.1 mg/kg/dose q4–6h PRN (maximum 5 mg/dose)

IV: 0.015 mg/kg/dose q4–6h PRN

Adolescents to adults: 1 to 2 mg/dose IV, IM, or SC q4–6h PRN; 1 to 4 mg PO q4–6h PRN

Notes:

Do not give to patients with known hypersensitivity to hydromorphone. Dose reduction recommended in renal insufficiency or severe hepatic impairment. Avoid use in neonates because of potential central nervous system effects. Use with caution in infants and young children. Causes less pruritus than morphine. Approximate 6:1 conversion from morphine (i.e., 6 mg morphine is equivalent to 1 mg dilaudid).

HYDROXYUREA

Hydrea, Droxia
Antineoplastic
Capsule: 500 mg (Hydrea); 200, 300, 400 mg (Droxia)

Pregnancy category D

Indications:

Treatment of malignancies including chronic myelogenous leukemia (CML), desmoid tumors, and brain tumors; adjunct in the management of sickle cell anemia to reduce pain events, acute chest syndrome, hospitalizations, transfusion needs, and mortality; utilized to treat hyperleukocytosis due to blast crisis in CML and in relapsed acute leukemias; treatment of hypereosinophilic syndrome.

Dosage:

Refer to individual protocol.

CML, hyperleukocytosis:

Initial dose 10 to 20 mg/kg PO once daily; adjust dose according to hematologic response and symptoms.

Sickle cell anemia:

Initial dose 15 mg/kg (range 10 to 20 mg/kg/day) once daily; increase dose in increments of 5 mg/kg/day every 12 weeks to a maximum of 35 mg/kg/day. Discontinue for bone marrow toxicity: ANC $<2\times10^9$/L, platelets $<80\times10^9$/L, reticulocyte count $<8\times10^9$/L, or hemoglobin <9 g/dL. Restart therapy after recovery at 2.5 mg/kg/day less than dose that produced toxicity.

Notes:

Do not give to patients with known hypersensitivity to hydroxyurea or those with severe anemia or severe bone marrow suppression. Use with caution in renal impairment.

IDARUBICIN

Idamycin, generic
Antineoplastic antibiotic, anthracycline
Injection: 5, 10 mg

Pregnancy category D

Indications:

Treatment of acute promyelocytic leukemia (APL), other types of acute myelogenous leukemia, and relapsed lymphoblastic leukemia.

Dosage:

Refer to individual protocol.

APL induction:

$12 \, mg/m^2/day$ IV as 4 doses on alternating days for 8 days

Notes:

Do not give to patients with known hypersensitivity to idarubicin, severe congestive heart failure, or cardiomyopathy. Avoid in preexisting bone marrow suppression unless the potential benefit warrants the risk. May need to reduce dosage with impaired renal or hepatic function. Irreversible myocardial toxicity may occur as the cumulative dosage approaches $550 \, mg/m^2$ (or $400 \, mg/m^2$ with chest irradiation or concomitant cyclophosphamide administration; based on anthracycline dose equivalents, see Chapter 30). This may be an acute or late effect and monitoring with ECHO or MUGA and ECG is required per protocol. Secondary leukemia has been reported.

IFOSFAMIDE

Ifex
Antineoplastic, alkylating agent

Injection: 1 g vial

Pregnancy category D

Indications:

Used in combination with certain other antineoplastics in the treatment of Hodgkin and non-Hodgkin lymphoma, acute lymphoblastic leukemia, osteosarcoma, rhabdomyosarcoma, Ewing sarcoma, and advanced Wilms tumor.

Dosage:

Refer to individual protocol.

Usual dose is 700 to $1800 \, mg/m^2/day$ for 5 days every 3 to 4 weeks

Notes:

Do not give to patients with known hypersensitivity to ifosfamide. Avoid in severe bone marrow suppression. Use with caution in impaired renal function; hydrate the patient prior to administration and ensure good urine flow (i.e., urine specific gravity ≤ 1.010). Ifosfamide may lead to syndrome of inappropriate antidiuretic hormone (SIADH) secretion. Mesna is used for uroprotection with higher doses to decrease risk of hemorrhagic cystitis. Urinalysis should be monitored closely for specific gravity and heme. May cause central nervous system toxicity including hallucination, somnolence, confusion, coma, or encephalopathy.

IMATINIB

Gleevec
Antineoplastic, tyrosine kinase inhibitor
Tablet: 100, 400 mg

Pregnancy category D

Indications:

Treatment of newly diagnosed Philadelphia chromosome positive (Ph$^+$) chronic myelogenous leukemia (CML) in chronic phase ages ≥2 years to adult; recurrent Ph$^+$ CML in chronic phase following stem cell transplantion; Ph$^+$ CML resistant to interferon alpha therapy; Ph$^+$ acute lymphoblastic leukemia (ALL) (relapsed or refractory); mastocytosis; desmoid tumor; gastrointestinal stromal tumors (GIST); hypereosinophilic syndrome or chronic eosinophilic leukemia; and myelodysplastic/myeloproliferative disease associated with platelet-derived growth factor receptor (PDGFR) gene rearrangements.

Dosage:

Refer to individual protocol.

Children ≥2 years: Ph$^+$ CML, chronic phase, new diagnosis: 340 mg/m^2/day divided q12–24h; maximum dose 600 mg/day

Ph$^+$ CML, chronic phase and recurrent after stem cell transplantion, resistant to interferon: 260 mg/m^2/day

May need to adjust dose with hepatic or hematologic toxicity.

The optimal duration of therapy for CML or ALL is not determined.

Notes:

Do not give to patients with known hypersensitivity to imatinib. May cause fluid retention, weight gain, edema, pleural effusion, pericardial effusion, and pulmonary edema. Use with caution in patients where fluid retention may be poorly tolerated such as congestive heart failure or left ventricular dysfunction. May cause Stevens-Johnson syndrome, hepatotoxicity, hemorrhage, and hematologic toxicity. Use with caution in patients with preexisting hepatic or renal impairment. Use with caution in patients receiving concurrent therapy that alters cytochrome P450 activity or requires metabolism by these isoenzymes. May cause photosensitivity, puritus, rash, gastrointestinal disturbance, bone or joint pain, and blurred vision.

IMMUNE GLOBULIN

Flebogamma 5% (50 mg/mL)
Gamunex 10% (100 mg/mL)
Gammagard 10% (100 mg/mL)
Octagam 5% (50 mg/mL)
Carimmune NF: 1, 3, 6, 12 g for reconstitution
Polygam S/D: 2.5, 5, 10 g for reconstitution
Immunoglobulins

Pregnancy category C

Indications:

Treatment of immunodeficiency states (e.g., human immunodeficiency virus, agammaglobulinemia), secondary immunodeficiencies (e.g., bone marrow transplant), immune thrombocytopenic purpura (ITP), Kawasaki disease, and lymphoproliferative disorders.

Dosage:

Immunodeficiency:
400 mg/kg/dose IV every 3 to 4 weeks.
Chronic lymphocytic leukemia:
400 mg/kg/dose IV every 3 weeks.
ITP:
800 to 1000 mg/kg IV for 1 to 2 consecutive days, then every 3 to 4 weeks based on clinical response and platelet count
HIV infection:
400 mg/kg IV every 4 weeks
HIV-associated thrombocytopenia:
500 to 1000 mg/kg/day IV for 1 to 5 days
Kawasaki disease:
2 g/kg IV as a single dose
Post-bone marrow transplant:
400 to 500 mg/kg q4 weeks (refer to protocol; based on desired IgG level, usually >400 mg/dL)

Notes:

Avoid in patients with hypersensitivity to immune globulin or blood products and in those with immunoglobulin A deficiency (except with the use of IgA-depleted products such as Gammagard or Polygam). May cause infusion-related toxicity requiring slower IV rate and premedication with acetaminophen and diphenhydramine. May lead to aseptic meningitis.

IRINOTECAN

Camptostar, generic
Antineoplastic, topoisomerase inhibitor
Injection: 20 mg/mL

Pregnancy category D

Indications:

Treatment of neuroblastoma, hepatoblastoma, brain tumors, Ewing sarcoma, and rhabdomyosarcoma.

Dosage:

Referral to individual protocol

Children: refractory solid tumor, low dose, protracted: 20 mg/m^2/day for 2 consecutive weeks, followed by a week of rest; repeat q3 weeks.

Children: refractory solid tumor or brain tumor: 50 mg/m^2/day for 5 days, repeat cycle q3 weeks.

Notes:

Do not give to patients with known hypersensitivity to irinotecan. Avoid concomitant administration with St. John's wort or ketoconazole and in patients with severe bone marrow failure. A new cycle of irinotecan should not begin until serious treatment-induced toxicity has recovered: ANC $\geq 1.5 \times 10^9$/L and platelet count $> 100 \times 10^9$/L. If the patient has not recovered following a 2 week rest, consider

discontinuing. May cause severe, dose-limiting, and potentially fatal diarrhea. Early diarrhea (during or shortly after infusion) may be accompanied by symptoms of rhinitis, increased salivation, flushing, miosis, lacrimation, diaphoresis, and abdominal cramping. Atropine 0.01 mg/kg IV (maximum dose 0.4 mg) may be used to prevent or treat symptoms.

Late diarrhea occurs >24 hours after therapy and can be prolonged leading to life-threatening dehydration and electrolyte imbalance. Treat promptly with loperamide until a normal pattern of bowel movements returns. Antibiotic support (cefixime or cefpodoxime has been used in children) as a prophylactic and treatment measure.

If the patient develops persistent diarrhea, ileus, fever, or severe neutropenia, interrupt or reduce subsequent doses. If grade 3 (7 to 9 stools/day, incontinence, and/or severe cramping) or grade 4 (≥ 10 stools/day, grossly bloody stool, and/or need for parenteral support) diarrhea occurs, interrupt treatment and reduce subsequent dosing.

May cause severe myelosuppression; halt for neutropenic fever. Use with caution in patients with renal or hepatic impairment.

IRON COMPLEX, POLYSACCHARIDE

Niferex-150, Fe-Tinic 150, Ferrex 150
Iron polysaccharide and ascorbic acid
Tablet: 50 mg
Capsule: 150 mg
Elixir: 100 mg/5 mL

Pregnancy category C

Indications:

Treatment of iron deficiency anemia.

Dosage:

See Ferrous Gluconate.

Notes:

See Ferrous Gluconate.

IRON DEXTRAN COMPLEX

Dexferrum, INFeD
Iron salt
Injection: 50 mg elemental iron/mL (2 mL)

Pregnancy category C

Indications:

Treatment of microcytic hypochromic anemia resulting from iron deficiency in patients in whom oral administration is not feasible or is ineffective. Approved in children $\geq$4 months.

Dosage:

Begin with a test dose 1 hour prior to starting iron dextran therapy:

Infants <10 kg: 10 mg (0.2 mL)

Children 10 to 20 kg: 15 mg (0.3 mL)

Children >20 kg to adult: 25 mg (0.5 mL)

Total replacement dose of iron dextran for iron deficiency anemia:

$$(mL) = 0.0442 \times LBW\ (kg) \times (Hgb_n - Hgb_o) + [0.26 \times LBW\ (kg)],$$

where

LBW = lean body weight

Males: 50 kg + 2.3 kg for every inch over 5 ft in height

Females: 45.5 kg + 2.3 kg for every inch over 5 ft in height

Hgb_n = desired hemoglobin (g/dL) = 12 if <15 kg or 14.8 if >15 kg

Hgb_o = measured hemoglobin (g/dL)

Total replacement dose of iron dextran for acute blood loss:

(Assumes 1 mL of normocytic, normochromic red cells = 1 mg elemental iron)

Replacement iron (mg) = blood loss (mL) × hematocrit

Maximum daily dose, IM/IV (United States):

Infants <5 kg: 25 mg (0.5 mL)

Children 5 to 10 kg: 50 mg (1 mL)

Children >10 kg to adults: 100 mg (2 mL)

Anemia of prematurity:

Neonates: 0.2 to 1 mg/kg/day or 20 mg/kg/week with epoietin alfa therapy

Anemia of chronic renal failure:

There is insufficient data to support IV iron if the ferritin level is >500 ng/mL.

Children: predialysis or peritoneal dialysis, as a single dose repeated as necessary (outside the United States):

<10 kg: 125 mg

10 to 20 kg: 250 mg

>20 kg: 500 mg

Children: hemodialysis, given during each dialysis for 10 doses:

<10 kg: 25 mg

10 to 20 kg: 50 mg

>20 kg: 100 mg

Parenteral administration:

IM: use Z-track technique (deep into upper outer quadrant of buttock); test dose at same site using the same method.

IV: infuse test dose over at least 5 minutes (Dexferrum) or 30 seconds (INFeD); dilute replacement dose in normal saline (50 to 100 mL) to maximum concentration of 50 mg/mL and infuse over 1 to 6 hours at a maximum rate of 50 mg/minute. Avoid dilution in dextrose due to an increased incidence of local pain and phlebitis.

Monitor vital signs and for symptoms of anaphylaxis during the IV infusion.

Notes:

Do not give to patients with known hypersensitivity to iron dextran (anaphylaxis may occur), in anemia not associated with iron deficiency, with hemochromatosis, or with hemolytic anemia. Use with caution in patients with histories of significant allergies, asthma, serious hepatic impairment, preexisting cardiac diseases, and rheumatoid arthritis (may cause an exacerbation of arthritis). Discontinue oral iron prior to initiating parenteral iron. Sweating, urticaria, arthralgia, fever, chills, dizziness, headache, and nausea may be delayed 24 to 48 hours after large doses of IV administered drug or 3 to 4 days following IM administration. The IV route is preferred for patients with chronic renal disease and cancer related anemia (adults).

Agents for treatment of acute anaphylaxis should be readily available. Adverse events are much more associated with the high molecular weight formulation (Dexferrum) than with the low molecular weight formulation (INFeD). *We recommend usage of only the low molecular weight formulation.*

Total-dose infusions have been used safely and are the preferred method of administration, though not currently approved in the United States. Must wait 14 days after a dose for reequilibration if retesting iron stores.

IRON SUCROSE

Venofer
Iron salt
Injection: 20 mg elemental iron/mL (5, 10 mL)

Pregnancy category B

Indications:

Treatment of microcytic, hypochromic anemia resulting from iron deficiency in chronic kidney disease patients, either dialysis-dependent or nondialysis-dependent, who may or may not be receiving erythropoietin

Dosage:

Children: end stage renal disease:

1 mg (elemental iron)/kg/dialysis treatment (repletion)

0.3 mg (elemental iron)/kg/dialysis treatment (maintenance)

Children: iron deficiency anemia (off-label use):

Calculation of iron deficit: body weight [kg] × (target Hgb-actual Hgb) [g/dL] × 2.4

Dose: 5 mg/kg/day IV until iron deficit is corrected

Adults: Hemodialysis dependent:

100 mg IV 1 to 3 times/week during dialysis, total of 10 doses (1000 mg); may continue to administer at lowest dose possible to maintain target hemoglobin and iron storage parameters

Adults: nondialysis-dependent chronic renal failure: 200 mg on 5 different days over a 2-week period (total dose 1000 mg)

Notes:

Do not give to patients with known hypersensitivity to iron formulations, anemia not associated with iron deficiency, hemochromatosis, hemolytic anemia, or iron overload. Use with caution in patients with history of significant allergies, asthma, hepatic impairment, or rheumatoid arthritis.

ITRACONAZOLE

Sporanox, generic
Antifungal
Capsule: 100 mg
Solution: 100 mg/10 mL

Pregnancy category C

Indications:

Treatment of susceptible systemic fungal infections including blastomycosis, coccidiomycosis, histoplasmosis, paracocciodiomycosis, and aspergillosis in patients who do not respond to or cannot tolerate amphotericin B;

treatment of oropharyngeal or esophageal candidiasis (oral solution only).

Dosage:

Children: limited data: 3 to 5 mg/kg/day PO once daily

Doses as high as 5 to 10 mg/kg/day divided q12–24h have been used in children with chronic granulomatous disease and for prophylaxis against *Aspergillus* infection; 6 to 8 mg/kg/day has been utilized in the treatment of disseminated histoplasmosis.

Notes:

Do not give to patients with known hypersensitivity to itraconzaole or other azole drugs. Do not use to treat onychomycosis in patients with evidence of left ventricular dysfunction, congestive heart failure (CHF) or a history of CHF, or women who are pregnant or intending to become pregnant. Use with caution in patients with renal or hepatic impairment. Many drug interactions exist; consult the Physician's Desk Reference. Avoid drinking grapefruit juice or soda while taking oral itraconazole due to altered absorption.

KETOROLAC TROMETHAMINE

Generic, previously available as Toradol
NSAID
Tablet: 10 mg
Injection: 15, 30 mg/mL

Pregnancy category C/D

Indications:

Short-term management of pain (up to 5 days for parenteral therapy, 5 to 14 days for oral therapy).

Dosage:

Loading dose: 1 mg/kg IM; maximum dose 60 mg (loading dose not necessary in IV administration)

Maintenance dose: 0.5 mg/kg/dose IM/IV q6h; maximum dose 30 mg q6h or 120 mg q24h

Children >50 kg and adults: 10 mg PO q6h PRN; maximum dose 40 mg/24 h

Notes:

Do not give to patients with known hypersensitivity to ketorolac or other NSAIDs, patients with active peptic ulcer disease, gastrointestinal bleeding or perforation, renal dysfunction, bleeding diathesis, thrombocytopenia, or cerebrovascular bleeding. Use with caution in patients with congestive heart failure, hypertension, or decreased renal or hepatic function. May cause impaired platelet function, nausea, dyspepsia, drowsiness, and interstitial nephritis.

LEUCOVORIN CALCIUM

Generic
Antidote, methotrexate; folic acid derivative
Tablets: 5, 10, 15, 25 mg
Injection: 50, 100, 200, 350 mg vials

Pregnancy category C

Indications:

Reduction of toxic effects (leucovorin rescue) of high-dose methotrexate, to counteract effects of impaired methotrexate elimination, or as an antidote for folic acid antagonist overdose. Indicated for the treatment of folate-deficient megaloblastic anemia of infancy, sprue, or pregnancy; treatment of nutritional deficiencies when oral folate therapy is not possible.

Dosage:

Rescue dose (following administration of high-dose methotrexate), see protocols:

15 mg/m^2 IV to start, then 15 mg/m^2 q6h; if serum creatinine 48 hours after the start of the methotrexate is elevated more than 50% or the serum methotrexate concentration is

$>5 \times 10^{-6}$ M, increase dose to 150 mg/m^2 dose q3h until serum methotrexate level is $<1 \times 10^{-7}$ M or per protocol (refer to published graphs for methotrexate clearance per protocol). If methotrexate clearance is delayed, continue leucovorin until level $<1 \times 10^{-7}$ M.

Folate-deficient megaloblastic anemia:

1 mg/day IM/IV

Megaloblastic anemia secondary to congenital deficiency of dihydrofolate reductase:

3 to 6 mg/day IM

Folic acid antagonist (e.g., pyrimethamine, trimethoprim) overdose:

5 to 15 mg/day PO for 3 days or until the blood counts are normal or 5 mg every 3 days; doses of 6 mg/day are needed for patients with platelet counts $<100 \times 10^9$/L.

Following intrathecal methotrexate (investigational):

12 mg/m^2 PO/IV as a single dose

Notes:

Do not give to patients with known hypersensitivity to leucovorin, pernicious anemia, or other megaloblastic anemia, such as secondary to vitamin B$_{12}$ deficiency. Do not administer intrathecal or intraventricular (may be harmful or fatal).

LOMUSTINE
CCNU
CeeNU
Antineoplastic, alkylating agent
Capsules: 10, 40, 100 mg

Pregnancy category D

Indications:

Treatment of primary or metastatic brain tumors and Hodgkin lymphoma.

Dosage:

Refer to individual protocol.

Usual dose is 75 to 130 mg/m^2 as a single dose every 6 weeks; subsequent doses adjusted per platelet and leukocyte counts.

Notes:

Do not give to patients with known hypersensitivity to lomustine. May need to adjust dose due to prolonged myelosuppression. Delayed pulmonary fibrosis may occur with high cumulative doses (e.g., ≥ 1 g/m^2).

MECLORETHAMINE
Mustargen
Antineoplastic, alkylating agent
Injection: 10 mg

Pregnancy category D

Indications:

Treatment of Hodgkin and non-Hodgkin lymphoma and brain tumors; sclerosing agent in intracavitary therapy of pleural, pericardial, and other malignant effusions.

Dosage:

Refer to individual protocol.

Children: MOPP regimen (Mustargen [mechlorethamine], Oncovin [vincristine], procarbazine, prednisone): 6 mg/m^2 IV on days 1 and 6 of a 28 day cycle

Brain tumors: MOPP regimen: 3 mg/m^2 IV on days 1 and 8 of a 28 day cycle

Intracavitary (adults): 10 to 30 mg or 0.2 to 0.4 mg/kg

Notes:

Do not give to patients with known hypersensitivity to mechlorethamine, preexisting profound myelosuppression, or pregnancy. Extravasation may result in severe tissue damage; treat promptly with cold compresses (6 to 12 hours) and sodium thiosulfate.

MELPHALAN

Alkeran
Antineoplastic, alkylating agent
Tablet: 2 mg
Injection: 50 mg

Pregnancy category D

Indications:

Treatment of neuroblastoma, rhabdomyosarcoma, brain tumors, acute myelogenous leukemia, Ewing sarcoma, medulloblastoma, Hodgkin lymphoma, and for conditioning prior to hematopoietic stem cell transplantation (HSCT).

Dosage:

Refer to individual protocol.

Children: rhabdomyosarcoma: 10 to 35 mg/m^2/dose IV every 21 to 28 days

High-dose therapy with HSCT conditioning: 70 to 100 mg/m^2 IV on days -7 and -6 prior to HSCT; *or* 140 to 220 mg/m^2 IV single dose prior to HSCT; *or* 50 mg/m^2/day × 4 days; *or* 70 mg/m^2/day × 3 days

Children: oral dosing: 4 to 20 mg/m^2/day days 1 to 21

Notes:

Do not give to patients with known hypersensitivity or to those whose disease was resistant to prior therapy. Long-term oral therapy and high cumulative doses (i.e., >600 mg) can increase the incidence of secondary leukemia. May lead to amenorrhea. Causes bone marrow suppression; use with caution in those with prior myelosuppressive chemotherapy or radiation therapy. Use with caution and consider dose reduction in patients with renal impairment. May increase the effects/levels of cyclosporine and carmustine.

MEPERIDINE HYDROCHLORIDE

Demerol, generic
Narcotic, analgesic
Tablets: 50, 100 mg
Elixir: 50 mg/5 mL
Injection: 10, 25, 50, 75, 100 mg/mL

Pregnancy category C/D

Indications:

Management of moderate to severe pain; used as an adjunct to anesthesia and preoperative sedation; treatment of rigors following administration of amphotericin B.

Dosage:

Children: 1 to 1.5 mg/kg/dose PO, IM, IV, or SC q3–4h PRN; maximum dose 100 mg

Adults: 50 to 150 mg/dose q3–4h PRN

Notes:

Do not give to patients with known hypersensitivity to meperidine. Avoid in patients receiving acyclovir, cimetidine, tricyclic antidepressants, and monoamine oxidase inhibitors within the past 14 days. Use with caution in renal or hepatic dysfunction, sickle cell disease, and seizure disorders. Accumulation of normeperidine metabolites may precipitate seizures. May cause central nervous system and respiratory depression, nausea, vomiting, constipation, bradycardia, hypotension, peripheral vasodilation, miosis, sedation, drowsiness, biliary or urinary tract spasm, increased intracranial pressure, and physical and psychological dependence. *Other narcotics are generally preferred for pain management.*

MERCAPTOPURINE

6-MP, 6-mercaptopurine
Purinethol

Antineoplastic, antimetabolite
Tablet: 50 mg

Pregnancy category D

Indications:

Used in conjunction with methotrexate for maintenance therapy in acute lymphoblastic leukemia; combination regimen in acute myelogenous and chronic myelogenous leukemias; non-Hodgkin lymphoma.

Dosage:

Refer to individual protocol.

50 to 100 mg/m^2 once daily

Notes:

Do not give to patients with known hypersensitivity to mercaptopurine, severe liver disease, or severe bone marrow suppression. Use with caution and adjust dose in patients with renal or hepatic dysfunction. Patients who receive allopurinol concurrently should have their mercaptopurine dose reduced by 33%.

MESNA

Mesnex
Prophylaxis, cyclophosphamide or ifosfamide-induced hemorrhagic cystitis.
Tablet: 400 mg
Injection: 100 mg/mL

Pregnancy category B

Indications:

Detoxifying agent used to inhibit hemorrhagic cystitis induced by ifosfamide and cyclophosphamide.

Dosage:

Refer to individual protocol.

Dose is dependent on which antineoplastic agent it is used with.

With ifosfamide and cyclophosphamide:

Mesna dose is 20% of alkylator dose IV 15 minutes before or combined with alkylator, followed by repeat doses 4 and 8 hours later; for high-dose alkylator therapy, give dose 15 minutes before alkylator then q3h for 3 to 6 doses. Total daily Mesna dose ranges from 60% to 160% of the daily alkylator dose.

IV continuous infusion of Mesna is given at doses equivalent to 60% to 100% of the ifosfamide or cyclophosphamide dose.

Mesna is given by IV infusion over 15 to 30 minutes or by continuous IV infusion, or per protocol.

Notes:

Do not give to patients with known hypersensitivity to Mesna or thiol compounds. May cause false positive urinary ketone measurements.

METHADONE HYDROCHLORIDE

Dolophine
Antidote, analgesic
Tablet: 5, 10 mg
Solution: 5 mg/5 mL, 10 mg/5 mL
Injection: 10 mg/mL (20 mL)
Pregnancy category B/D

Indications:

Management of severe pain; used in narcotic detoxification maintenance programs and for the treatment of iatrogenic narcotic dependency.

Dosage:

Children: analgesia:

0.7 mg/kg/24 hour divided q4–6h PRN PO, SC, IM, or IV

Adults: analgesia:

2.5 to 10 mg PO, IM, IV, or SC q3–4h PRN, up to 5 to 20 mg q6–8h

Detoxification: see Physician's Desk Reference: 15 to 40 mg/day PO

Notes:

Do not give to patients with known hypersensitivity to methadone. Use with caution in patients with respiratory disease as respiratory depression lasts longer than analgesic effects. May cause cardiac arrhythmias, sedation, increased intracranial pressure, hypotension, and bradycardia, in addition to respiratory depression. Prolonged half-life; average 19 hours in children and 35 hours in adults. Repeated use can result in cumulative effects necessitating adjustment to the dose and frequency of administration. Conversion from other narcotics to methadone can be quite challenging; discussion with a provider with experience in this area is warranted (see Chapter 28).

METHOTREXATE

Rheumatrex, Trexall, generic
Antineoplastic, antimetabolite, antirheumatic
Tablet (Trexall): 2.5, 5, 7.5, 10, 15 mg
Injection: 1 g vial

Pregnancy category X

Indications:

Treatment of acute lymphoblastic leukemia (ALL; including meningeal leukemia), trophoblastic neoplasms, osteosarcoma, non-Hodgkin lymphoma, rheumatoid arthritis, dermatomyositis, and psoriasis.

Dosage:

Refer to individual protocol.

Acute lymphoblastic leukemia (refer to protocol, phase):

7.5 to 30 mg/m^2 once per week or every 2 weeks PO/IM; 10 to 18,000 mg/m^2 bolus

dosing or by continuous infusion IV over 6 to 42 hours (dependent on phase of therapy); 50 to 400 mg/m^2 IV bolus every 10 days

Doses 100 to 500 mg/m^2 may require leucovorin and doses >500 mg/m^2 require leucovorin rescue.

Osteosarcoma/solid tumors:

Children <12 years: 12 g/m^2 IV over 4 hours (dose range 12 to 18 g) + leucovorin rescue

Children ≥12 years: 8 g/m^2 IV over 4 hours (maximum dose 18 g) + leucovorin rescue

Non-Hodgkin lymphoma:

200 to 500 mg/m^2 IV; repeat every 4 weeks, as per protocol.

Meningeal leukemia (and prophylaxis):

10 to 15 mg/m^2 intrathecal (IT) (maximum 15 mg) per protocol; dosed by age:

Children <1 year: 6 mg

Children 1 to <2 years: 8 mg

Children 2 to <3 years: 10 mg

Children ≥3 years: 12 to 15 mg

Dilute in 4 to 6 mL 0.9% NaCl or Elliotts B solution.

Intrathecal methotrexate may be combined with other agents for IT administration (i.e., cytarabine, hydrocortisone).

Trophoblastic neoplasms (adults):

15 to 30 mg/day PO/IM for 5 days; repeat weekly for three to five courses.

Notes:

Do not give to patients with known hypersensitivity to methotrexate, severe renal or hepatic impairment, or preexisting profound bone marrow suppression. High-dose methotrexate (>1 g/m^2) should not be administered to patients with a creatinine clearance of less than 50% to 75% of normal. Patients should receive alkaline fluids to maintain urine pH of 7 or higher while receiving high-dose methotrexate. Follow serum levels per protocol and administer leucovorin rescue per protocol; follow methotrexate degradation curve per protocol. Methotrexate has been associated with acute and severe chronic hepatotoxicity, severe bone marrow suppression, and renal failure with delayed clearance, high-dose administration, concurrent nephrotoxic drugs, or inadequate hydration. Intrathecal and parenteral administration of methotrexate have been associated with acute neurotoxicity. Severe dermatologic reactions and radiation dermatitis have been reported. May accumulate in fluid collections (pleural effusions, ascites) increasing local toxicity.

Ensure no TMP-SMX, penicillin, NSAIDs, or PPIs are given until the methotrexate level is $<1 \times 10^{-7}M$ due to competitive excretion and risk of toxicity secondary to delayed methotrexate clearance.

Intrathecal drugs should be prepared and administered separately from other chemotherapeutic drugs to avoid inappropriate administration.

Recommend giving patients one pill size only to avoid accidental overdose with dose modifications during maintenance therapy for ALL.

METHYLENE BLUE

Urolene blue, generic
Antidote, drug-induced methemoglobinemia
Tablet (Urolene Blue): 65 mg
Injection: 10 mg/mL

Pregnancy category C/D

Indications:

Antidote for cyanide poisoning and drug-induced methemoglobinemia; treatment of NADPH-methemoglobin reductase deficiency; treatment and prevention of ifosfamide-induced encephalopathy (adults).

Dosage:

Children:

Methemoglobinemia: 1 to 2 mg/kg (25 to 50 mg/m^2) IV as a single dose; may be repeated after 1 hour as necessary

NADPH-methemoglobin reductase deficiency: 1 to 1.5 mg/kg/day PO (maximum dose 300 mg/day) given with ascorbic acid 5 to 8 mg/kg/day

Notes:

Use with caution in patients with G6PD deficiency or renal insufficiency. May cause nausea, vomiting, dizziness, headache, abdominal pain, diaphoresis, phototoxicity, and skin staining. May cause transient blue-green coloration of urine and stool. At high doses, may cause methemoglobinemia.

METHYLPREDNISOLONE

Medrol, Medrol dose pack, Depo-Medrol, Solu-Medrol
Corticosteroid
Tablets: 2, 4, 8, 16, 24, 32 mg
Tablets (dose pack): 4 mg
Injection, sodium succinate (Solu-Medrol): 40, 125, 500, 1000, 2000 mg (IV/IM)
Injection (acetate) (Depo-Medrol): 20, 40, 80 mg/mL (IM)

Pregnancy category C

Indications:

Anti-inflammatory or immunosuppressive agent used to treat a variety of diseases of hematologic, allergic, inflammatory, neoplastic, and autoimmune origin.

Dosage:

Anti-inflammatory/immunosuppressive:

0.5 to 1.7 mg/kg/24 hours PO, IM, or IV divided q6–12h

Chemotherapy:

Refer to individual protocols for dosing (in lieu of prednisone; convert dose for steroid potency, 80% of prednisone dose).

Notes:

Do not give to patients with hypersensitivity to methylprednisolone. Do not administer with live-virus vaccines or during active infection with varicella or herpes zoster. Avoid use in patients with systemic fungal infections. May cause hypertension, glucose intolerance, gastrointestinal bleeding, osteoporosis, pseudotumor cerebri, Cushing's syndrome, adrenal axis suppression, and acne. May increase levels of cyclosporine and tacrolimus.

METOCLOPRAMIDE

Reglan, Maxolon, generic
Antiemetic
Tablets: 5, 10 mg
Syrup: 5 mg/5 mL
Injection: 5 mg/mL

Pregnancy category B

Indications:

Treatment of gastroesophageal reflux (GER) and prevention of nausea and vomiting associated with chemotherapy.

Dosage:

GER or gastrointestinal (GI) dysmotility:

Infants and children: 0.1 to 0.2 mg/kg/dose up to QID, PO, IV, or IM; maximum dose 0.8 mg/kg/24 hours

Adults: 10 to 15 mg/dose on awakening and at night, IM, PO, or IV

Antiemetic:

1 to 2 mg/kg/dose q2–6h PO, IV, or IM. Give first dose 30 minutes prior to emetogenic drug. Premedicate with diphenhydramine to reduce incidence of extrapyramidal symptoms.

Notes:

Do not give to patients with known hypersensitivity to metoclopramide, GI obstruction, pheochromocytoma, or history of seizure disorder. Sedation, headache, anxiety, depression, leukopenia, and diarrhea may occur.

MICAFUNGIN

Mycamine
Antifungal, echinocandin
Injection: 50, 100 mg

Pregnancy category C

Indications:

Treatment of patients with candidemia, esophageal candidiasis, disseminated candidiasis; prophylaxis of *Candida* infections in patients undergoing hematopoietic stem cell transplantation; treatment of invasive *Aspergillosis*. Not effective against cryptococcus, fusariosis, and zygomycosis.

Dosage:

Not FDA approved for use in children. Guidelines are per pharmacokinetic studies, short duration trials, and case reports.

Prophylaxis of Candida infections in HSCT recipients:

Infants, children, and adolescents: 1.5 to 2 mg/kg/day IV daily

Adults: 50 mg IV daily

Disseminated candidiasis:

Neonates <1000 g: 10 mg/kg/day IV daily

Neonates ≥1000 g: 7 mg/kg/day IV daily

Infants, children, and adolescents: 2 to 4 mg/kg/day IV daily (maximum dose 200 mg)

Adults: 100 mg IV daily

Aspergillosis, esophageal candidiasis:

Neonates: 8 to 12 mg/kg/IV daily

Infants, children, and adolescents: 4 to 8.6 mg/kg IV daily (maximum dose 325 mg)

Adults: 150 mg IV once daily

Notes:

Do not give to patients with known hypersensitivity to micafungin or other echinocandins. Use with caution in patients with renal or hepatic impairment and in patients receiving concomitant hepatotoxic drugs; monitor for evidence of worsening. May cause electrolyte disturbances, cytopenias, skin rash, central nervous system, and cardiovascular effects.

MITOXANTRONE

Novantrone, generic
Antineoplastic, anthracenedione
Injection, solution: 2 g/mL

Pregnancy category D

Indications:

Treatment of acute myelogenous leukemia; active in pediatric sarcoma, Hodgkin and non-Hodgkin lymphoma, acute lymphoblastic leukemia, and myelodysplastic syndrome.

Dosage:

Leukemia: children ≤2 years: 0.4 mg/kg IV daily for 3 to 5 days

Children >2 years and adults: 12 mg/m^2 IV daily for 2 to 3 days; acute leukemia in relapse: 8 to 12 mg/m^2 IV daily for 5 days; AML: 10 mg/m^2 IV daily for 3 to 5 days

Solid tumors: children: 18 to 20 mg/m^2 IV q3–4 weeks or 5 to 8 mg/m^2 IV weekly

Adults: 12 to 14 mg/m^2 IV q3–4 weeks (maximum total 80 to 120 mg/m^2)

Notes:

Do not give to patients with known hypersensitivity to mitoxantrone. May cause severe myelosuppression; use with caution in patients with preexisting myelosuppression. Irreversible myocardial toxicity may occur as the cumulative dosage approaches 550 mg/m^2 (or 400 mg/m^2 with chest irradiation or concomitant cyclophosphamide administration; based on anthracycline dose equivalents, see Chapter 30). This may be an acute or late effect and monitoring with ECHO or MUGA and ECG is required per protocol. Extravasation may lead to severe tissue damage. Dosage may need to be reduced in patients with impaired hepatobiliary function, preexisting bone marrow suppression, or previous treatment with cardiotoxic drugs or chest radiation.

MORPHINE SULFATE

Roxanol, Oramorph SR, MS Contin
Narcotic, analgesic
Tablets: 15, 30 mg
Controlled-release tablets: 15, 30, 60 mg (100 and 200 mg for opioid tolerant patients)
Extended-release capsules: 30 mg (60, 90, 120 mg for opioid tolerant patients)
Sustained-release pellets in capsules: 10, 20, 30, 50, 60 mg (100, 200 mg for opioid tolerant patients)
Solution: 10, 20, 100 mg/5 mL
Suppository: 5, 10, 20, 30 mg
Injection: 0.5, 1, 2, 3, 4, 5, 8, 10, 15, 25, 50 mg/mL

Pregnancy category C/D

Indications:

Relief of moderate to severe pain, acute and chronic, after nonnarcotic analgesics have failed; preanesthetic medication; relief of dyspnea from acute left ventricular failure and pulmonary edema.

Dosage:

Dose should be titrated to effect.

Neonates:

0.1 to 0.2 mg/kg IV q3–4h; q6h dosing may be appropriate for extremely premature infants or infants with hepatic dysfunction

Infants and children:

Tablet and solution (immediate release): 0.2 to 0.5 mg/kg/dose PO q4–6h PRN

Tablet (controlled release): 0.3 to 0.6 mg/kg/ dose PO q12h

Injection: 0.05 to 0.2 mg/kg/dose IM, IV, or SC q2–4h PRN; maximum 15 mg/dose

Adults:

Tablets and solution (immediate release): 10 to 30 mg PO q4h PRN

Tablet (controlled release): 15 to 30 mg PO q8–12h PRN

Injection: 2 to 15 mg/dose IV, IM, or SC

Patient-controlled analgesia (PCA) dosing guidelines:

PCA (on demand) dose: 0.01 to 0.04 mg/kg

Suggested lock out (between PCA doses): 10 to 20 minutes

Continuous dose:

Neonate 0.01 to 0.02 mg/kg/h

Infant/child: 0.01 to 0.07 mg/kg/h

Adult: 0.8 to 10 mg/h (higher doses with tolerance)

Bolus (loading): 0.03 to 0.1 mg/kg

The one hour maximum is 0.1 to 0.15 mg/kg (6 to 8 mg/h in tolerant adults), and typically equals the continuous dose plus 2 to 3 PCA bolus doses.

Notes:

Do not give to patients with severe renal or liver insufficiency. May cause severe pruritus, urinary retention, respiratory depression, central nervous system depression, constipation, and ileus. Prolonged use can result in physical and psychological dependence. Consider nighttime low continuous dose infusion of 0.01 to 0.02 mg/kg/h without a change in lock out so as to allow sleep. Avoid narcotization with sedation and respiratory depression. Monitor vitals and encourage use of incentive spirometry and ambulation with repetitive dosing or PCA use.

MYCOPHENOLATE MOFETIL (MMF)

CellCept, Myfortic, generic (capsule, tablet)
Immunosuppressive agent
Capsule, as mofetil or CellCept: 250 mg
Tablet, as mofetil or CellCept: 500 mg
Tablet, delayed release, as mycophenolic acid, Myfortic: 180, 360 mg (not recommended for children whose total body surface area [TBSA] is $<1.19\,m^2$)
Injection, as mofetil or CellCept: 500 mg
Powder for oral suspension, CellCept: 200 mg/mL

Pregnancy category D

Indications:

Used as an immunosuppressant drug frequently in combination with other immunosuppressants (e.g., cyclosporine, corticosteroids) for the prophylaxis of organ rejection (renal, hepatic, cardiac, and bone marrow transplants), chronic graft-versus-host disease, myasthenia gravis, proliferative lupus nephritis, and relapsing nephrotic syndrome.

Dosage:

Limited data are available for pediatric dosing. Pharmacokinetic studies have indicated that doses based on body surface area result in a more appropriate area under the curve than doses based on body weight.

Children: 600 mg/m^2/dose BID *or*
by TBSA:

1.25 to 1.5 mg/m^2: 750 mg BID

$>1.5\,m^2$: 1 g BID

Notes:

Do not give to patients with known hypersensitivity to mycophenolate mofetil. Risk appears to be associated with the intensity and duration of immunosuppression; may result in an increased incidence of lymphoma or other malignancies especially in combination with other immunosuppressants. Patients should avoid excessive exposure to sunlight and should use sun protection factor. Use with caution and adjust dose in patients with renal impairment.

NALOXONE

Narcan, generic
Narcotic antagonist
Injection: 0.4 mg/mL

Pregnancy category C

Indications:

Used to reverse central nervous system and respiratory depression in suspected narcotic overdose; treatment of coma of unknown etiology.

Dosage:

Treatment of opiate intoxication:

Neonates, children <5 years or <20 kg: 0.1 mg/kg/dose; repeat q2–3 minutes PRN IM, IV, SC, or via ETT

Children >5 years or ≥20 kg: 2 mg/dose; if no response, repeat q2–3 minutes PRN IM, IV, SC, or via ETT

Adults: 0.4 to 2.0 mg/dose q2–3 minutes PRN IM, IV, SC, or via ETT. Use in 0.1 to 0.2 mg increments in opioid-dependent patients. If no response and cumulative dose >10 mg, reevaluate diagnosis.

IV continuous infusion: 0.005 mg/kg loading dose, then 0.0025 to 0.16 mg/kg/h. Taper gradually to avoid relapse.

Patient-controlled analgesia side effect reversal (pruritus and/or urinary retention with morphine):

IV continuous infusion: begin with 1 mcg/kg/ h, then titrate up or down to 0.25 to 2 mcg/ kg/h to abate opioid-related side effects; taper infusion gradually over 2 to 4 hours when discontinuing.

Notes:

Do not give to patients with known hypersensitivity to naloxone. The dose for pediatric postoperative narcotic reversal is one-tenth of the dose for opiate intoxication. Endotracheal administration can be done safely by diluting in 1 to 2 mL of normal saline. Will produce narcotic withdrawal in patients with dependence. Use with caution in patients with chronic heart disease. Abrupt reversal of narcotic dependency may result in nausea, vomiting, diaphoresis, tachycardia, hypertension, and tremulousness.

NELARABINE

Arranon, ara-G
Antineoplastic, antimetabolite
Injection: 5 mg/mL

Pregnancy category D

Indications:

Treatment of T-cell acute lymphoblastic leukemia and T-cell lymphoblastic lymphoma.

Dosage:

Refer to individual protocol.

Children: 650 mg/m^2 daily, days 1 to 5; repeat cycle q21 days

Adults: 1500 mg/m^2/dose on days 1, 3, and 5; repeat cycle q21 days

Notes:

Do not give to patients with known hypersensitivity to nelarabine. May cause severe neurotoxicity, including severe somnolence, seizure, and peripheral neuropathy. Observe closely for neurotoxicity. Adverse effects associated with demyelination or similar to Guillain–Barré syndrome (ascending peripheral neuropathies) have been reported. Neurotoxicity is dose limited and may not reverse completely. Risk of neurotoxicity may increase in patients with concurrent intrathecal chemotherapy or history of cranial irradiation. May cause bone marrow suppression. Use with caution in patients with renal or hepatic impairment. Monitor blood counts, electrolytes, renal function, and transaminases frequently.

OCTREOTIDE ACETATE

Sandostatin, generic
Antidiarrheal, antidote, antihemorrhagic, antisecretory, somatostain analog
Injection: 0.2, 1 mg/mL
Injection, preservative free: 0.05, 0.1, 0.5 mg/mL

Pregnancy category B

Indications:

Treatment of secretory diarrhea in patients with metastatic carcinoid or vasoactive intestinal peptide-secreting tumors, chemotherapy-induced diarrhea, graft-versus-host disease associated diarrhea, and esophageal varices/gastrointestinal (GI) bleeding.

Dosage:

Infants and children: (data limited to small studies): diarrhea: 1 to 10 mcg/kg IV/SC q12h; begin at low dose and titrate to effect *or* IV continuous infusion 1 mcg/kg bolus followed by continuous infusion 1 mcg/kg/h.

Esophageal varices/GI bleeding: 1 to 2 mcg/kg initial IV bolus followed by 1 to 2 mcg/kg/h continuous infusion; titrate to response, taper doses by 50% q12h when no active bleeding occurs for 24 hours, may discontinue dose when at 25% of initial dose.

Notes:

Do not give to patients with known hypersensitivity to octreotide. May need to adjust dose for patients with diabetes; may alter insulin requirements. Use with caution in patients with renal or hepatic impairment or a history of cardiac arrhythmias. Long term use may increase the incidence of gallstones or sludge formation. May cause neuromuscular, central nervous system, or cardiovascular toxicities. May decrease level/effects of cyclosporine. Do not give with meals; may decrease absorption of vitamin B_{12} and dietary fats.

ONDANSETRON

Zofran
Antiemetic, serotonin 5-HT$_3$ antagonist
Tablets: 4, 8, 16, 24 mg
Tablets (ODT, orally disintegrating): 4, 8 mg
Solution: 4 mg/5 mL
Injection: 2 mg/mL
Injection, premixed in D5W: 32 mg/50 mL

Pregnancy category B

Indications:

Prevention of nausea and vomiting associated with initial and repeat courses of emetogenic cancer chemotherapy or radiation, prevention of postoperative nausea and vomiting, treatment of emesis induced by acute gastroenteritis.

Dosage:

Prevention of chemotherapy-induced nausea and vomiting:

IV: 0.15 mg/kg/dose 30 minutes prior to the start of emetogenic chemotherapy, with subsequent doses administered 4 and 8 hours after the first dose or every 8 hours until the chemotherapy is complete. For highly emetogenic drugs, give 0.45 mg/kg as a single dose 30 minutes prior to the start of chemotherapy, followed by 0.15 mg/kg/dose q4h PRN. Maximum single dose 32 mg.

Oral: Dose based on total body surface area (TBSA), weight, or age:

TBSA:

<0.3 m^2: 1 mg TID PRN

0.3 to 0.6 m²: 2 mg TID PRN

0.6 to 1 m²: 3 mg TID PRN

>1 m²: 4 to 8 mg TID PRN

Weight:

Same as IV dosing; round to closest convenient dose

Age:

<11 years: dose based on TBSA

Children ≥11 years and adults: 8 mg TID PRN; first dose 30 minutes prior to start of chemotherapy

Notes:

Do not give to patients with known hypersensitivity to ondansetron. Ondansetron is a substrate for the cytochrome P450 enzyme system, so inducers or inhibitors of this system may affect the elimination of ondansetron. Data are limited for use in children under 3 years of age. May need to adjust dose and interval for severe hepatic impairment. Side effects are usually mild, with headache, sedation, constipation, and dry mouth being the most common. May also cause bronchospasm, tachycardia, hypokalemia, seizures, lightheadedness, diarrhea, transient increases in bilirubin or transaminases, and transient blindness (minutes to 48 hours). ECG changes (QT prolongation) have been reported. Data are not available for use in children with radiation-induced nausea and vomiting. However, based on efficacy in adults and safety in children, it is commonly used. Give 1 to 2 hours prior to radiation; may need round the clock dosing for abdominal radiation.

OXALIPLATIN

Eloxatin, generic
Antineoplastic, alkylating agent
Injection: 5 mg/mL

Pregnancy category D

Indications:

Treatment of relapsed or refractory solid tumors, brain tumors, and non-Hodgkin lymphoma.

Dosage:

Refer to individual protocol.

Children: ≤1 year: 4.3 mg/kg IV over 2 hours q3 weeks

Children: >1 year: 130 mg/m² IV over 2 hours q3 weeks

Notes:

Do not give to patients with known hypersensitivity to oxaliplatin, in pregnancy, or in those with grade 3 or 4 neuropathy (usually due to prior exposure). Anaphylaxis may occur within minutes of administration; appropriate supportive and resuscitative medications and equipment should be available. Two different types of neuropathy may occur: (1) an acute (within 2 days) reversible (resolves within 14 days) sensory neuropathy with peripheral symptoms that are often exacerbated by cold (may include pharyngolaryngeal dysesthesia), and (2) persistent (over 14 days) sensory neuropathy that presents with paresthesias, dysesthesias, hypoesthesias, and impaired proprioception that interferes with activities of daily living. Symptoms may improve with discontinuing treatment. May cause pulmonary fibrosis or hepatotoxicity. When administered as sequential infusions, taxane derivatives should be administered before platinum derivatives to limit myelosuppression and enhance efficacy.

PENTAMIDINE ISETHIONATE

Pentam 300, NebuPent
Antibiotic, antiprotozoal
Injection: 300 mg vial (Pentam 300)
Inhalation: 300 mg vial (NebuPent)

Pregnancy category C

Indications:

Treatment of *Pneumocystis jiroveci pneumonia* (PCP) in patients who cannot tolerate or who fail to respond to trimethoprim-sulfamethoxazole, prevention of PCP infection in immunocompromised hosts, treatment of African trypanosomiasis, and treatment of visceral and cutaneous leishmaniasis caused by *Leishmania donovani*.

Dosage:

Prophylaxis for PCP:

4 mg/kg/24 hours IM/IV (over 1 to 2 hours) every 2 to 4 weeks

Inhalation (≥5 years): 300 mg in 6 mL water via inhalation qmonth (use with Respirgard II nebulizer)

Maximum single dose 300 mg

Treatment of PCP:

4 mg/kg/dose IM/IV daily for 14 to 21 days (preferably IV)

Notes:

Do not give to patients with known hypersensitivity to pentamidine isethionate. Adjust dose in renal impairment. Use with caution in patients with diabetes mellitus, renal or hepatic dysfunction, hypertension, or hypotension. Additive toxicity may occur with aminoglycosides, amphotericin B, cisplatin, and vancomycin. Can see Jarisch-Herxheimer-like reaction (fever, chills, headache, myalgia). Inhalation therapy may cause irritation of the airway, bronchospasm, cough, oxygen desaturation, dyspnea, and loss of appetite. May cause hypoglycemia, hyperglycemia, hypotension (with infusion <2 hours), nausea, vomiting, fever, mild hepatotoxicity, pancreatitis, hypocalcemia, megaloblastic anemia, granulocytopenia, and nephrotoxicity.

POSACONAZOLE

Noxafil
Antifungal

Suspension: 40 mg/mL

Pregnancy category C

Indications:

Prophylaxis of invasive *Aspergillus* and *Candida* infections in high risk, severely immunocompromised patients (e.g., hematopoietic stem cell transplant recipient, graft-versus-host disease, hematologic malignancy with prolonged chemotherapy-induced neutropenia); treatment of oropharyngeal candidiasis (including those refractory to itraconzaole and/or fluconazole); treatment of serious invasive fungal infections including zygomycosis and coccidioidomycosis in patients intolerant or refractory to other antifungal therapy.

Dosage:

Children ≥13 years and adults:

Prophylaxis of invasive Aspergillus and Candida infections: 200 mg TID

Treatment of refractory, invasive fungal infections: 800 mg/day in divided doses (given BID to QID)

Treatment of orophargyngeal candidiasis:

Initial: 100 mg BID on day 1, then 100 mg daily for 13 days

Refractory: 400 mg BID

Notes:

Do not give to patients with known hypersensitivity to posaconazole and avoid concurrent administration with ergot alkaloids. Cross sensitivity reactions with other azoles have not yet been studied but may exist. May cause hepatotoxicity, and frequent monitoring is recommended. May alter drug levels of cyclosporine (also tacrolimus and sirolimus) resulting in nephrotoxicity, leukoencephalopathy, and death. Use with caution in neonates (oral solution contains sodium benzoate, a metabolite of benzyl alcohol, which has been associated with a potentially fatal toxicity).

PREDNISONE

Deltasone, Liquid Pred, Orasone, generic
Corticosteroid
Tablets: 1, 2.5, 5, 10, 20, 50 mg
Solution: 1, 5 mg/mL

Pregnancy category C/D

Indications:

Management of adrenocortical insufficiency; used for anti-inflammatory or immunosuppressant effects in autoimmune diseases such as immune thrombocytopenia purpura; chemotherapy for acute lymphoblastic leukemia and Hodgkin and non-Hodgkin lymphoma.

Dosage:

Dose is dependent on condition being treated and response of patient. Consider alternate day dosing for long-term therapy. Discontinuation of long-term therapy requires gradual tapering.

Anti-inflammatory or immunosuppressant (includes immune thrombocytopenic purpura, aplastic anemia):

0.5 to 2 mg/kg/day PO divided 1–3 times daily

Chemotherapy:

40 to 180 mg/m^2/day, as per protocol

Notes:

Avoid use in patients with life-threatening infections (except septic shock or tuberculous meningitis), systemic fungal infections, varicella, and in those with hypersensitivity to prednisone. Use with caution in patients with hypothyroidism, cirrhosis, hypertension, congestive heart failure, ulcerative colitis, gastrointestinal bleeding, and thromboembolic disorders. May cause adrenal axis suppression, hypertension, hyperglycemia, irritability, gastritis, skin atrophy, osteoporosis, cataracts, fluid retention, mood lability, nausea, diarrhea, bone pain, acne, and weight gain. Consider use of antacid in long-term therapy. Avascular necrosis and growth retardation are seen in patients with long-term or repeated high-dose therapy. Ensure patients are aware of risk of varicella infection in non-immune states.

PROCARBAZINE HYDROCHLORIDE

Matulane
Antineoplastic, alkylating agent
Capsule: 50 mg

Pregnancy category D

Indications:

Treatment of Hodgkin lymphoma and brain tumors.

Dosage:

Refer to individual protocol.

50 to 100 mg/m^2 daily for 10 to 14 days

Notes:

Avoid in patients with known hypersensitivity to procarbazine or with preexisting bone marrow aplasia. May cause nausea, vomiting, dry mouth, constipation, headache, dizziness, and hair loss. Use with caution and reduce dose in patients with renal or hepatic impairment or marrow suppression. May potentiate central nervous system depression when used with phenothiazine derivatives, barbiturates, narcotics, alcohol, tricyclic antidepressants, and methyldopa. Drug (e.g., monoamine oxidase inhibitors) and food interactions are common. Avoid food with high tyramine content (i.e., aged cheese or meats, tea, dark beer, coffee, cola drinks, wine, soybean products, peanuts, avocadoes, bananas) because hypertensive crisis, tremor, excitation, cardiac palpitations, and angina may occur.

RASBURICASE
Elitek
Recombinant urate oxidase, uric acid lowering agent, antigout agent
Injection: 1.5, 7.5 mg vials

Pregnancy category C

Indications:
Initial management or prevention of hyperuricemia in high risk patients with leukemia, lymphoma, or a select group of patients with solid tumors at risk for tumor lysis syndrome with initiation of chemotherapy. Indicated only for short-term use; maximum of 5 days.

Dosage:
0.15 to 0.2 mg/kg/dose IV over 30 minutes (round down to nearest 1.5 mg). May repeat q24h PRN up to 4 additional doses. Administer until the uric acid is normal and the patient is stable. Most patients respond to 1 dose.

Give prior to chemotherapy if expected massive tumor lysis and/or renal involvement/dysfunction (e.g., Burkitt lymphoma with bulky disease).

Notes:
Do not give to patients with known hypersensitivity to rasburicase. Contraindicated in patients with G6PD deficiency (may cause hemolysis) or severe asthma. Methemoglobinemia has been reported with use. May cause vomiting, nausea, fever, headache, abdominal pain, constipation, diarrhea, and rash. When measuring serum uric acid levels, ensure tubes are prechilled and samples are placed in an ice water bath and analyzed within 4 hours. Collection at room temperature may lead to spuriously low uric acid levels due to continued degradation by rasburicase in the sample.

RHD IMMUNE GLOBULIN
WinRho SDF, Rhophylac
Immune globulin
Injection: 600, 1500, 2500, 5000, 15,000 IU (1 mcg = 5 IU)

Pregnancy category C

Indications:
Treatment of immune thrombocytopenic purpura (ITP) in nonsplenectomized RhD-positive patients; suppression of RhD isoimmunization in an RhD-negative individual exposed to RhD-positive blood or during delivery (or pregnancy) of an RhD-positive infant (if father known to be RhD-positive or status unknown).

Dosage:
ITP:
Hemoglobin $\geq 10\,g/dL$: 50 mcg/kg IV (250 IU/kg), administer dose over 3 to 5 minutes

Hemoglobin $< 10\,g/dL$: 25 to 40 mcg/kg IV (125 to 200 IU/kg)

New onset ITP: 75 mcg/kg (375 IU/kg) as a single dose has been used safely and efficaciously in pediatric patients with platelets $\leq 20 \times 10^9/L$

Dose frequency is dependent on duration of response, clinical symptoms, and adverse effects; may be given q2–4 weeks.

Notes:
Avoid in patients with known hypersensitivity to immunoglobulins or thimerosal and in patients with IgA deficiency. Use with extreme caution in patients with a hemoglobin less than 8 g/dL. Adverse events

associated with administration in ITP include headache, chills, fever, and reduction in hemoglobin (resulting from the destruction of RhD-positive red cells). May interfere with immune response to live-virus vaccines. Causes acute hemolysis with an average hemoglobin decrease of 1.5 to 2 g/dL at 1 week. Do not use in patients with active bleeding. Current FDA guidelines strongly recommend that patients be monitored in a health care center for 8 hours after a dose of RhD immune globulin, with urinalyses at baseline and 2, 4, and 8 hours after administration due to risk of severe hemolysis.

RITUXIMAB

Rituxan

Antineoplastic, monoclonal antibody

Injection: 10 mg/mL

Pregnancy category C

Indications:

Treatment of relapsed or refractory low grade or follicular CD20 positive, B-cell non-Hodgkin lymphoma; first-line therapy for diffuse large B-cell non-Hodgkin lymphoma in combination with other chemotherapeutics; systemic autoimmune disorders including autoimmune hemolytic anemia and immune thrombocytopenia purpura; posttransplant lymphoproliferative disorder; rheumatoid arthritis; refractory graft-versus-host disease; refractory systemic lupus erythematosis.

Dosage:

Refer to individual protocol.

Children and adults: 375 mg/m² IV qweek for 4 weeks (range 3 to 6 weeks)

Courses may be repeated for treatment of malignancies or recurrent symptoms with autoimmune disorders.

Notes:

Rare cases of progressive multifocal leukoencephalopathy due to Creutzfeldt–Jakob virus have been reported. Infusional toxicity is common and primarily avoided with a slow infusion and premedication. Most common, infusional toxicity is seen with the first infusion and reactions may include development of hives, bronchospasm, hypoxia, hypotension, pulmonary infiltrates, and respiratory distress syndrome. Some reactions have been fatal. Close monitoring is required for all infusions and appropriate resuscitative medications and equipment must be close by. In the case of mild reactions, temporary cessation of the infusion is indicated with acetaminophen, diphenhydramine, and fluids as indicated. Hydrocortisone may also be indicated. If symptoms resolve, reinitiate the infusion at a 50% reduced rate and monitor closely. Subsequent infusions should run slowly and the patient should be premedicated. Rituximab should be discontinued altogether following a life-threatening reaction. Use with caution in patients with preexisting pulmonary or cardiac conditions and in those at risk for development of tumor lysis syndrome. Causes immunosuppression. Quantitative immunoglobulins and specific antibody response should be checked prior to and following treatment with rituximab to determine if immunoglobulin infusions might be needed post treatment until recovery of immune function. Reactivation of hepatitis B has been noted (mainly in adult patients); thus, immune status to hepatitis B virus should be documented. Although specific to B-cells, *Pneumocystis jiroveci* pneumonia (PCP) infection after rituximab has been reported; therefore, patients should receive PCP prophylaxis for 6 months or until recovery of immune function is documented.

SARGRAMOSTIM

GM-CSF
Leukine
Colony-stimulating factor
Injection: 250, 500 mcg

Pregnancy category C

Indications:

Accelerates myeloid recovery and engraftment after autologous or allogeneic hematopoietic stem cell transplantation (HSCT); mobilizes hematopoietic progenitor cells into peripheral blood for collection by leukapheresis; increases neutrophil counts in patients receiving myelosuppressive chemotherapy; used in neonatal neutropenia.

Dosage:

Neonates with neutropenia and sepsis:

10 mcg/kg/day IV/SC for 5 days

Children and adults (no FDA approved dosing in children) after HSCT:

250 mcg/kg/day IV/SC for 21 days, beginning 2 to 4 hours after marrow infusion on day 0 of HSCT or not sooner than 24 hours after chemotherapy. Administer as a 30-minute, 2-hour, or 6-hour infusion. Reduce dose to 125 mcg/kg if adverse effect (after resolution).

Administer daily until the absolute neutrophil count is $\geq 5.0 \times 10^9$/L for 1 day or until day +21 post-HSCT, whichever comes first (or per protocol).

Do not administer within 24 hours prior to or after chemotherapy or 12 hours prior to radiation therapy.

Notes:

May lead to excessive immature myeloid cells in the peripheral blood or bone marrow (>10%). Avoid in patients with a history of immune thrombocytopenic purpura, known hypersensitivity to granulocyte-macrophage colony-stimulating factors, or yeast-derived products. Use with caution in patients with autoimmune or chronic inflammatory conditions, hypertension, cardiovascular disease, pulmonary disease, or renal or hepatic impairment.

SIROLIMUS

Rapamune
Immunosuppressant agent
Solution: 1 mg/mL
Tablet: 1, 2 mg

Pregnancy category C

Indications:

Graft-versus-host disease prophylaxis in hematopoietic stem cell transplant recipients; prophylaxis and treatment of rejection in renal transplant patients; primary immunosuppression in other organ transplant.

Dosage:

Refer to individual protocol.

Children ≥ 13 years of age and <40 kg: Loading dose 3 mg/m^2 on day 1 followed by maintenance 1 mg/m^2/day divided q12h or once daily; adjust dose to achieve target sirolimus trough blood concentration.

Notes:

Do not give to patients with known hypersensitivity to sirolimus. Immunosuppression may result in increased susceptibility to infection. May increase risk for development of lymphoma or other malignancy. Avoid excessive sun exposure and use sun protection factor. Severe hypersensitivity and skin reactions have been reported. Monitor renal and hepatic function; dose reduction may be necessary. Use with caution in the perioperative period due to an increased risk of surgical complications from wound dehiscence and impaired wound and tissue healing. Prophylaxis against *Pneumocystis jiroveci* and cytomegalovirus is recommended.

SODIUM THIOSULFATE

Versiclear
Antidote, extravasation of mechlorethamine, cisplatin, or cyanide; antifungal agent (topical)
Injection: 100, 250 mg/mL

Indications:

Treatment of extravasations of selected chemotherapeutic agents.

Dosage:

Chemotherapy infiltration: children and adults:

Mechlorethamine: use 2 mL for each mg infiltrated

Notes:

Do not give to patients with known hypersensitivity to sodium thiosulfate. Inject slowly, over at least 10 minutes; rapid administration may cause hypotension.

SUCCIMER

Chemet (2,3-dimercaptosuccinic acid; DMSA)
Antidote (lead toxicity), chelating agent
Capsule: 100 mg

Pregnancy category C

Indications:

Treatment of lead poisoning in asymptomatic children with blood levels between 45 and 69.9 mcg/dL. Can be considered at lower lead levels (20 to 44.9 mcg/dL) if aggressive environmental interventions have not impacted level although not noted to improve neurocognitive outcome.

Dosage:

Lead chelation, children:
10 mg/kg/dose (350 mg/m^2/dose) PO q8h for 5 days, followed by 10 mg/kg/dose PO q12h for 14 days. Repeat courses separated by a minimum of 2 weeks may be necessary to treat rebound lead concentrations (resulting from mobilization of lead from bone stores).

Notes:

Do not give to patients with known hypersensitivity to succimer. Use with caution in impaired hepatic or renal function. May see gastrointestinal symptoms, increased transaminases, rash, headache, and dizziness. Do not administer with other chelators. Treat iron deficiency and eliminate environmental exposure to lead. Monitor lead levels. May sprinkle contents of the capsules on food if unable to swallow.

TACROLIMUS

Prograf, generic
Immunosuppressant agent
Capsule: 0.5, 1, 5 mg
Injection: 5 mg/mL

Indications:

Prevention of organ rejection in solid organ transplant patients; prevention or treatment of graft-versus-host disease (GVHD) in allogeneic hematopoietic stem cell transplantation.

Dosage:

Children: younger children usually require higher dosing on a mg/kg basis than older children.

Solid organ transplant: initial dose 0.15 to 0.3 mg/kg/day PO divided q12h; may give IV continuous infusion 0.01 to 0.06 mg/kg/day (refer to specific organ protocol)

Prevention of GVHD: initial 0.03 mg/kg/day (based on lean body weight) as IV continuous infusion. Begin 24 hours prior to stem cell infusion and continue until oral medication can be tolerated. May occasionally be given as a q12h IV infusion.

Conversion from IV to PO dose (1:4 ratio): Multiply total daily IV dose by 4 and administer in two divided oral doses per day.

Notes:

Do not give to patients with known hypersensitivity to tacrolimus, castor oil, or any component. Immunosuppression may increase risk of infection or development of lymphoma or other malignancies. Risk is related to intensity and duration of use. May cause nephrotoxicity and neurotoxicity. Do not administer concurrently with cyclosporine. Monitor electrolytes. Monitor tacrolimus drug levels and adjust dosages per protocol.

TEMOZOLOMIDE

Temodar
Antineoplastic, alkylating agent
Capsule: 5, 20, 100, 140, 180, 250 mg
Injection: 100 mg

Pregnancy category D

Indications:

Treatment of refractory anaplastic astrocytoma; treatment of newly diagnosed glioblastoma multiforme; active against recurrent . glioblastoma multiforme, metastatic melanoma, brain stem glioma, ependymoma, medulloblastoma, primitive neuroectodermal tumor (PNET), neuroblastoma, and anaplastic oligodendroglioma.

Dosage:

Refer to individual protocol.

Children: 100 to 200 mg/m^2 IV/PO once daily for 5 days every 28 days

Metronomic dosing: 75 mg/m^2/day 5 days/week, 21 to 42 day cycles

May also be administered concurrently with radiation therapy.

Notes:

Do not give to patients with known hypersensitivity to temozolomide, dacarbazine, or any component. Thrombocytopenia and neutropenia are dose-limiting toxicities and may occur late in the treatment cycle and take 14 days to resolve. Monitor blood counts and ensure platelet count $\geq 100 \times 10^9$/L and ANC $\geq 1.5 \times 10^9$/L prior to initiation of each cycle of therapy. Rare cases of aplastic anemia, myelodysplasia, and secondary malignancies have been reported. Prophylaxis against *Pneumocystis jiroveci* is required, especially with concurrent administration of irradiation. Avoid in pregnancy; may cause fetal harm.

THIOGUANINE

6-TG, 6-Thioguanine
Antineoplastic, antimetabolite
Tablet (scored): 40 mg

Pregnancy category D

Indications:

Remission induction and consolidation phases in acute myelogenous leukemia; delayed intensification phase in acute lymphoblastic leukemia.

Dosage:

Refer to individual protocol.

Infants and children <3 years: 3.3 mg/kg/day PO divided q12h for 4 days

Children ≥3 years and adults: 50 to 200 mg/m^2/day PO divided q12–24h for 4 to 14 days or per protocol

Notes:

Do not give to patients with known hypersensitivity to thioguanine. Use with caution and reduce dosage in patients with renal or hepatic impairment. May cause nausea, vomiting, anorexia, stomatitis, diarrhea, myelosuppression, and veno-occlusive disease (sinusoidal obstructive syndrome). Increases busulfan toxicity.

THIOTEPA

Thioplex, generic
Antineoplastic, alkylating agent
Powder for injection: 15, 30 mg

Pregnancy category D

Indications:

Treatment of superficial tumors of the bladder, brain tumors, and other meningeal neoplasms (including intrathecal administration); control of pleural, pericardial, or peritoneal effusions caused by metastatic tumors; also used in high-dose regimens with autologous hematopoietic stem cell transplantation (HSCT).

Dosage:

Refer to individual protocol.
Children, HSCT: 300 mg/m^2/dose over 3 hours IV; repeat q24h for 3 doses. Maximum tolerated dose over 3 days is 900 to 1125 mg/m^2.
Intrathecal: 5 to 11.5 mg/m^2 per dose weekly for 2 to 7 doses

Notes:

Do not give to patients with known hypersensitivity to thiotepa or severe myelosuppression. Reduce dose in patients with renal, hepatic, or bone marrow dysfunction. May cause central nervous system changes, skin hyperpigmentation, nausea, vomiting, hematuria, and elevation of liver transaminases and bilirubin.

THROMBIN, TOPICAL

Evithrom, Recothrom, Thrombi-Gel, Thrombi-Pad, Thrombin-JMI (epistaxis kit, spray kit)
Hemostatic agent
Powder (Recothrom): 5000, 20,000 unit vials
Powder, topical (bovine, Thrombin-JMI): available in epistaxis kit 5000 IU, spray 20,000 IU
Solution, topical (Evithrom): 800 to 1200 IU/mL
Sponge, topical (Thrombi-Gel): ≥1000, ≥2000 IU
Pad, topical (bovine, Thrombi-Pad): ≥200 IU

Pregnancy category C

Indications:

Hemostasis for minor bleeding from accessible capillaries and small venules.

Dosage:

Apply powder directly to the site of bleeding or on oozing surface, or use 1000 to 2000 IU/mL of solution where bleeding is profuse. May be diluted with NS to other concentrations as needed. Use 100 IU/mL for bleeding from skin or mucosal surfaces. May utilize epistaxis/spray kit for mucosal/nose bleeds.

Notes:

Avoid in patients with known hypersensitivity to thrombin. Some forms are of human or bovine origin. May cause fever or allergic reactions. Topical use only. Not for administration systemically or directly into sites of brisk arterial bleeding. Avoid in patients with factor V deficiency due to cross-reactivity.

TOPOTECAN

Hycamtin
Antineoplastic, camptothecin, topoisomerase inhibitor
Capsule: 0.25, 1 mg

Injection: 4 mg

Pregnancy category D

Indications:

Treatment of pediatric solid tumors, including sarcoma and neuroblastoma.

Dosage:

Refer to individual protocol.

Children:

Pediatric solid tumors: 1 mg/m^2/day (range 0.75 to 1.9 mg/m^2/day) for 3 days as a continuous IV infusion; repeat q3 weeks

Single agent therapy for refractory solid tumors or hematologic malignancy: 2.4 mg/m^2/day once daily for 5 days of a 21 day course

Combination therapy for solid tumors: 0.75 mg/m^2/dose once daily for 5 days every 21 days in combination with cyclophosphamide

Notes:

Do not give to patients with known hypersensitivity to topotecan. Bone marrow toxicity is dose limiting, primarily neutropenia. Has been associated with neutropenic colitis; should be a strong consideration in patients with neutropenia, fever, and abdominal pain. Severe diarrhea has been reported, may require dose adjustment. May cause fetal harm; must ensure contraception to avoid pregnancy. Use with caution in patients with renal or hepatic impairment.

TRANEXAMIC ACID

Cyklokapron, Lysteda
Antifibrinolytic, antihemophilic, hemostatic agent
Tablet (Lysteda): 650 mg
Injection (Cyklokapron): 100 mg/mL

Pregnancy category B

Indications:

Short-term use (2 to 8 days) in hemophilia or von Willebrand disease patients for mucosal bleeding (including tooth extraction) to reduce or prevent hemorrhage and reduce need for factor replacement. May be used to treat primary menorrhagia or recurrent epistaxis, to prevent gastrointestinal or ocular hemorrhage following trauma, and to decrease perioperative blood loss and need for transfusion in patients undergoing congenital heart disease or scoliosis surgery.

Dosage:

Children and adults:

Tooth extraction in patients with hemophilia:

10 mg/kg immediately before oral surgery IV, then 10 mg/kg/dose IV/PO q6–8h; may be used for 2 to 8 days

Menorrhagia:

1300 mg PO TID for up to 5 days during monthly menstruation

Notes:

Do not use in patients with known subarachnoid hemorrhage, active intravascular clotting process, or acquired defective color vision. Use with caution in patients with cardiovascular or cerebrovascular disease. Dose modification is required in patients with renal impairment. May cause hypotension, thromboembolic complications, headache, and visual abnormalities (seen in animals). Do not administer concomitantly with factor IX and prothrombin complex concentrates or hormonal contraception due to increased risk of thrombosis. Use with caution in patients with upper urinary tract bleeding due to potential for clot formation and ureteral obstruction. Use with extreme caution in patients with disseminated intravascular coagulation.

TRIMETHOPRIM/
SULFAMETHOXAZOLE

Bactrim, Septra, Co-trimoxazole, Sulfatrim, TMP-SMX, generic
Antibiotic, sulfonamide derivative
Tablet, single strength: 80 mg trimethoprim (TMP) and 400 mg sulfamethoxazole (SMX)
Tablet, double strength: 160 mg TMP and 800 mg SMX
Suspension: 40 mg TMP/200 mg SMX per 5 mL
Injection: 16 mg TMP/80 mg SMX per mL

Pregnancy category C/D

Indications:

Oral treatment of urinary tract infection (UTI) and otitis media; prophylaxis for *Pneumocystis jiroveci* pneumonia (PCP); IV treatment of documented or suspected PCP infection in immunocompromised patients.

Dosage:

Dosage recommendations are based on the TMP component. May be given PO or IV.

Children >2 months of age:

Minor/moderate infection:

8 to 12 mg TMP/kg/day PO divided q12h

Serious infection/PCP:

20 mg TMP/kg/day divided q6–8h PO/IV

UTI or otitis media prophylaxis:

2 to 4 mg TMP/kg once daily

Prophylaxis for PCP:

5 mg TMP/kg/day divided q12h 2 to 3 consecutive days a week (maximum dose 320 mg TMP/day)

Notes:

Do not give to patients with known hypersensitivity to sulfa drugs or any component, porphyria, or megaloblastic anemia due to folate deficiency. Do not use in infants under 2 months of age. Use with caution in patients with G6PD deficiency and impaired renal or hepatic impairment. Serious adverse reactions include Stevens-Johnson syndrome, toxic epidermal necrolysis, hepatic necrosis, agranulocytosis, aplastic anemia, and other blood dyscrasias. Discontinue with rash. May need to be held temporarily in oncology patients who are on TMP-SMX for PCP prophylaxis and subsequently develop neutropenia. Numerous drug interactions are reported. TMP-SMX decreases the clearance of warfarin and methotrexate, decreases serum cyclosporine concentrations, and increases the effect of sulfonylureas, phenytoin, and thiopental. *Do not give to patients within 24 hours of receiving high-dose methotrexate and until level is $<1 \times 10^{-7} M$ due to competitive excretion and increased risk of methotrexate toxicity due to delayed clearance.*

VALACYCLOVIR

Valtrex, generic
Antiviral
Caplet: 500 mg, 1 g

Pregnancy category B

Indications:

Treatment of herpes zoster and herpes simplex virus (HSV) in immunocompromised patients; treatment of varicella zoster virus (VZV) in immunocompetent children (ages 2 to 18 years); treatment of HSV labialis in adolescents and adults.

Dosage:

Children:

Varicella, immunocompetent: 2 years to <18 years: 20 mg/kg/dose PO TID for 5 days (maximum 1 g TID); initiate within 24 hours of onset of rash

Herpes labialis (cold sores): >12 years: 2 g q12h for 1 day; initiated at earliest symptoms

Immunocompromised children at risk for HSV or VZV infection with normal renal

function: (limited data) 15 to 30 mg/kg/dose PO TID (maximum 2 g/dose)

Notes:

Do not give to patients with known hypersensitivity to valacyclovir or acyclovir. Use with caution in patients with renal impairment or those receiving concomitant nephrotoxic drugs. Adjust dose in patients with renal impairment. Monitor renal function.

VINBLASTINE SULFATE

Velban, generic
Antineoplastic, mitotic inhibitor
Injection: 10 mg vial

Pregnancy category D

Indications:

Treatment of Hodgkin and non-Hodgkin lymphoma, pediatric brain tumors (gliomas), Langerhans cell histiocytosis, choriocarcinoma, and advanced testicular germ cell tumors.

Dosage:

Refer to individual protocol.

Hodgkin lymphoma:

2.5 to 6 mg/m^2/dose IV once every 1 to 2 weeks for 3 to 6 cycles; maximum weekly dose 12.5 mg/m^2

Langerhans cell histiocytosis:

6 mg/m^2/dose IV once every 1 to 3 weeks

Brain tumors:

6 mg/m^2/dose IV weekly

Notes:

Do not give to patients with known hypersensitivity to vinblastine or with severe leukopenia. Dose modification may be needed in patients with hepatic impairment or neurotoxicity. Extravasation may cause local severe tissue damage. May cause peripheral neuropathy, myelosuppression, jaw pain, myalgia, paresthesia, constipation, abdominal pain, ileus, and mild alopecia. *Intrathecal administration is fatal.*

VINCRISTINE SULFATE

Vincasar, generic
Antineoplastic, mitotic inhibitor
Injection: 1, 2 mg vials (1 mg/mL)

Pregnancy category D

Indications:

Treatment of acute lymphoblastic leukemia (ALL), Hodgkin and non-Hodgkin lymphoma, neuroblastoma, Wilms tumor, and rhabdomyosarcoma.

Dosage:

Refer to individual protocol.

Children ≤10 kg or total body surface area (TBSA) <1 m^2:

0.05 mg/kg/dose IV once weekly; maximum single dose 2 mg

Children >10 kg or TBSA ≥1 m^2:

1 to 2 mg/m^2 IV; may repeat weekly for 3 to 6 weeks. Maximum single dose is 2 mg (some protocols allow for higher dosing in Hodgkin lymphoma and high risk ALL).

Neuroblastoma:

IV continuous infusion with doxorubicin: 1 mg/m^2/day for 72 hours

Notes:

Do not give to patients with known hypersensitivity to vincristine. Avoid in patients with the demyelinating form of Charcot-Marie-Tooth disease. Asparaginase may decrease clearance of vincristine. Dose modification may be required in patients with impaired hepatic function, preexisting neuromuscular disease, or severe side effects of treatment with vincristine. Extravasation may cause local severe tissue damage.

May cause peripheral neuropathy, paresthesias, ileus, jaw pain, cranial nerve paralysis (ptosis), vocal cord paralysis, hyponatremia, syndrome of inappropriate antidiuretic hormone (SIADH) secretion, alopecia, and constipation.

Intrathecal administration is fatal. Vincristine should never be taken into the procedure room for a patient undergoing a lumbar puncture for instillation of intrathecal chemotherapy.

VITAMIN K₁/PHYTONADIONE

AquaMEPHYTON, Mephyton
Vitamin, water soluble
Tablet: 5 mg
Suspension: 1 mg/mL
Injection: 2, 10 mg/mL

Pregnancy category C

Indications:

Prevention and treatment of hypoprothrombinemia caused by anticoagulants or drug-induced vitamin K deficiency; hemorrhagic disease of the newborn.

Dosage:

Hemorrhagic disease of the newborn:

Prophylaxis: 0.5 to 1 mg IM within 1 hour of birth

Treatment: 1 to 2 mg/24 hours IM, SC, or IV

Oral anticoagulant overdose:

Infants and children: 0.5 to 5 mg/dose PO, IM, IV, or SC (give 5 mg for major bleeding, 0.5 to 2.5 mg for minor bleeding)

Adults: 2.5 to 10 mg/dose PO, IM, IV, or SC

Dose may be repeated 12 to 48 hours after PO dose or 6 to 8 hours after parenteral dose

Vitamin K deficiency (due to drugs, malabsorption, or decreased synthesis of vitamin K by the liver):

Infants and children: 2.5 to 5 mg/24 hours PO or 1 to 2 mg/dose IM/IV/SC as a single dose

Adults: 2.5 to 5 mg/24 hours PO or 10 mg/dose IM/SC/IV

Notes:

Do not give to patients with known hypersensitivity to phytonadione. Antagonizes action of warfarin. Protect product from light. Parenteral dosing may cause flushing, dizziness, cardiac or respiratory arrest, hypotension, or anaphylaxis. High doses (10 to 20 mg) in neonates may cause hyperbilirubinemia and severe hemolytic anemia. Monitor prothrombin time (PT), activated partial thromboplastin time (APTT); blood coagulation factors may increase within 6 to 12 hours after oral dosing and within 1 to 2 hours after parenteral dosing.

VORICONAZOLE

VFEND
Antifungal agent
Injection: 200 mg
Powder for suspension: 200 mg/5 mL
Tablet: 50, 200 mg

Pregnancy category D

Indications:

Treatment of invasive aspergillosis, especially in immunocompromised patients; treatment of candidemia in nonneutropenic patients; deep tissue *Candida* infections including esophageal; treatment of serious fungal infections caused by *Scedosporium apiospermum* or *Fusarium* species in patients intolerant or refractory to conventional antifungal therapy.

Dosage:

Limited information on pediatric dosing; children ≤12 years of age appear to require higher dosing than adults.

Children 2 to 11 years: loading dose 6 mg/kg/dose IV q12h for 2 doses on day 1 followed by maintenance dose 4 mg/kg/dose IV q12h

(approximates exposure of adult dose of 3 mg/kg/dose)

Infectious Diseases Society of America (IDSA) guidelines: invasive aspergillosis: maintenance dose 5 to 7 mg/kg/dose IV q12h

Children ≥ 12 years and adults: loading dose 6 mg/kg/dose IV q12h for 2 doses on day 1; followed by maintenance dose:

Invasive aspergillosis and other deep tissue fungal infections: 4 mg/kg/dose IV q12h

Candidemia: 3 to 4 mg/kg/dose IV q12h

Notes:

Do not give to patients with known hypersensitivity to voriconazole. Use with caution in patients with known hypersensitivity to azoles; cross-reactivity studies have not been done. Tablets may contain lactose and should be used with caution in patients with lactose intolerance. Avoid concurrent administration with rifampin, CYP3A4 substrates, and ergot alkaloids. Voriconazole is metabolized by cytochrome P450 enzymes and many drug interactions exist. May cause severe hepatic toxicity, visual changes, cardiac arrhythmias, auditory hallucinations, and photosensitivity. May cause fetal harm; must ensure contraception to avoid pregnancy. Use with caution in neonates; oral suspension contains sodium benzoate, a metabolite of benzyl alcohol, which may cause a potentially fatal toxicity. Use with caution in patients with renal or hepatic toxicity; dose adjustment may be necessary.

WARFARIN SODIUM

Coumadin, Jantoven, generic
Anticoagulant
Tablets: 1, 2, 2.5, 3, 4, 5, 6, 7.5, 10 mg
Injection: 5 mg

Pregnancy category X

Indications:

Prophylaxis and treatment of venous thromboembolic disorders; prevention of arterial thromboembolism in patients with prosthetic heart valves or atrial fibrillation; prevention of death, venous thromboembolism, and recurrent myocardial infarction (MI) after acute MI.

Dosage:

Infants and children (to maintain an international normalized ratio [INR] between 2 and 3):

Initial dose: 0.2 mg/kg PO for 1 to 2 days; maximum dose 10 mg

Maintenance dose: 0.1 mg/kg/24 hours PO daily; range 0.05 to 0.34 mg/kg/24 hours (consult published charts based on INR)

Adults: 5 to 10 mg PO daily × 2 to 5 days, adjust for desired INR; maintenance dose range 2 to 10 mg/day PO

Onset of action is within 36 to 72 hours and peak effects occur within 5 to 7 days. Monitor INR after 5 to 7 days of new dosage; high risk patients may require more frequent monitoring.

Usual duration of therapy for first venous thrombotic event is 3 months (depending on elimination of procoagulant factor and based on resolution of clot).

Notes:

Do not give to patients with known hypersensitivity to warfarin, severe liver or kidney disease, uncontrolled bleeding, gastrointestinal (GI) ulcers, status-post neurosurgical procedures, and malignant hypertension. Concomitant use with vitamin K may decrease anticoagulant effect. Concomitant use with aspirin, nonsteroidal anti-inflammatory drugs, or indomethacin may increase warfarin's anticoagulant effect and cause severe GI irritation. May cause fever, skin lesions, necrosis (especially in protein C deficiency), hemorrhage, hemoptysis, anorexia, nausea, vomiting, and diarrhea. Many drug interactions exist; review all medications prior to initiation of therapy. The INR is the recommended test to monitor anticoagulant effect. The absolute INR desired is dependent on the indication and has been extrapolated from adults. An INR of 2 to 3 has been recommended for prophylaxis and treatment of deep vein thrombosis, pulmonary emboli, and bioprosthetic heart valves. Younger children may require higher dosing. Certain foods and medications may alter levels and should be reviewed in detail with the patient. *Antidote is vitamin K and prothrombin complex concentrates (PCC; fresh frozen plasma if PCC unavailable).*

References

Taketomo CK, Hodding JH, Kraus DM. Pediatric Dosage Handbook. 17th ed. Hudson, OH: Lexi-Comp, 2010.

Physicians' Desk Reference, 65th ed. Montvale, NJ: Medical Economics Company, Inc., 2011.

Custer JW, Rau RE. The Johns Hopkins Hospital: The Harriet Lane Handbook, A Manual for Pediatric House Officers, 18th ed. Philadelphia, PA: Elsevier-Mosby, 2009.

Index